ATLAS OF
Regional Anesthesia

ATLAS OF
Regional Anesthesia

Fifth Edition

Ehab Farag MD, FRCA
Professor, Department of Anesthesiology,
Director of Clinical Research
Cleveland Clinic Learner College of Medicine,
Staff Anesthesiologist, Cleveland Clinic, Cleveland, OH

Loran Mounir-Soliman MD
Staff, Departments of Pain Management,
Anesthesiology and Pediatric Anesthesiology,
Cleveland Clinic, Cleveland, OH

With David L. Brown
Professor of Anesthesiology
Cleveland Clinic Learner College of Medicine
Chairman of Anesthesiology Institute
Cleveland Clinic
Cleveland, OH

ILLUSTRATIONS BY
Joe Kanasz (fifth edition)
Jo Ann Clifford (fourth edition)

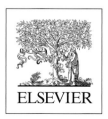

ELSEVIER

ELSEVIER

1600 John F. Kennedy Blvd.
Ste 1800
Philadelphia, PA 19103-2899

ATLAS OF REGIONAL ANESTHESIA   ISBN 978-0-323-35490-5

Library of Congress Cataloging in Publication Data

A catalog record for this book is available from the Library of Congress

your source for books,
journals and multimedia
in the health sciences
www.elsevierhealth.com

Working together
to grow libraries in
developing countries

www.elsevier.com • www.bookaid.org

The publisher's policy is to use **paper manufactured from sustainable forests**

Executive Content Strategist: Bill Schmitt
Content Development Specialist: Carole McMurray
Project Manager: Julie Taylor
Illustrations Manager: Karen Giacomucci
Designer: Christian Bilbow

Printed in China

Last digit is the print number: 9   8   7   6   5   4   3   2   1

Dedicated to

To my wife, Abeer, who has been my best friend and support system through all my endeavors.
Ehab Farag

I dedicate this book to an amazing woman, my wife Dalia, whose relentless support is my real strength. To Natalie, Krista and Nicole, the true joys of my life, and last but not least, my mom whose prayers bless my steps.
Loran Mounir-Soliman

Contributors

Kenneth C. Cummings III, MD
Department of General Anesthesiology
Cleveland Clinic
Cleveland, Ohio

Ibrahim Farid, MD
Associate Professor of Anesthesiology, NEOMED
Chair, Department of Anesthesia and Pain Medicine
Director, Pediatric Pain Center
Akron Children's Hospital
Akron, Ohio

Rami Edward Karroum, MD
Department of Pediatric Anesthesiology
Akron Children's Hospital
Akron, Ohio

Kamal Maheshwari, MD
Department of General Anesthesiology
Cleveland Clinic
Cleveland, Ohio

Wael Ali Sakr Esa, MD, PhD
Assistant Professor of Anesthesiology
General Anesthesiology, Pain Management,
Director Orthopedic Anesthesia
Anesthesiology Institute
CCLCM, Case Western Reserve University
Cleveland, Ohio

John Seif, MD
Department of Pediatric Anesthesiology
Cleveland Clinic
Cleveland, Ohio

Brian D. Sites, MD
Associate Professor of Anesthesiology and Orthopedics
Dartmouth Medical School, Hanover; Director of
Regional Anesthesiology and Orthopedics, Department of
Anesthesiology, Dartmouth-Hitchcock Medical Center
Lebanon, New Hampshire

Brian C. Spence, MD
Assistant Professor of Anesthesiology, Dartmouth
Medical School, Hanover; Director of Same-Day Surgery
Program, Department of Anesthesiology, Dartmouth-
Hitchcock Medical Center, Lebanon, New Hampshire

Maria Yared, MD
Department of General Anesthesiology
Cleveland Clinic
Cleveland, Ohio

Preface to the Fifth Edition

Regional anesthesia is one of the fundamental pillars of modern anesthesia. *The Atlas of Regional Anesthesia* by Dr. David Brown has become a classic textbook for regional anesthesia since its first edition in 1991. Since the last edition published in 2010, the use of ultrasound has changed the map of the practice of regional anesthesia. In this new edition, now *Brown's Atlas of Regional Anesthesia*, we combined the classical techniques from the original atlas with updated techniques and blocks using ultrasound. We believe the eyes do not see what the brain does not recognize. Therefore we felt it was important to include a number of ultrasound images and figures that identify the optimal position of the needle, as well as the best position of the patient and the anesthesiologist during the procedure. We have tried to retain the simplicity of the original atlas through self-explanatory figures and a few purposeful pearls to demonstrate the block performance. We tried to limit the techniques to the most commonly used and routinely adopted in our practice. Moreover, we have added videos of real patients for better clarification, showing real-time blocks performance in addition to advanced techniques using peripheral nerve catheters. Our aim is to transform the atlas into a virtual workshop that enables the reader to feel comfortable with the procedures after reading the text and watching the video. In this new edition we did rewrite all the blocks using ultrasound and added new blocks like subcostal, quadratus lumborum, paravertebral, adductor canal, and many more. We have added new chapters on regional anesthesia pharmacology and on regional anesthesia using ultrasound in pediatric patients. We hope this new edition will be useful to anyone interested in learning regional anesthesia or in mastering regional anesthesia.

We would like to thank Mr. Joe Kanasz for his extraordinary medical illustrations; Mrs. Mariela Madrilejos, our editorial assistant; Ms. Carole McMurray; and Mr. William Schmitt from Elsevier for their help and incessant support during the production process of this edition.

Editors
Ehab Farag, MD, FRCA
Loran Mounir-Soliman, MD

Introduction to the Fourth Edition

The necessary, but somewhat artificial, separation of anesthetic care into regional or general anesthetic techniques often gives rise to the concept that these two techniques should not or cannot be mixed. Nothing could be further from the truth. To provide comprehensive regional anesthesia care, it is absolutely essential that the anesthesiologist be skilled in all aspects of anesthesia. This concept is not original: John Lundy promoted this idea in the 1920s when he outlined his concept of "balanced anesthesia." Even before Lundy promoted this concept, however, George Crile had written extensively on the concept of anociassociation.

It is often tempting, and quite human, to trace the evolution of a discipline back through the discipline's developmental family tree. When such an investigation is carried out for regional anesthesia, Louis Gaston Labat, MD, often receives credit for being central in its development. Nevertheless, Labat's interest and expertise in regional anesthesia were nurtured by Dr. Victor Pauchet of Paris, France, to whom Dr. Labat was an assistant. The real trunk of the developmental tree of regional anesthesia consists of the physicians willing to incorporate regional techniques into their early surgical practices. In Labat's original 1922 text, *Regional Anesthesia: Its Technique and Clinical Application,* Dr. William Mayo in the foreword stated:

The young surgeon should perfect himself in the use of regional anesthesia, which increases in value with the increase in the skill with which it is administered. The well equipped surgeon must be prepared to use the proper anesthesia, or the proper combination of anesthesias, in the individual case. I do not look forward to the day when regional anesthesia will wholly displace general anesthesia; but undoubtedly it will reach and hold a very high position in surgical practice.

Perhaps if the current generation of both surgeons and anesthesiologists keeps Mayo's concept in mind, our patients will be the beneficiaries.

It appears that these early surgeons were better able to incorporate regional techniques into their practices because they did not see the regional block as the "end all." Rather, they saw it as part of a comprehensive package that had benefit for their patients. Surgeons and anesthesiologists in that era were able to avoid the flawed logic that often seems to pervade application of regional anesthesia today. These individuals did not hesitate to supplement their blocks with sedatives or light general anesthetics; they did not expect each and every block to be "100%." The concept that a block has failed unless it provides complete anesthesia without supplementation seems to have occurred when anesthesiology developed as an independent specialty. To be successful in carrying out regional anesthesia, we must be willing to get back to our roots and embrace the concepts of these early workers who did not hesitate to supplement their regional blocks. Ironically, today some consider a regional block a failure if the initial dose does not produce complete anesthesia; yet these same individuals complement our "general anesthetists" who utilize the concept of anesthetic titration as a goal. Somehow, we need to meld these two views into one that allows comprehensive, titrated care to be provided for all our patients.

As Dr. Mayo emphasized in Labat's text, it is doubtful that regional anesthesia will "ever wholly displace general anesthesia." Likewise, it is equally clear that general anesthesia will probably never be able to replace the appropriate use of regional anesthesia. One of the principal rationales for avoiding the use of regional anesthesia through the years has been that it was "expensive" in terms of operating room and physician time. As is often the case, when examined in detail, some accepted truisms need rethinking. Thus it is surprising that much of the renewed interest in regional anesthesia results from focusing on health care costs and the need to decrease the length and cost of hospitalization.

If regional anesthesia is to be incorporated successfully into a practice, there must be time for anesthesiologist and patient to discuss the upcoming operation and anesthetic prescription. Likewise, if regional anesthesia is to be effectively used, some area of an operating suite must be used to place the blocks before moving patients to the main operating room. Immediately at hand in this area must be both anesthetic and resuscitative equipment (such as regional trays), as well as a variety of local anesthetic drugs that span the timeline of anesthetic duration. Even after successful completion of the technical aspect of regional anesthesia, an anesthesiologist's work is really just beginning: it is as important to use appropriate sedation intraoperatively as it was preoperatively while the block was being administered.

Contents

The videos accompanying this text can be accessed at www.expertconsult.com and include more than 25 ultrasound scans of procedures discussed in the book. The videos should be used in conjunction with the text and not as a standalone product.

SECTION I

Introduction

Pharmacology and Ultrasound 1

Kamal Maheshwari, David L. Brown and Loran Mounir-Soliman
with contributions from Brian D. Sites and Brian C. Spence

Regional anesthesia is a fast-growing field with application in a wide range of surgical procedures. Better technique with the help of ultrasound, better and safer local anesthetics, and better drug delivery systems for continuous anesthesia all helped in gaining the current status. Far too often, those unfamiliar with regional anesthesia regard it as complex because of the long list of local anesthetics available and the varied techniques described. The goal throughout this book is to simplify regional anesthesia by providing specific information about various elements involved in decision making.

One of the first steps in simplifying regional anesthesia is to understand the two principal decisions necessary in prescribing a regional technique. First, the *appropriate technique* needs to be chosen for the patient, the surgical procedure, and the physicians involved. Second, the *appropriate local anesthetic and potential additives* must be matched to patient, procedure, regional technique, and physician. This book will detail how to integrate these concepts into your practice.

DRUGS

Numerous local anesthetic drugs are used in varied concentration and with different additives. The decision to choose one particular local anesthetic is influenced by patient factors, surgical factors, and the available resources (cost factors). Not all procedures are created equal in terms of the amount of time needed to complete an operation, and the severity or nature of pain will be different. If anesthesiologists are to use regional techniques effectively, they must be able to choose a local anesthetic that lasts the right amount of time and provides effective anesthesia and analgesia. To do this, they need to understand the local anesthetic timeline from the shorter-acting to the longer-acting agents (Fig. 1-1) and the effect of additives. Also, they need to understand the factors associated with successful continuous nerve block management.

All local anesthetics share the basic structure of aromatic end, intermediate chain, and amine end (Fig. 1-2). This basic structure is subdivided clinically into two classes of drugs: the amino esters and the amino amides. The *amino esters* possess an ester linkage between the aromatic end and the intermediate chain. These drugs include cocaine, procaine, 2-chloroprocaine, and tetracaine (Figs. 1-3 and 1-4). The *amino amides* contain an amide link between the

aromatic end and the intermediate chain. These drugs include lidocaine, prilocaine, etidocaine, mepivacaine, bupivacaine, and ropivacaine (see Figs. 1-3 and 1-4).

AMINO ESTERS

Cocaine was the first local anesthetic used clinically, and it is used today primarily for topical airway anesthesia. It is unique among the local anesthetics in that it is a vasoconstrictor rather than a vasodilator. Some anesthesia departments have limited the availability of cocaine because of fears of its abuse potential. In those institutions, mixtures of lidocaine and phenylephrine rather than cocaine are used to anesthetize the airway mucosa and shrink the mucous membranes.

Procaine was synthesized in 1904 by Einhorn, who was looking for a drug that was superior to cocaine and other solutions in use. Currently, procaine is seldom used for peripheral nerve or epidural blocks because of its low potency, slow onset, short duration of action, and limited power of tissue penetration. It is an excellent local anesthetic for skin infiltration, and its 10% form can be used as a short-acting (i.e., lasting <1 hour) spinal anesthetic.

Chloroprocaine has a rapid onset and a short duration of action. Its principal use is in producing epidural anesthesia for short procedures (i.e., lasting <1 hour). Its use declined during the early 1980s after reports of prolonged sensory and motor deficits resulting from unintentional subarachnoid administration of an intended epidural dose. Since that time, the drug formulation has changed. Short-lived yet annoying back pain may develop after large (>30 mL) epidural doses of 3% chloroprocaine.

	Procaine	Chloroprocaine	Lidocaine	Mepivacaine	Tetracaine	Ropivacaine	Etidocaine	Bupivacaine
Infiltration	45–60		75–90					180–360
+ epi	60–90		90–180					200–400
Peripheral			90–120	100–150		360–480		480–780
+ epi			120–180	120–220		480–600		600–900
SAB*	60–75		60		70–90			90–110
+ epi	75–90		75–100		100–150			100–150
phenylephrine†	90–120				200–300			
Epidural		45–50	80–120	90–140		140–200	120–200	165–225
+ epi		60–90	120–180	140–200		160–220	150–225	180–240

Figure 1-1. Local anesthetic timeline (length in minutes of surgical anesthesia).

*Subarachnoid block.
†For lower extremity surgery.

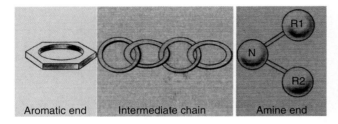

Aromatic end   Intermediate chain   Amine end

Figure 1-2. Basic local anesthetic structure.

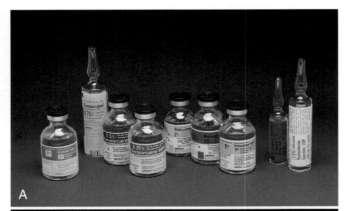

A

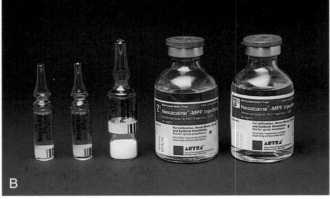

B

Figure 1-3. Local anesthetics commonly used in the United States. A, Amides. B, Esters.

Tetracaine, first synthesized in 1931, has become widely used in the United States for spinal anesthesia. It may be used as an isobaric, hypobaric, or hyperbaric solution for spinal anesthesia. Without epinephrine, it typically lasts 1.5 to 2.5 hours, and with the addition of epinephrine, it may last up to 4 hours for lower extremity procedures. Tetracaine is also an effective topical airway anesthetic, although caution must be used because of the potential for systemic side effects. Tetracaine is available as a 1% solution for intrathecal use or as anhydrous crystals that are reconstituted as tetracaine solution by adding sterile water immediately before use. Tetracaine is not as stable as procaine or lidocaine in solution, and the crystals undergo deterioration over time. Nevertheless, when a tetracaine spinal anesthetic is ineffective, one should question technique before "blaming" the drug.

AMINO AMIDES

Lidocaine was the first clinically used amide local anesthetic, having been introduced by Lofgren in 1948. Lidocaine has become the most widely used local anesthetic in the world because of its inherent potency; rapid onset; tissue penetration; and effectiveness during infiltration, peripheral nerve block, and both epidural and spinal blocks. During peripheral nerve block, a 1% to 1.5% solution is often effective in producing an acceptable motor blockade, whereas during epidural block, a 2% solution seems most effective. In spinal anesthesia, a 5% solution in dextrose is most commonly used, although it may also be used as a 0.5% hypobaric solution in a volume of 6 to 8 mL. Others use lidocaine as a short-acting 2% solution in a volume of 2 to 3 mL. The suggestion that lidocaine causes an unacceptable frequency of neurotoxicity with spinal use needs to be balanced against its long history of use. We believe that the basic science research may not completely

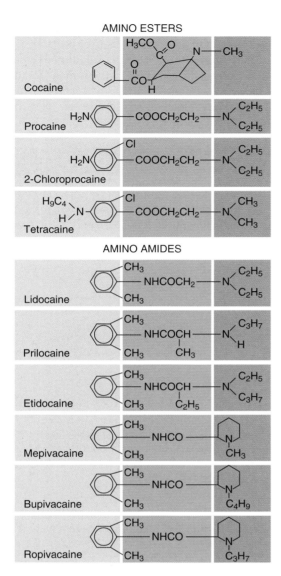

Figure 1-4. Chemical structure of commonly used amino ester and amino amide local anesthetics.

reflect the typical clinical situation. In any event, we have reduced the total dose of subarachnoid lidocaine we administer to less than 75 mg per spinal procedure, inject it more rapidly than in the past, and no longer use it for continuous subarachnoid techniques. Patients often report that lidocaine causes the most common local anesthetic allergies. However, many of these reported allergies are simply epinephrine reactions resulting from intravascular injection of the local anesthetic epinephrine mixture, often during dental injection.

Prilocaine is structurally related to lidocaine, although it causes significantly less vasodilation than lidocaine and thus can be used without epinephrine. Prilocaine is formulated for infiltration, peripheral nerve block, and epidural anesthesia. Its anesthetic profile is similar to that of lidocaine, although in addition to producing less vasodilation, it has less potential for systemic toxicity in equal doses. This

attribute makes it particularly useful for intravenous regional anesthesia. Prilocaine is not more widely used because, when metabolized, it can produce both orthotoluidine and nitrotoluidine, agents in methemoglobin formation.

Etidocaine is chemically related to lidocaine and is a long-acting amide local anesthetic. Etidocaine is associated with profound motor blockade and is best used when this attribute can be of clinical advantage. It has a more rapid onset of action than bupivacaine, but is used less frequently. Those clinicians using etidocaine often use it for the initial epidural dose and then use bupivacaine for subsequent epidural injections.

Mepivacaine is structurally related to lidocaine, and the two drugs have similar actions. Overall, mepivacaine is slightly longer acting than lidocaine, and this difference in duration is accentuated when epinephrine is added to the solutions.

Bupivacaine is a long-acting local anesthetic that can be used for infiltration, peripheral nerve block, and epidural and spinal anesthesia. Useful concentrations of the drug range from 0.125% to 0.75%. By altering the concentration of bupivacaine, sensory and motor blockade can be separated. Lower concentrations provide sensory blockade principally, and as the concentration is increased, the effectiveness of motor blockade increases with it. If an anesthesiologist had to select a single drug and a single drug concentration, 0.5% bupivacaine would be a logical choice because at that concentration it is useful for peripheral nerve block, subarachnoid block, and epidural block. Cardiotoxicity during systemic toxic reactions with bupivacaine became a concern in the 1980s. Although it is clear that bupivacaine alters myocardial conduction more dramatically than lidocaine, the need for appropriate and rapid resuscitation during any systemic toxic reaction cannot be overemphasized. Levobupivacaine is the single enantiomer (L-isomer) of bupivacaine and appears to have a systemic toxicity profile similar to that of ropivacaine, and clinically it has effects similar to those of racemic bupivacaine.

Ropivacaine is another long-acting local anesthetic, similar to bupivacaine; it was introduced in the United

States in 1996. It may offer an advantage over bupivacaine because experimentally it appears to be less cardiotoxic. Initial studies also suggest that ropivacaine may produce less motor block than that produced by bupivacaine, with similar analgesia. Ropivacaine may also be slightly shorter acting than bupivacaine, with useful drug concentrations ranging from 0.25% to 1%. Many practitioners believe that ropivacaine may offer particular advantages for postoperative analgesic infusions and obstetric analgesia.

Levobupivacaine is a pure S enantiomer of bupivacaine with lower cardiac toxicity profile but similar pharmacokinetic profile. Levobupivacaine potency is less than bupivacaine and more than ropivacaine. It can be used for all peripheral nerve blocks and neuraxial blocks.

DepoBupivacaine (Exparel) is a new drug that utilizes the DepoFoam technology developed by Pacira Pharmaceuticals, Inc. (Parsippany, NJ, USA). The bupivacaine is encapsulated in multivesicular liposomes, from which sustained release of the drug happens in the infiltrated areas for up to 72 hours. The drug is approved by the Food and Drug Administration (FDA) for postoperative pain control when used for local surgical wound infiltration.

VASOCONSTRICTORS

Vasoconstrictors are often added to local anesthetics to prolong the duration of action and improve the quality of the local anesthetic block. Although it is still unclear whether vasoconstrictors actually allow local anesthetics to have a longer duration of block or are effective because they produce additional antinociception through α-adrenergic action, their clinical effect is not in question.

$$HO-\bigcirc-CH-CH_2-NH-CH_3$$
$$\quad\quad\quad | $$
$$\quad\quad\quad OH$$
(with HO substituents on the ring)

Epinephrine is the most common vasoconstrictor used; overall, the most effective concentration, excluding spinal anesthesia, is a 1 : 200,000 concentration. When epinephrine is added to local anesthetic in the commercial production process, it is necessary to add stabilizing agents because epinephrine rapidly loses its potency on exposure to air and light. The added stabilizing agents lower the pH of the local anesthetic solution into the 3 to 4 range and, because of the higher pKas of local anesthetics, slow the onset of effective regional block. Thus if epinephrine is to be used with local anesthetics, it should be added at the time the block is performed, at least for the initial block. In subsequent injections made during continuous epidural block, commercial preparations of local anesthetic–epinephrine solutions can be used effectively.

$$\bigcirc-CH-CH_2-NH-CH_3$$
$$\quad | $$
$$\quad OH$$
$$OH$$

Phenylephrine also has been used as a vasoconstrictor, principally with spinal anesthesia; effective prolongation of block can be achieved by adding 2 to 5 mg of phenylephrine to the spinal anesthetic drug. Norepinephrine also has been used as a vasoconstrictor for spinal anesthesia,

although it does not appear to be as long lasting as epinephrine or to have any advantages over it. Because most local anesthetics are vasodilators, the addition of epinephrine often does not decrease blood flow as many fear it will; rather, the combination of local anesthetic and epinephrine results in tissue blood flow similar to that before injection.

LOCAL ANESTHETIC TOXICITY

Local anesthetic can cause direct nerve injury and/or systemic toxicity. If systemic toxicity is suspected, it should be treated swiftly with intralipid. See Table 1-1 for the local anesthetic systemic toxicity (LAST) management protocol.

Table 1-1

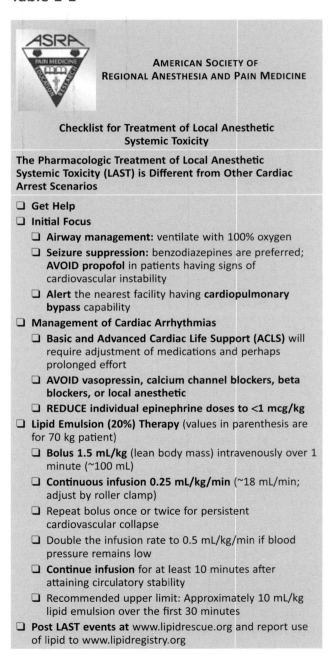

AMERICAN SOCIETY OF REGIONAL ANESTHESIA AND PAIN MEDICINE

Checklist for Treatment of Local Anesthetic Systemic Toxicity

The Pharmacologic Treatment of Local Anesthetic Systemic Toxicity (LAST) is Different from Other Cardiac Arrest Scenarios

- ❑ **Get Help**
- ❑ **Initial Focus**
  - ❑ **Airway management:** ventilate with 100% oxygen
  - ❑ **Seizure suppression:** benzodiazepines are preferred; **AVOID propofol** in patients having signs of cardiovascular instability
  - ❑ **Alert** the nearest facility having **cardiopulmonary bypass** capability
- ❑ **Management of Cardiac Arrhythmias**
  - ❑ **Basic and Advanced Cardiac Life Support (ACLS)** will require adjustment of medications and perhaps prolonged effort
  - ❑ **AVOID vasopressin, calcium channel blockers, beta blockers, or local anesthetic**
  - ❑ **REDUCE individual epinephrine doses to <1 mcg/kg**
- ❑ **Lipid Emulsion (20%) Therapy** (values in parenthesis are for 70 kg patient)
  - ❑ **Bolus 1.5 mL/kg** (lean body mass) intravenously over 1 minute (~100 mL)
  - ❑ **Continuous infusion 0.25 mL/kg/min** (~18 mL/min; adjust by roller clamp)
  - ❑ Repeat bolus once or twice for persistent cardiovascular collapse
  - ❑ Double the infusion rate to 0.5 mL/kg/min if blood pressure remains low
  - ❑ **Continue infusion** for at least 10 minutes after attaining circulatory stability
  - ❑ Recommended upper limit: Approximately 10 mL/kg lipid emulsion over the first 30 minutes
- ❑ **Post LAST events** at www.lipidrescue.org and report use of lipid to www.lipidregistry.org

Data reproduced from: American Society of Regional Anesthesia and Pain Medicine Checklist for Managing Local Anesthetic Systemic Toxicity: 2012 Version. Neal, Joseph; Mulroy, Michael; Weinberg, Guy with permission.

NEEDLES, CATHETERS, AND SYRINGES

Effective regional anesthesia requires comprehensive knowledge of equipment—that is, the needles, syringes, and catheters that allow the anesthetic to be injected into the desired area. In early years, regional anesthesia found many variations in the method of joining needle to syringe. Around the turn of the century, Schneider developed the first all-glass syringe for Hermann Wolfing-Luer. Luer is credited with the innovation of a simple conical tip for easy exchange of needle to syringe, but the "Luer-Lok" found in use on most syringes today is thought to have been designed by Dickenson in the mid-1920s. The Luer fitting became virtually universal, and both the Luer slip tip and the Luer-Lok were standardized in 1955.

In almost all disposable and reusable needles used in regional anesthesia, the bevel is cut on three planes. The design theoretically creates less tissue laceration and discomfort than the earlier styles did, and it limits tissue coring. Many needles that are to be used for deep injection during regional block incorporate a security bead in the shaft so that the needle can be easily retrieved on the rare occasions when the needle hub separates from the needle shaft. Figure 1-5 contrasts a blunt-beveled, 25-gauge needle with a 25-gauge "hypodermic" needle. Traditional teaching holds that the short-beveled needle is less traumatic to neural structures. There is little clinical evidence that this is so, and experimental data about whether sharp or blunt needle tips minimize nerve injury are equivocal.

Figure 1-6 shows various spinal needles. The key to their successful use is to find the size and bevel tip that allow one to cannulate the subarachnoid space easily without causing repeated unrecognized puncture. For equivalent needle size, rounded needle tips that spread the dural fibers are associated with a lesser incidence of headache than are those that cut fibers. The past interest in very-small-gauge spinal catheters to reduce the incidence of spinal headache, with controllability of a continuous technique, faded during the controversy over lidocaine neurotoxicity.

Figure 1-7 depicts epidural needles. Needle tip design is often mandated by the decision to use a catheter with the epidural technique. Figure 1-8 shows two catheters available for either subarachnoid or epidural use. Although each has advantages and disadvantages, a single–end-hole catheter appears to provide the highest level of certainty of catheter tip location at the time of injection, whereas a multiple–side-hole catheter may be preferred for continuous analgesia techniques.

Continuous Infusion Dosage With the advent of ultrasound and better training, more and more continuous nerve block catheters are performed to help patients. Current practice is to limit continuous infusion at 0.4/mg/kg/hr

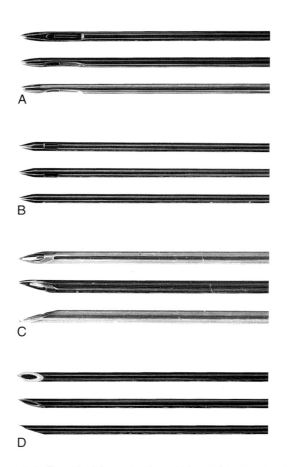

Figure 1-5. Frontal, oblique, and lateral views of regional block needles. A, Blunt-beveled, 25-gauge axillary block needle. B, Long-beveled, 25-gauge ("hypodermic") block needle. C, 22-gauge ultrasonography "imaging" needle. D, Short-beveled, 22-gauge regional block needle. *(From Brown DL: Regional Anesthesia and Analgesia. Philadelphia, WB Saunders, 1996. By permission of the Mayo Foundation, Rochester, Minn.)*

Figure 1-6. Frontal, oblique, and lateral views of common spinal needles. A, Sprotte needle. B, Whitacre needle. C, Greene needle. D, Quincke needle. *(From Brown DL: Regional Anesthesia and Analgesia. Philadelphia, WB Saunders, 1996. By permission of the Mayo Foundation, Rochester, Minn.)*

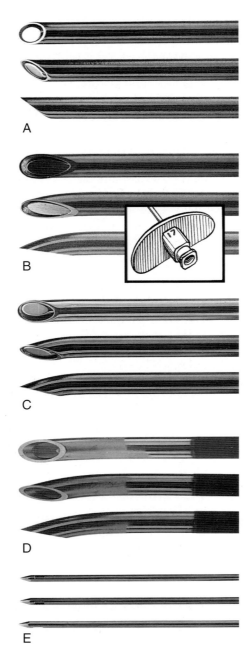

Figure 1-7. Frontal, oblique, and lateral views of common epidural needles. A, Crawford needle. B, Tuohy needle; the *inset* shows a winged hub assembly common to winged needles. C, Hustead needle. D, Curved, 18-gauge epidural needle. E, Whitacre, 27-gauge spinal needle. *(From Brown DL: Regional Anesthesia and Analgesia. Philadelphia, WB Saunders, 1996. By permission of the Mayo Foundation, Rochester, Minn.)*

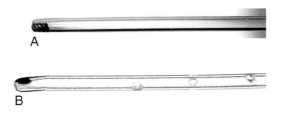

Figure 1-8. Epidural catheter designs. A, Single distal orifice. B, Closed tip with multiple side orifices. *(From Brown DL: Regional Anesthesia and Analgesia. Philadelphia, WB Saunders, 1996. By permission of the Mayo Foundation, Rochester, Minn.)*

(bupivacaine/ropivacaine). See Table 1-2 for specific block recommendations.

NERVE STIMULATORS

In recent years, use of nerve stimulators has increased from occasional use to common use and is often of critical importance. The growing emphasis on techniques that use either multiple injections near individual nerves or placement of stimulating catheters has provided impetus for this change. The primary impediment to successful use of a nerve stimulator in a clinical practice is that it is at least a three-handed or two-individual technique (Fig. 1-9), although there are devices allowing control of the stimulator current using a foot control, eliminating the need for a third hand or a second individual. In those situations requiring a second set of hands, correct operation of contemporary peripheral nerve stimulators is straightforward and easily taught during the course of the block. There are a variety of circumstances in which a nerve stimulator is helpful, such as in children and adults who are already anesthetized when a decision is made that regional block is an appropriate technique, in individuals who are unable to report paresthesias accurately, in performing local anesthetic administration on specific nerves, and in placement of stimulating catheters for anesthesia or postoperative analgesia. Another group that may benefit from the use of a nerve stimulator is patients with chronic pain, in whom accurate needle placement and reproduction of pain with electrical stimulation or elimination of pain with accurate administration of small volumes of local anesthetic may improve diagnosis and treatment.

When nerve stimulation is used during regional block, insulated needles are most appropriate because the current from such needles results in a current sphere around the needle tip, whereas uninsulated needles emit current at the tip as well as along the shaft, potentially resulting in less precise needle location. A peripheral nerve stimulator should allow between 0.1 and 10 milliamperes (mA) of current in pulses lasting approximately 200 msec at a frequency of 1 or 2 pulses per second. The peripheral nerve stimulator should have a readily apparent readout of when a complete circuit is present, a consistent and accurate current output over its entire range, and a digital display of the current delivered with each pulse. This facilitates generalized location of the nerve while stimulating at 2 mA and allows refinement of needle positioning as the current pulse is reduced to 0.5 to 0.1 mA. The nerve stimulator should have the polarity of the terminals clearly identified because peripheral nerves are most effectively stimulated by using the needle as the cathode (negative terminal). Alternatively, if the circuit is established with the needle as anode (positive terminal), approximately four times as much current is necessary to produce equivalent stimulation. The positive lead of the stimulator should be placed in a site remote from the site of stimulation by connecting the lead to a common electrocardiographic electrode (see Fig. 1-9).

The use of a nerve stimulator is not a substitute for a complete knowledge of anatomy and careful site selection for needle insertion; in fact, as much attention should be

Table 1-2 Dosage Chart for Common Continuous Nerve Blocks

Block type	Local anesthetic	Continuous rate (mL/hr)	Bolus dose (mL)	Lock-out interval (min)	Number of doses per hour
Interscalene	0.25 % Bupivacaine or 0.2 % ropivacaine	8	12	60	1
Supraclavicular	0.25 % Bupivacaine or 0.2 % ropivacaine	8	12	60	1
Popliteal	0.25 % Bupivacaine or 0.2 % ropivacaine	8	12	60	1
Femoral*	0.12 % Bupivacaine or 0.1 % ropivacaine	8	0	—	—

Adapted from: Local Anesthetics. 2015. Pharmacology and Physiology in Anesthesia Practice. Robert K. Stoelting.

Lower concentration used for femoral block to reduce the chances of motor blockade and to prevent falls.

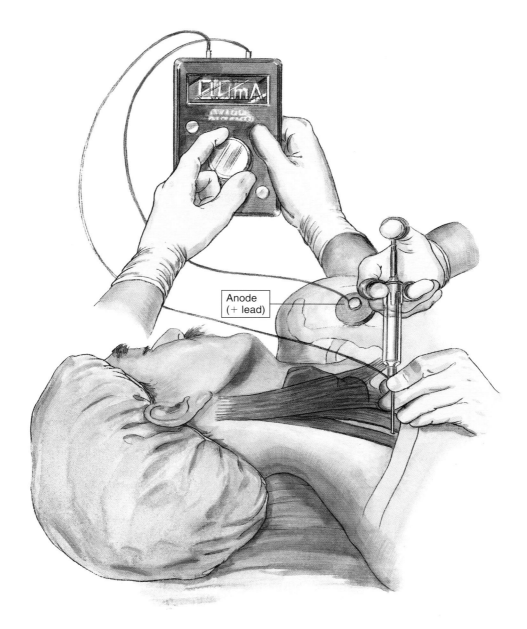

Figure 1-9. Nerve stimulator technique.

paid to the anatomy and technique when using a nerve stimulator as when not using it. Large myelinated motor fibers are stimulated by less current than are smaller unmyelinated fibers, and muscle contraction is most often produced before patient discomfort. The needle should be carefully positioned to a point where muscle contraction can be elicited with 0.5 to 0.1 mA. If a pure sensory nerve is to be blocked, a similar procedure is followed; however, correct needle localization will require the patient to report a sense of pulsed "tingling or burning" over the cutaneous distribution of the sensory nerve. Once the needle is in the final position and stimulation is achieved with 0.5 to 0.1 mA, 1 mL of local anesthetic should be injected through the needle. If the needle is accurately positioned, this amount of solution should rapidly abolish the muscle contraction or the sensation with pulsed current.

ULTRASONOGRAPHY

(see Video 1: Introduction to Ultrasound on the Expert Consult Website)

In the last decade, image-guided peripheral nerve blocks have become the norm for anesthesiologists at the forefront of regional anesthesia innovation. The dominant method of imaging is ultrasonography. Ultrasonographic imaging devices are noninvasive, portable, and moderately priced. Most work has been done using scanning probes with frequencies in the range of 5 to 10 megahertz (MHz). These devices are capable of identifying vascular and bony structures but not nerves. Contemporary devices using high-resolution probes (12 to 15 MHz) and compound imaging allow clear visualization of nerves, vessels, catheters, and local anesthetic injection and can potentially improve the techniques of ultrasonography-assisted peripheral nerve block. Use of these devices is limited by their cost, the need for training in their use and familiarity with ultrasonographic image anatomy, and the extra set of hands required. They work best with superficial nerve plexuses and can be limited by excessive obesity or anatomically distant structures. One of the keys to using this technology effectively is a sound understanding of the physics behind ultrasonography. A corollary to understanding the physics is the need for study and appreciation of the relevant human anatomy.

WAVELENGTH AND FREQUENCY

Ultrasound is a form of acoustic energy defined as the longitudinal progression of pressure changes (Fig. 1-10). These pressure changes consist of areas of compression and relaxation of particles in a given medium. For simplicity, an ultrasound wave is often modeled as a sine wave. Each ultrasound wave is defined by a specific wavelength (λ) measured in units of distance, amplitude (h) measured in decibels (dB), and frequency (f) measured in hertz (Hz) or cycles per second. Ultrasound is defined as a frequency of more than 20,000 Hz. Current transducers used for ultrasonography-guided regional anesthesia generate waves in the 3- to 13-MHz range (or 30,000 to 130,000 Hz).

ULTRASOUND GENERATION

Ultrasound is generated when multiple piezoelectric crystals inside a transducer rapidly vibrate in response to an alternating electric current. Ultrasound then travels into the body where, on contact with various tissues, it can be reflected, refracted, and scattered (Fig. 1-11).

To generate a clinically useful image, ultrasound waves must reflect off tissues and return to the transducer. The transducer, after emitting the wave, switches to a receive mode. When ultrasound waves return to the transducer, the piezoelectric crystals will vibrate once again, this time transforming the sound energy back into electrical energy. This process of transmission and reception can be repeated over 7000 times per second and, when coupled with computer processing, results in the generation of a real-time, two-dimensional image that appears seamless. By convention, whiter (hyperechoic) objects represent a larger degree of reflection and higher signal intensities, whereas darker (hypoechoic) images represent less reflection and weaker signal intensities.

CLINICAL ISSUES RELATED TO PHYSICS

Resolution. Resolution refers to the ability to clearly distinguish two structures lying beside one another. Although there are several different types of resolution, anesthesiologists are mostly concerned with lateral resolution (left–right distinction) and axial resolution (front–back distinction). Ultrasonography systems with higher frequencies have better resolution and can effectively

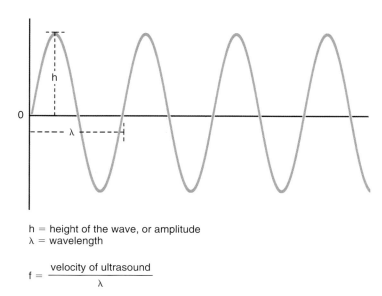

h = height of the wave, or amplitude
λ = wavelength

$$f = \frac{\text{velocity of ultrasound}}{\lambda}$$

Figure 1-10. Ultrasound wave basics.

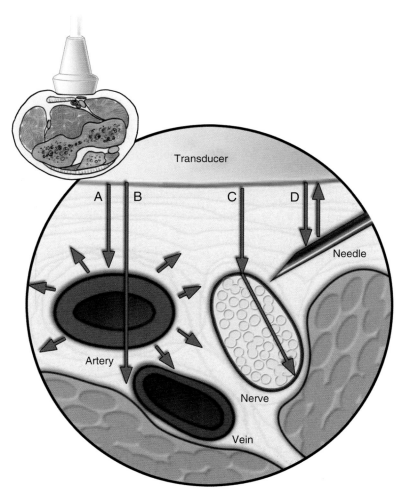

Figure 1-11. Production of an ultrasonographic image. This figure demonstrates the many responses that an ultrasound wave produces when traveling through tissue. A, Scatter reflection: the ultrasound wave is deflected in several random directions both toward and away from the probe. Scattering occurs with small or irregular objects. B, Transmission: the ultrasound wave continues through the tissue away from the probe. C, Refraction: when an ultrasound wave contacts the interface between two media with different propagation velocities, the wave is refracted (bent) to an extent depending on the difference in velocities. D, Specular reflection: a large, smooth object (e.g., the needle) returns (reflects) the ultrasound wave toward the probe when it is perpendicular to the ultrasound beam.

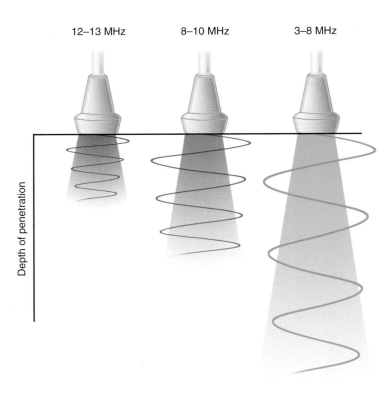

Figure 1-12. Probe frequency and depth of tissue penetration. Higher-frequency ultrasound attenuates to a larger degree at more superficial depths, although it provides more image detail.

discriminate closely spaced peripheral neural structures. However, because of a process known as *attenuation*, high-frequency ultrasound cannot penetrate into deep tissue (Fig. 1-12). Attenuation is the loss of ultrasound energy into the surrounding tissue, primarily as heat. For superficial blocks between 1 and 4 cm in depth, frequencies greater than 10 MHz are preferred. For blocks at depths greater than 4 cm, frequencies less than 8 MHz should result in adequate tissue penetration, with a predictable degradation in resolution.

Focus.   Although axial resolution is related simply to the frequency of ultrasound, lateral resolution also depends on beam thickness. Any maneuver that generates a narrow beam will increase the lateral resolution. Most ultrasonography machines have an electronic focus that generates a focal point (narrowest part of the beam) that can be placed directly over the target of interest. However, this increases the divergence of the beam beyond the region of the focus point (far field), resulting in image degradation of structures beyond this focal point. Thus the beam focus should be placed at the level of the object that is being assessed to provide the clearest possible picture of the object (Fig. 1-13).

Gain.   The overall gain and time gain compensation (TGC) controls allow the operator to increase or decrease the signal intensity. In clinical terms, the gain controls the "brightness" of the ultrasonographic image. The TGC control allows the operator to adjust gain at specific depths of the image. By increasing the overall gain or the TGC, one can compensate for the darker aspects of the ultrasonographic image, which are simply the result of ultrasound attenuation. Inappropriately low gain settings may result in the apparent absence of an existing structure (i.e., "missing structure" artifact), whereas inappropriately high gain settings can easily obscure existing structures.

COLOR DOPPLER

Color-flow Doppler ultrasonography relies on the fact that if an ultrasound pulse is sent out and strikes moving red blood cells, the ultrasound that is reflected back to the transducer will have a frequency that is different from the original emitted frequency. This change in frequency is known as the *Doppler shift*. It is this frequency change that can be used in cardiac and vascular applications to calculate both blood flow velocity and blood flow direction. The Doppler equation states that

$$\text{Frequency shift} = 2 \times V \times Ft \times \text{cosine } \Phi/c$$

where V is velocity of the moving object, Ft is the transmitted frequency, Φ is the angle of incidence of the ultrasound beam and the direction of blood flow, and c is the speed of ultrasound in the medium. The direction of blood flow is not as crucial for regional anesthesia as it is for cardiovascular anesthesia. What is most important is being able to positively identify blood vessels by visualizing color flow. This is especially important when interrogating a projected

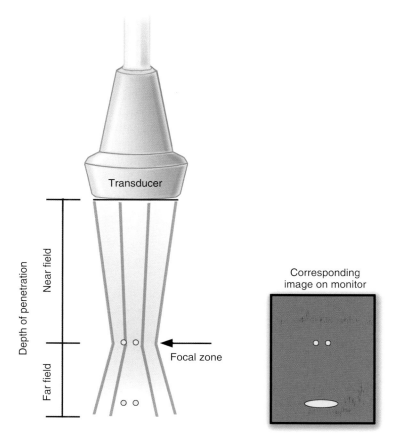

Figure 1-13. Basics of ultrasonographic probe focusing.

trajectory of the needle when placing a block. By placing color-flow Doppler over the expected needle path, the clinician should be able to screen for and avoid any unanticipated vasculature.

GENERAL PRINCIPLES OF AN ULTRASONOGRAPHY-GUIDED NERVE BLOCK

During ultrasonographic needle guidance, most nerves are imaged in cross-section (short axis). Alternatively, if the transducer is moved 90 degrees from the short-axis view, the long-axis view is generated. The short-axis view is generally preferred because it allows the operator to assess the lateromedial perspective of the target nerve, which is lost in the long-axis view (Fig. 1-14).

Two techniques have emerged regarding the orientation of the needle with respect to the ultrasound beam (Fig. 1-15). The in-plane approach generates a long-axis view of the needle, allowing full visualization of the shaft and tip of the needle. The out-of-plane view generates a short-axis view of the needle. One disadvantage of the in-plane approach is the challenge of maintaining needle imaging with a very thin ultrasound beam. A limitation of the out-of-plane view is that it generates a short-axis view of the block needle, which may be very hard to visualize. With the

Short-axis image

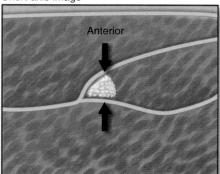

Long-axis image

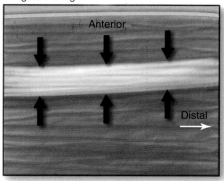

Figure 1-14. Short-axis *(top)* and long-axis *(bottom)* imaging of the median nerve.

out-of-plane view, the operator cannot confirm that the needle tip (rather than part of the shaft) is being imaged, and therefore the needle location is often inferred from tissue movement or small injections of solution.

Two main types of ultrasound probes are used for regional anesthesia:

A- Linear probe (usually higher frequency probe) that allows better resolution and more accurate identification of the margins for the target structure, with narrower ultrasonographic window.

B- Curvilinear probe (generally with lower frequency), which makes it more suitable for deeper structures, providing wider view to detect important structures adjacent to the target nerve. The caveat with the curvilinear probe is a lower degree of resolution (Figures 1-16, 1-17A, and 1-17B).

Regardless of the machine or transducer selected, there are four basic transducer manipulation techniques, which can be described as the "PART" of scanning:

Pressure (P): Various degrees of pressure are applied to the transducer that are translated onto the skin.

Alignment (A): Sliding the transducer defines the lengthwise course of the nerve and reference structures.

Rotation (R): The transducer is turned in either a clockwise or counterclockwise direction to optimize the image (either long or short axis) of the nerve and needle.

Tilting (T): The transducer is tilted in both directions to maximize the angle of incidence of the ultrasound beam to the target nerve, thereby maximizing reflection and optimizing image quality.

The primary objective of PART maneuvers is to optimize the amount of ultrasound that reflects off an object and returns to the transducer (Fig. 1-18).

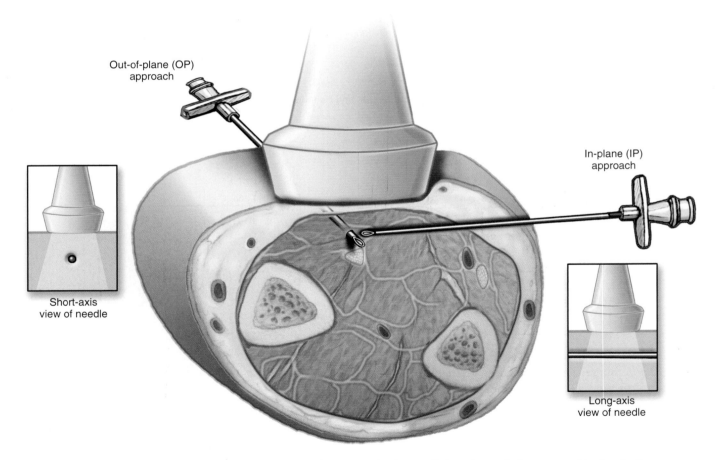

Out-of-plane (OP) approach

Short-axis view of needle

In-plane (IP) approach

Long-axis view of needle

Figure 1-15. The in-plane *(right)* and out-of-plane *(left)* needle approaches for needle insertion and ultrasonographic visualization.

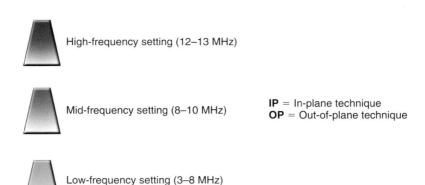

High-frequency setting (12–13 MHz)

Mid-frequency setting (8–10 MHz)

IP = In-plane technique
OP = Out-of-plane technique

Low-frequency setting (3–8 MHz)

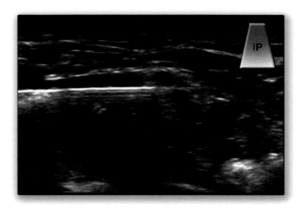

Figure 1-16. Our system for ultrasonographic needle guidance recommendations. For a block for which we would recommend a high-frequency setting with the in-plane (IP) technique of needle visualization, a red scan plane with an "IP" inside the plane is shown. For a low-frequency setting with the out-of-plane (OP) technique for needle visualization, we show a green scan plane with an "OP" in the plane. The midfrequency setting is indicated by a blue scan plane. An example is shown in the upper right of the figure. In this case, we recommend starting with a high-frequency probe setting and an in-plane technique for needle visualization.

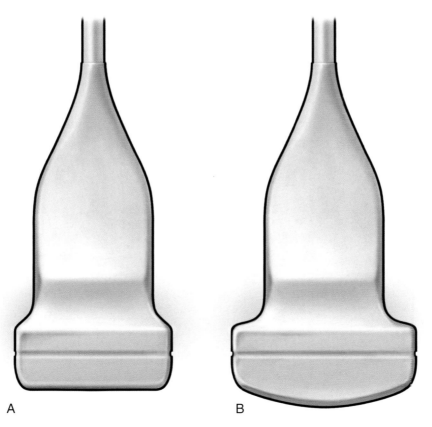

A   B

Figure 1-17. A, Linear probe; B, Curvilinear probe.

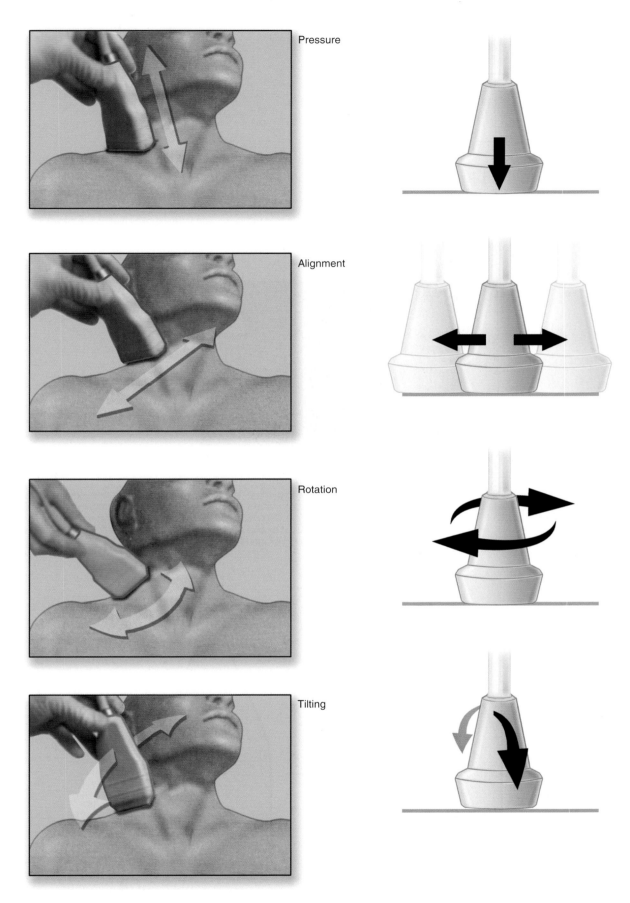

Pressure

Alignment

Rotation

Tilting

Figure 1-18. PART maneuvers: pressure, alignment, rotation, and tilting.

Pharmacology of Local Anesthetics in Pediatrics 2

Ibrahim Farid and Rami Edward Karroum

Key Points

Neonates and infants are more prone to developing systemic toxicity to local anesthetics (LAs), particularly amides LAs, compared with older children and adults. This is due to reduced plasma concentration of α_1-acid glycoprotein with higher unbound fraction and decreased clearance of amides LAs.

Higher baseline heart rates in neonates and infants predispose them to increased sensitivity for bupivacaine-induced cardiotoxicity compared with adults. This is due to the strong affinity of bupivacaine for the fast sodium channels, resulting in prolonged blockade of these channels in the cardiac conduction system and a profound decrease in ventricular conduction velocity.

Chloroprocaine is the LA of choice for epidural infusion in neonates and small infants due to its very low risk of systemic toxicity and accumulation compared with amide LAs in this age group, as well as easier dosing and pump programming.

Regional anesthesia is usually performed under general anesthesia, which may mask the earliest signs of systemic toxicity, particularly central nervous system (CNS) signs. Therefore refractory cardiovascular collapse may be the first and only sign in pediatric patients.

It is recommended to use an epinephrine-containing test dose in all regional blocks before giving the full bolus dose. Order of sensitivity for detection of unintentional intravascular injection in pediatric patients when a test dose of LAs mixed with epinephrine is given, from most to least sensitive, is:

Increase T wave amplitude and ST segment

changes > increase in systolic blood pressure

more than 10% > increase in heart rate 10%

to 15% above baseline heart rate

before administration of test dose.

Total doses of LAs should not exceed the maximum allowable dose under any circumstances. The dose should be based on the lean body weight rather than the actual body weight, particularly in obese patients.

INTRODUCTION

Local anesthetics (LAs) are divided into two main chemical compounds: the amides and the esters.

Amide LAs are metabolized exclusively in the liver by cytochrome P450 enzymes. These enzymes reach adult activity level by 9 months to 1 year of age. Therefore neonates and infants have a decreased clearance of amide LAs. Amide LAs bind to serum proteins. α_1-acid glycoprotein is the major serum protein that binds amide LAs. Albumin has a very low affinity to bind amide LAs. However, being the most abundant protein in serum, albumin binding capacity to amide LAs is not insignificant.

Infants have a decreased level of α_1-acid glycoprotein and albumin. Adult levels of protein binding are reached at about 1 year of age. Therefore neonates and infants are more prone to developing toxicity from amide LAs due to a higher serum-free fraction and lower clearance rate. The susceptibility to cardiac toxicity is amplified by increased heart rates. Due to their higher baseline heart rates, neonates and infants are more sensitive than adults to amide LA-induced cardiotoxicity.

Neonates and infants have a relatively larger volume of distribution (VD) of amide LAs compared with adults. Toxicity will be more likely to occur following repeated doses and/or continuous infusion. This can be explained by the fact that larger VD prevents high serum drug concentrations from occurring after a slow incremental injection of a single dose of amide LAs.

Commonly used amide LAs in children include lidocaine, ropivacaine, bupivacaine, its L-enantiomer levobupivacaine, and eutectic mixture of local anesthetics (EMLA) cream.

Ester LAs are degraded in plasma by cholinesterases. Although neonates and infants have a lower level of cholinesterases, this has not been shown to be of clinical significance. Commonly used ester LAs in children include tetracaine and 2% to 3% chloroprocaine. Chloroprocaine use for continuous epidural analgesia in neonates and infants has been on the rise due to its rare incidence of systemic toxicity.

AMIDE LOCAL ANESTHETICS

BUPIVACAINE

This is the most commonly used amide LA for regional blockade in pediatric anesthesia. Its long duration of action is related to its high binding to plasma proteins. Adding epinephrine will not result in further prolongation of the duration of action. However, epinephrine will reduce the rate of systemic absorption and the peak plasma concentration of bupivacaine. Its relatively slow onset of action is due to its high pKa of 8.1. It is a racemic mixture of levorotatory (L) and dextrorotatory (D) enantiomers; the L-enantiomer is the bioactive form, and the D-enantiomer is responsible for its toxicity. Toxicity from bupivacaine can be serious, ranging from central nervous system (CNS) excitation to cardiovascular collapse. Direct cardiac toxicity is due to prolonged blockade of the sodium channels in the cardiac conduction system, resulting in a profound decrease in ventricular conduction velocity. This phenomenon is markedly amplified by tachycardia due to the strong affinity of bupivacaine for the fast sodium channels. Stereoselectivity of the sodium channel in the open state, however, has not been demonstrated.

The threshold for toxicity occurs at a bupivacaine level of 2 to 4 mcg/mL. The maximum dose of bupivacaine is 2.5 to 3 mg/kg. The most commonly used concentrations for single-shot peripheral nerve block and caudal epidural is 0.25% (Table 2-1). After a single administration, analgesia usually lasts for 3 to 4 hours. For an epidural catheter, the loading dose is 0.05 mL/kg/spinal segment or between 0.5 and 1 mL/kg, not to exceed the maximum dose of 2.5 mg/kg. For continuous epidural infusion, a concentration ranging from 0.0625% to 0.125% is used and usually runs at a dose of 0.2 to 0.4 mg/kg/hr (Table 2-2).

LIPOSOMAL BUPIVACAINE

Recently, a liposome bupivacaine has been approved by the Food and Drug Administration (FDA) for use in adults as a local anesthetic injected into the surgical site for postsurgical pain relief. The liposome bupivacaine formulation incorporates liposome-encapsulated bupivacaine (Depo-Foam) and a small amount of extraliposomal bupivacaine.

The liposome-encapsulated component permits bupivacaine release over an extended period. The extraliposomal component allows for rapid release and relatively rapid onset of action. There are some recent studies evaluating its use in the epidural space in adults as an alternative to continuous bupivacaine infusion through an indwelling epidural catheter. Liposomal bupivacaine is not currently approved for use in children. If approved, it may offer an attractive alternative in children in whom an indwelling catheter is not an option, but in whom prolonged regional blockade provided by liposome bupivacaine formulation may be beneficial.

LEVOBUPIVACAINE (L-ENANTIOMER OF BUPIVACAINE)

Levobupivacaine has almost the same blocking properties and pharmacokinetics as its racemic counterpart bupivacaine. The effect on the cardiac conduction system is stereospecific, with the L-enantiomer having much less effect than the D-enantiomer present in the racemic mixture of bupivacaine. As a result, levobupivacaine carries a reduced risk of cardiac toxicity compared with bupivacaine. It is currently unavailable in the United States.

ROPIVACAINE

This exists as an L-enantiomer. It is chemically similar to bupivacaine, but with a difference of having a propyl (three-carbon) side chain, whereas bupivacaine has a butyl (four-carbon) side chain. In an equipotent dose, it carries a lower risk of cardiac and neurological toxicities compared with bupivacaine. This makes ropivacaine an attractive alternative to bupivacaine in pediatric patients. The data

Table 2-1 Single-Shot Caudal Epidural Dose of LAs

Local Anesthetics	Concentration	Dose (mg/kg)	Dose (mL/kg)
Bupivacaine	0.25% (2.5 mg/mL)	2.5 mg/kg	1 mL/kg
Ropivacaine	0.2% (2 mg/mL)	2 mg/kg	1 mL/kg

Table 2-2 Suggested Epidural Infusion Concentrations and Rates for Pediatric Patients

LAs	Maximum Rate of Infusion and Suggested Infusion Concentration (conc.)		
	Neonates and infants up to 6 months	Infants (6 months to 1 year)	Children older than 1 year
Chloroprocaine*	Conc. of 2%. Rate of 5 to 15 mg/kg/hr	N/A***	N/A***
Bupivacaine	Conc. of 0.0625%. Rate of 0.2 mg/kg/hr for no more than 48 hours.	Conc. of 0.0625% to 0.125%. Rate of 0.3 to 0.4 mg/kg/hr. Reduce the infusion rate 30% after 48 hours and discontinue after 72 hours.	Conc. of 0.0625% to 0.125%. Rate of 0.4 mg/kg/hr.
Ropivacaine**	Conc. of 0.1%. Rate of 0.2 mg/kg/hr for no more than 72 hours. Reduce the infusion rate 30% after 48 hours.	Conc. of 0.1% to 0.2%. Rate of 0.3 to 0.4 mg/kg/hr. Reduce the infusion rate 30% after 48 hours.	Conc. of 0.1% to 0.2%. Rate of 0.4 mg/kg/hr.

*Chloroprocaine is the first choice for epidural infusion in neonates due to reduced risk of systemic toxicity compared with amide LAs.

**Ropivacaine is the second choice for epidural infusion in neonates due to its better toxicity profile compared with bupivacaine.

***N/A = nonapplicable. Chloroprocaine is not usually used in this age group and is replaced by amide LAs.

available from studies on infants and children do not report greater sparing of motor function following ropivacaine blockade compared with bupivacaine. Adult studies are conflicting in this regard.

The most commonly used concentration for single-shot caudal and single-shot peripheral nerve block is 0.2 % (see Table 2-1). For an epidural catheter, the loading dose is 0.05 mL/kg/spinal segment or between 0.5 and 1 mL/kg, not to exceed the maximum dose of 3 mg/kg. For continuous infusion, the concentration range is from 0.1% to 0.2% and usually runs at a dose of 0.2 to 0.5 mg/kg/hr (see Table 2-2).

LIDOCAINE

Lidocaine is not commonly used in pediatrics due to its short duration of analgesia. The amides ropivacaine and bupivacaine are more commonly used instead.

EMLA CREAM

This is a eutectic mixture of equal quantities of lidocaine 2.5% and prilocaine 2.5%. It is commonly used to provide transdermal local anesthesia in pediatric patients. Methemoglobinemia has been reported with the use of EMLA cream. Therefore the maximum total surface area to which the cream is applied should be calculated in advance, and the maximum allowable dose should never be exceeded (Table 2-3). This is particularly important in neonates. However, close attention should also be paid to the dose used in infants and toddlers. EMLA cream should be applied only to intact skin, and the dose should be reduced in case it is applied to mucous membranes. Other reported side effects include blanching and rash at the site of application. The duration of action is 1 to 2 hours.

Table 2-3 Maximum Recommended Doses and Application Areas for EMLA Cream

Body Weight and Age	Maximum Total Dose	Maximum Surface Area
0 to 3 months or <5 kg	1 g	10 cm^2
3 to 12 months and 5 to 10 kg	2 g	20 cm^2
1 to 6 years and 10 to 20 kg	10 g	100 cm^2
7 to 12 years and >20 kg	20 g	200 cm^2

LIDOCAINE AND TETRACAINE (SYNERA) TRANSDERMAL PATCH

This is a combination of lidocaine, an amide LA, and tetracaine, an ester LA. The drug formulation is an emulsion in which the oil phase is a 1 : 1 eutectic mixture of lidocaine 7% and tetracaine 7%. Each patch contains 70 mg lidocaine and 70 mg tetracaine and has a total skin contact area of 50 cm, and an active drug-containing area of 10 cm^2. The eutectic mixture has a melting point below room temperature, and therefore both LAs exist as a liquid oil rather

than as crystals. The patch has a heating component that begins to heat once the patch is removed from the pouch and is exposed to oxygen in the air. It increases skin temperature slightly to increase blood flow into the area and speeds up delivery of LAs to provide anesthesia to a depth of almost 7 mm. It is used to facilitate venipuncture, intravenous cannulation, and some superficial dermatological procedures. It should be applied only to intact skin. Methemoglobinemia has been reported, and caution should be exercised in patients with congenital or idiopathic methemoglobinemia. Caution should be exercised in patients with pseudocholinesterase deficiency, as they are at greater risk of tetracaine toxicity.

If being used with other products containing an LA, consider the potential for additive effects. The heating component contains iron powder and must be removed before magnetic resonance imaging (MRI). Application of the patch for a longer duration than recommended, or simultaneous or sequential application of multiple patches, is not recommended because of the risk for increased drug absorption and possible adverse reactions. Cutting the patch or removing the top cover could cause the patch to heat to temperatures that could result in thermal injury. On the other hand, covering the holes on the top side of the patch could cause the patch not to heat. The most common side effects are local skin reactions such as redness of the skin and swelling; these reactions are generally mild and resolve spontaneously after discontinuation of the patch. Safety and effectiveness of the patch have been established in patients 3 years of age and older. Apply the patch for 20 to 30 minutes prior to venipuncture or intravenous cannulation. For superficial dermatological procedures such as superficial excision or shave biopsy, apply the patch for 30 minutes prior to the procedure. A topical cream of lidocaine and tetracaine (Pliaglis) also exists, but is indicated only for adult use.

ESTER LOCAL ANESTHETICS

TETRACAINE

Tetracaine is the most commonly used LA for spinal anesthesia in children. Some centers use spinal anesthesia with tetracaine as the sole anesthetic for inguinal hernia repair in premature or ex-premature neonates. This practice is most relevant for those premature neonates who are less than 60 weeks postconceptual age at the time of surgery. This population is at risk for developing postoperative apnea, and the use of spinal anesthesia may decrease the incidence of such complication.

Neonates have a larger total volume of cerebrospinal fluid (CSF) compared with adults (4 mL/kg compared with 2 mL/kg, respectively). In addition, 50% of the total CSF volume is in the spinal portion of the subarachnoid space compared with only 25% of the total CSF volume in adults. Also, neonates have a more rapid turnover of CSF than adults. As a result, neonates require larger doses of LAs for spinal anesthesia, and the duration of the spinal block is shorter.

Tetracaine is used in a concentration of 1% (10 mg/mL), and the calculated dose is mixed in an equivalent volume

Table 2-4 Tetracaine Dose for Spinal Anesthesia for Inguinal Hernia Repair

Local Anesthetic	Age and Weight	Dose	Duration of Action
Tetracaine 1% in 10% dextrose (1:1 dilution) (hyperbaric)	Neonates and less than 5 kg* Infants and 5 to 15 kg Children and greater than 15 kg	0.5 to 0.6 mg/kg 0.3 to 0.4 mg/kg 0.2 to 0.3 mg/kg	90 to 120 minutes**

*Maximum dose of 1 mg/kg can be used to achieve mid to high thoracic level dermatomes.

**Duration can be extended by 30% with the addition of epinephrine.

of dextrose 10% to make the solution hyperbaric. The final concentration of tetracaine is 0.5% (5 mg/mL). For inguinal hernia repair, neonates less than 5 kg require the largest dose of 0.5 to 0.6 mg/kg. For infants 5-15 kg, the dose is 0.3 to 0.4 mg/kg, and for children greater than 15 kg, the dose is 0.2 to 0.3 mg/kg (Table 2-4).

The duration of the block is 90 to 120 minutes. This can be extended by 30% with the addition of epinephrine 1:100,000. If a higher block level is desired in neonates, the dose can be increased up to a maximum of 1 mg/kg. This dose can result in a block that extends to a dermatome height in the mid to upper thoracic region.

CHLOROPROCAINE

Chloroprocaine is increasingly used to provide continuous epidural infusion for postoperative pain control in neonates. It is rapidly metabolized by cholinesterases, with an elimination half-life of few minutes. Although neonates have a reduced level of plasma esterases compared with adults, this is clinically insignificant. Therefore the incidence of systemic toxicity is rare and the risk of accumulation is minimal. This safety profile allows better analgesia in neonates, as it allows the use of higher infusion rates and thus wider dermatomal coverage compared with amide LAs. Chloroprocaine has a rapid onset of action (5 to 10 minutes) because of its high tissue penetrance. It has a short duration of action (45 minutes) that can be prolonged to 70 to 90 minutes with addition of epinephrine. Its potency is 25% that of bupivacaine or tetracaine. Epidural anesthesia is achieved by administering up to 1 mL/kg of 2% to 3% chloroprocaine with epinephrine 1:200,000 (maximum dose of chloroprocaine: 20 to 30 mg/kg). For continuous epidural analgesia rates, refer to Table 2-2.

TOXICITY OF LOCAL ANESTHETICS

DIRECT NEUROTOXICITY

All LAs are potentially capable of producing direct neurotoxicity. This complication is rare, and conclusive human studies are still lacking in this field. However, animal studies show that the risk is higher on the developing nervous system and is directly related to the concentration of the LA. Therefore neonates and infants are at higher risk since their nervous system is still developing. It is recommended to avoid the use of a high concentration of LAs in this age group.

SYSTEMIC TOXICITY

Predisposing Factors

Neonates and infants are more prone to developing systemic toxicity to LAs, particularly amide LAs, compared with older children and adults. This is due to:

- Reduced plasma concentration of α_1-acid glycoprotein in this age group, resulting in higher unbound fraction of amide LAs, which is responsible for toxicity.
- Decreased clearance of amide LAs in neonates and infants due to decreased metabolism in the liver by cytochrome P450 enzymes.
- Regional anesthesia is usually performed under general anesthesia, which may mask the earliest signs of systemic toxicity, particularly CNS signs. Therefore refractory cardiovascular collapse may be the first and only sign.
- Higher baseline heart rates in neonates and infants predispose them to increased sensitivity for bupivacaine-induced cardiotoxicity compared with adults.

Clinical Picture

- Systemic toxicity can result from accidental intravascular injection of LAs or secondary to systemic absorption of LAs from the regional block site, particularly when maximum recommended doses are exceeded.
- Systemic toxicity is consistent with signs of CNS and cardiac toxicity.
- Regional anesthesia is usually performed under general anesthesia in pediatric patients. Although general anesthesia with inhalational agents raises the threshold for seizure, it will also lower the threshold for cardiac toxicity. Therefore, general anesthesia may confound the diagnosis of systemic toxicity, and the first sign may be cardiovascular collapse.
- The bupivacaine threshold for cardiac toxicity is lower than its CNS toxicity in pediatrics. Therefore in pediatrics, signs of cardiac toxicity may precede signs of CNS toxicity or may be the only sign of systemic toxicity. This is different from adults, where signs of CNS toxicity usually precede cardiac toxicity.
- Signs of systemic toxicity under general anesthesia may be nonspecific and consist of muscle rigidity,

unexplained hypoxemia, unexplained tachycardia, dysrhythmias, and cardiovascular collapse.

- When bupivacaine is mixed with epinephrine (usually in a 1 : 200,000 dilution), the earliest and most reliable sign of unintentional intravascular injection is increase in the T wave amplitude of more than 50% compared with baseline, with associated ST segment changes. These electrocardiogram (EKG) changes are very sensitive. They occur within 60 seconds from injection. If only a small test dose is given, these changes are transient and brief and do not progress into cardiovascular collapse.
- Following a test dose of bupivacaine and epinephrine, tachycardia is not a sensitive sign for unintentional intravascular injection in pediatrics.
- Order of sensitivity for detection of unintentional intravascular injection in pediatrics, from most to least sensitive, is:

  Increase T wave amplitude and ST segment changes
  > increase in systolic blood pressure more than 10%
  > increase in heart rate 10% to 15% above baseline heart rate before administration of test dose.

- After the age of 8 years, T wave changes are less sensitive for the detection of intravascular injection.
- If a bolus dose of bupivacaine is unintentionally injected intravascularly, cardiac arrhythmias and subsequent cardiovascular collapse develop rapidly.

Prevention/Reducing the Risk

- Careful calculation of total doses of LAs administered.
- Total doses of LAs should not exceed the maximum allowable dose under any circumstances (Table 2-5).
- The dose should be based on the lean body weight rather than the actual body weight, particularly in obese patients. Lean body weight can be extrapolated by knowing actual body weight and ideal body weight.
- The dose should be reduced in pediatric patients with associated comorbidities such as patients with liver failure or congestive heart failure (CHF).
- Decrease bolus dose of amide LAs by 30% for all infants younger than 6 months of age.
- Limit the duration of amide LA infusion to no more than 48 hours for bupivacaine and 72 hours for ropivacaine for all infants and neonates less than 6 months of age (see Table 2-2).

Table 2-5 Maximum Recommended Doses of Commonly Used LAs

LAs	Dose (mg/kg)
Bupivacaine	2.5 to 3
Ropivacaine	3
Levobupivacaine	3
Lidocaine / lidocaine + epinephrine	4/7
2-chloroprocaine	20

- Chloroprocaine is the LA of choice for epidural infusion in neonates and small infants due to its very low risk of systemic toxicity and accumulation compared with amide LAs in this age group.
- When mixing two different LAs, toxicity is additive. So when mixing equivalent amounts of two different LAs, the maximum dose for each should be reduced by 50%.
- Using ropivacaine or levobupivacaine instead of bupivacaine may reduce the risk of cardiotoxicity.
- When performing an epidural block, aspiration of blood or CSF through the needle or catheter may indicate that the tip is within a vessel or subarachnoid space, respectively. However, a false-negative aspiration test tends to occur frequently in pediatric patients. This is related to the fact that even the smallest applied negative pressure can result in collapse of the thin-walled vessels.
- It is recommended to use an epinephrine-containing test dose in all regional blocks before giving the full bolus dose. This will help detect unintentional intravascular injections as mentioned earlier.
- The only exception for the use of an epinephrine-containing test dose is the block that involves an end artery, such as penile and digital blocks.
- Slow and intermittent injection of all bolus doses should occur over several minutes. Rapid injection can result in systemic toxicity even if the maximum allowable dose is not exceeded and the injection is not intravascular. This results from a rapid surge of LAs in the blood beyond the protein-carrying capacity of neonates and infants.
- Absorption of LAs from the site of regional block from higher to lower is:

  Intercostal > caudal > lumbar epidural > thoracic epidural > brachial > femoral > sciatic

- Ilioinguinal/iliohypogastric nerve blocks, particularly in children less than 15 kg, are associated with alarming levels of bupivacaine in the blood, even when half the maximum recommended dose is used. Therefore this block should be performed under ultrasound guidance, as it can limit the required volume needed to perform the block. A volume of 0.2 mL/kg of ropivacaine 0.2% is used in an ultrasound-guided block compared with the anatomic landmark method that may require the use of up to 1 mL/kg.
- Whenever a regional block is performed in pediatric patients, all resuscitation equipment should be immediately available.

Treatment

Effective CPR

- This is the first line of treatment in conjunction with Intralipid administration.
- This includes securing the airway and ensuring adequate breathing and circulation through the performance of quality chest compression.

Intralipid 20%

- This is recommended as the next line of treatment for cardiotoxicity induced by bupivacaine and ropivacaine.
- Give immediately and without delay *in conjunction* with cardiopulmonary resuscitation (CPR).
- Acts as a "lipid sink" by promoting dissociation of bupivacaine from the myocardium and therefore shortens the duration of bupivacaine-induced asystole.
- Pediatric dose is similar to adult doses and consists of a bolus of 1.5 mL/kg over 1 minute. Repeat bolus dose can be given in 3 to 5 minutes with a maximum of 3 mL/kg. This is followed by a maintenance infusion of 0.25 mL/kg/min until the circulation is restored.

Prevention and Treatment of Seizure

- Should only occur after securing the airway and ensuring adequate breathing and oxygenation, because the majority of cases of morbidity that occurs with seizure are related to airway complications such as aspiration and hypoxia.
- Midazolam 0.05 to 0.2 mg/kg IV is the agent of choice.
- Propofol 1 to 2 mg/kg may be also used to control seizure; however, this should be used with caution and in the absence of hypotension or cardiovascular instability.
- Mild hyperventilation can help raise the seizure threshold by inducing respiratory alkalosis
- Some case reports suggest the use of Intralipid 20% to treat CNS toxicity of LAs, even in the absence of cardiotoxicity and suggests its use as a first line of treatment in this context.

Support the Circulation

- Intravenous fluid bolus with 10 to 20 mL/kg of isotonic fluids such as lactated Ringer's.
- Phenylephrine infusion starting at a rate of 0.1 mcg/kg/min to support the vascular tone antagonizes the LA-induced vasodilatation.
- Successful use of cardiopulmonary bypass has been also reported.

Suggested Reading

Amory C, Mariscal A, Guyot E, et al. Is ilioinguinal/iliohypogastric nerve block always totally safe in children? *Paediatr Anaesth* 2003;13:164–166.

Bardsley H, Gristwood R, Baker H, et al. A comparison of the cardiovascular effects of levobupivacaine and rac-bupivacaine following intravenous administration to healthy volunteers. *Br J ClinPharmacol* 1998;46:245–249.

Berde CB. Toxicity of local anesthetics in infants and children. *J Pediatr* 1993;122:S14–S20.

Cook DR. Paediatric anaesthesia: pharmacological considerations. *Drugs* 1976;12:212–221.

Coté CJ, Lerman J, Todres ID, editors. *A practice of anesthesia for infants and children.* 5th ed. Philadelphia: Saunders Elsevier; 2013 Chapter 41: Regional anesthesia.

Gorfine SR, Onel E, Patou G, Krivokapic ZV. Bupivacaine extended-release liposome injection for prolonged postsurgical analgesia in patients undergoing hemorrhoidectomy: a multicenter, randomized, double-blind, placebo-controlled trial. *Dis Colon Rectum* 2011;54:1552–1559.

Gourrier E, Karoubi P, el Hanache A, et al. Use of EMLA cream in a department of neonatology. *Pain* 1996;68:431–434.

Hodgson PS, Neal JM, Pollock JE, Liu SS. The neurotoxicity of drugs given intrathecally (spinal). *Anesth Analg* 1999;88: 797–809.

Krane EJ, Haberkern CM, Jacobson LE. Postoperative apnea, bradycardia, and oxygen desaturation in formerly premature infants: prospective comparison of spinal and general anesthesia. *Anesth Analg* 1995;80:7–13.

Litz RJ, Roessel T, Heller AR, Stehr SN. Reversal of central nervous system and cardiac toxicity after local anesthetic intoxication by lipid emulsion injection. *Anesth Analg* 2008;106: 1575–1577.

Mauch JY, Spielmann N, Hartnack S, Weiss M. Electrocardiographic and haemodynamic alterations caused by three different test solutions of local anaesthetics to detect accidental intravascular injection in children. *Br J Anaesth* 2012;108: 283–289.

McCloskey JJ, Haun SE, Deshpande JK. Bupivacaine toxicity secondary to continuous caudal epidural infusion in children. *Anesth Analg* 1992;75:287–290.

Mirtallo J. State of the art review: intravenous fat emulsions: current applications, safety profile, and clinical implications. *Ann Pharmacother* 2010;44:688–700.

Rice LJ, DeMars PD, Whalen TV, et al. Duration of spinal anesthesia in infants less than one year of age. Comparison of three hyperbaric techniques. *Reg Anesth* 1994;19:325–329.

Ward RM, Mirkin BL. Perinatal/neonatal pharmacology. In: Brody TM, Larner J, Minneman KP, editors. *Human pharmacology: molecular to clinical.* 3rd ed. St Louis: Mosby-Year Book; 1998. p. 873–883.

Weinberg GL. Treatment of local anesthetic systemic toxicity (LAST). *Reg Anesth Pain Med* 2010;35:188–193.

Weinberg G, Lin B, Zheng S, et al. Partitioning effect in lipid resuscitation: further evidence for the lipid sink. *Crit Care Med* 2010;38:2268–2269.

Willschke H, Marhofer P, Bosenberg A, et al. Ultrasonography for ilioinguinal/iliohypogastric nerve blocks in children. *Br J Anaesth* 2005;95:226–230.

SECTION II
Upper Extremity Blocks

Upper Extremity Block Anatomy 3

David L. Brown

Man uses his arms and hands constantly ... as a result he exposes his arms and hands to injury constantly. ... Man also eats constantly. ... Man's stomach is never really empty. ... The combination of man's prehensibility and his unflagging appetite keeps a steady flow of patients with injured upper extremities and full stomachs streaming into hospital emergency rooms. This is why the brachial plexus is so frequently the anesthesiologist's favorite group of nerves.

Classical Anesthesia Files, David Little, 1963

The late David Little's appropriate observations do not always lead anesthesiologists to choose a regional anesthetic for upper extremity surgery. However, those selecting regional anesthesia recognize that there are multiple sites at which the brachial plexus block can be induced. If anesthesiologists are to deliver comprehensive anesthesia care, they should be familiar with brachial plexus blocks. Familiarity with these techniques demands an understanding of brachial plexus anatomy. One problem with understanding this anatomy is that the traditional wiring diagram for the brachial plexus is unnecessarily complex and intimidating.

Figure 3-1 illustrates that the plexus is formed by the ventral rami of the fifth to eighth cervical nerves and the greater part of the ramus of the first thoracic nerve. In addition, small contributions may be made by the fourth cervical and the second thoracic nerves. The intimidating part of this anatomy is what happens from the time these ventral rami emerge from between the middle and anterior scalene muscles until they end in the four terminal branches to the upper extremity: the musculocutaneous, median, ulnar, and radial nerves. Most of what happens to the roots on their way to becoming peripheral nerves is not clinically essential information for an anesthesiologist. There are some broad concepts that may help clinicians understand the brachial plexus anatomy; throughout, my goal in this chapter is to simplify this anatomy.

After the roots pass between the scalene muscles, they reorganize into trunks—superior, middle, and inferior. The trunks continue toward the first rib. At the lateral edge of the first rib, these trunks undergo a primary anatomic division into ventral and dorsal divisions. This is also the point at which understanding of brachial plexus anatomy gives way to frustration and often unnecessary complexity. This anatomic division is significant because nerves destined to supply the originally ventral part of the upper extremity separate from those that supply the dorsal part. As these divisions enter the axilla, the divisions give way to cords. The posterior divisions of all three trunks unite to form the posterior cord; the anterior divisions of the superior and middle trunks form the lateral cord; the un-united, anterior division of the inferior trunk forms the medial cord. These cords are named according to their relationship to the second part of the axillary artery.

At the lateral border of the pectoralis minor muscle (which inserts onto the coracoid process), the three cords reorganize to give rise to the peripheral nerves of the upper extremity. Simplified, the branches of the lateral and medial cords are all "ventral" nerves to the upper extremity. The posterior cord, in contrast, provides all "dorsal" innervation to the upper extremity. Thus the radial nerve supplies all the dorsal musculature in the upper extremity below the shoulder. The musculocutaneous nerve supplies muscular innervation in the arm while providing cutaneous innervation to the forearm. In contrast, the median and ulnar nerves are nerves of passage in the arm, but in the forearm and hand they provide the ventral musculature with motor innervation. These nerves can be further categorized: the median nerve innervates more heavily in the forearm, whereas the ulnar nerve innervates more heavily in the hand.

Some writers have focused anesthesiologists' attention on the fascial investment of the brachial plexus. As the brachial plexus nerve roots leave the transverse processes, they do so between prevertebral fascia that divides to invest both the anterior and the middle scalene muscles. Many suggest that this prevertebral fascia surrounding the brachial plexus is tubular throughout its course, thus allowing needle placement within the "sheath" to produce brachial plexus block easily. There is no question that the brachial plexus is invested with prevertebral fascia; however, the fascial covering is discontinuous, with septa subdividing portions of the sheath into compartments that clinically may prevent adequate spread of local anesthetics. Ultrasonographic observation of injections near the brachial plexus confirms our earlier clinical impressions of fascial discontinuity. My clinical impression is that the discontinuity of the "sheath" increases as one moves from transverse process to axilla.

Most upper extremity surgery is performed with the patient resting supine on an operating table with the arm extended on an arm board. Thus anesthesiologists must

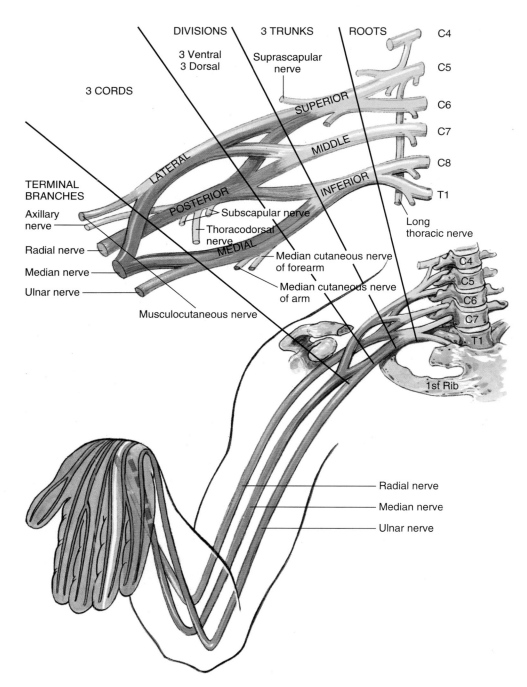

Figure 3-1. Brachial plexus anatomy.

understand and clearly visualize the innervation of the upper extremity while the patient is in this position. Figures 3-2 through 3-7 illustrate these features with the arm in the supinated and pronated positions for the cutaneous nerves and dermatomal and osteotomal patterns, respectively.

An additional clinical "pearl" that will help anesthesiologists check brachial plexus block before initiation of the surgical procedure is the "four Ps." Figure 3-8 shows how the mnemonic "push, pull, pinch, pinch" can help an anesthesiologist remember how to check the four peripheral nerves of interest in the brachial plexus block. By having the patient resist the anesthesiologist's pulling the forearm away from the upper arm, motor innervation to the biceps muscle is assessed. If this muscle has been weakened, one can be certain that local anesthetic has reached the musculocutaneous nerve. Likewise, by asking the patient to

attempt to extend the forearm by contracting the triceps muscle, one assesses the radial nerve. Finally, pinching the fingers in the distribution of the ulnar or median nerve—that is, at the base of the fifth or second digit, respectively—helps the anesthesiologist develop a sense of the adequacy of block of both the ulnar and median nerves. Typically, if these maneuvers are performed shortly after brachial plexus block, motor weakness will be evident before sensory block. As a historical highlight, this technique for checking the upper extremity was developed during World War II to allow medics a method of quick analysis of injuries to the brachial plexus.

Although some of the brachial plexus neural anatomy of interest to anesthesiologists has been outlined, there are some anatomic details that should be highlighted (Fig. 3-9). As the cervical roots leave the transverse processes on their

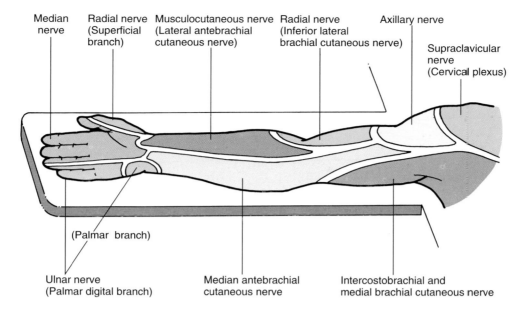

Median nerve · Radial nerve (Superficial branch) · Musculocutaneous nerve (Lateral antebrachial cutaneous nerve) · Radial nerve (Inferior lateral brachial cutaneous nerve) · Axillary nerve · Supraclavicular nerve (Cervical plexus)

(Palmar branch)

Ulnar nerve (Palmar digital branch) · Median antebrachial cutaneous nerve · Intercostobrachial and medial brachial cutaneous nerve

Figure 3-2. Upper extremity peripheral nerve innervation with arm supinated on arm board.

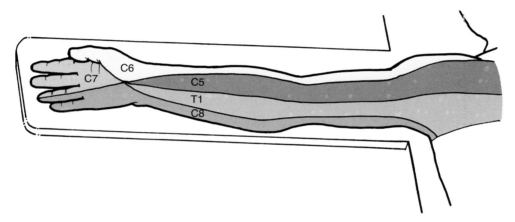

C6 · C7 · C5 · T1 · C8

Figure 3-3. Upper extremity dermatome innervation with arm supinated on arm board.

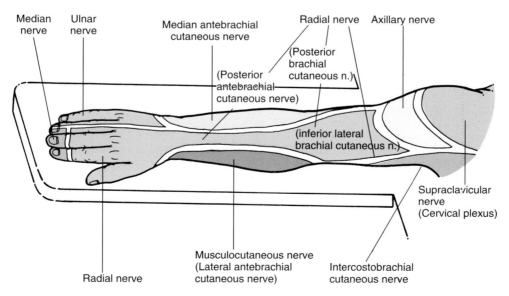

Median nerve · Ulnar nerve · Median antebrachial cutaneous nerve · Radial nerve · Axillary nerve · (Posterior brachial cutaneous n.) · (Posterior antebrachial cutaneous nerve) · (inferior lateral brachial cutaneous n.) · Supraclavicular nerve (Cervical plexus)

Radial nerve · Musculocutaneous nerve (Lateral antebrachial cutaneous nerve) · Intercostobrachial cutaneous nerve

Figure 3-4. Upper extremity peripheral nerve innervation with arm pronated on arm board.

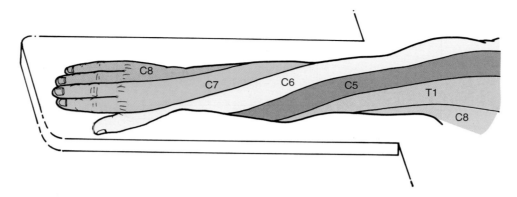

Figure 3-5. Upper extremity dermatome innervation with arm pronated on arm board.

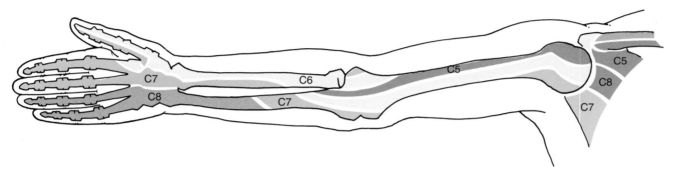

Figure 3-6. Upper extremity osteotomes with arm supinated.

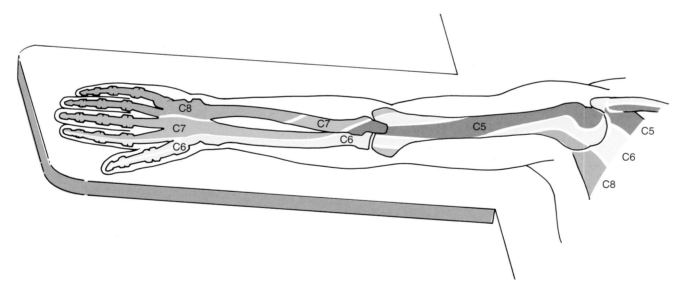

Figure 3-7. Upper extremity osteotomes with arm pronated on arm board.

way to the brachial plexus, they exit in the gutter of the transverse process immediately posterior to the vertebral artery. The vertebral arteries leave the brachiocephalic and subclavian arteries on the right and left, respectively, and travel cephalad, normally entering a bony canal in the transverse process at the level of C6 and above. Thus, one must be constantly aware of needle tip location in relationship to the vertebral artery. It should be remembered that the vertebral artery lies anterior to the roots of the brachial plexus as they leave the cervical vertebrae.

Another structure of interest in the brachial plexus anatomy is the phrenic nerve. It is formed from branches of the third, fourth, and fifth cervical nerves and passes through the neck on its way to the thorax on the ventral surface of the anterior scalene muscle. It is almost always blocked during interscalene block and less frequently with supraclavicular techniques or with cervical paravertebral block. Avoidance of phrenic blockade is important in only a small percentage of patients, although phrenic nerve location should be kept in mind for those with significantly decreased pulmonary function—that is, those whose day-to-day activities are limited by their pulmonary impairment.

Another detail of the brachial plexus anatomy that needs amplification is the organization of the brachial plexus nerves (divisions) as they cross the first rib. Textbooks often

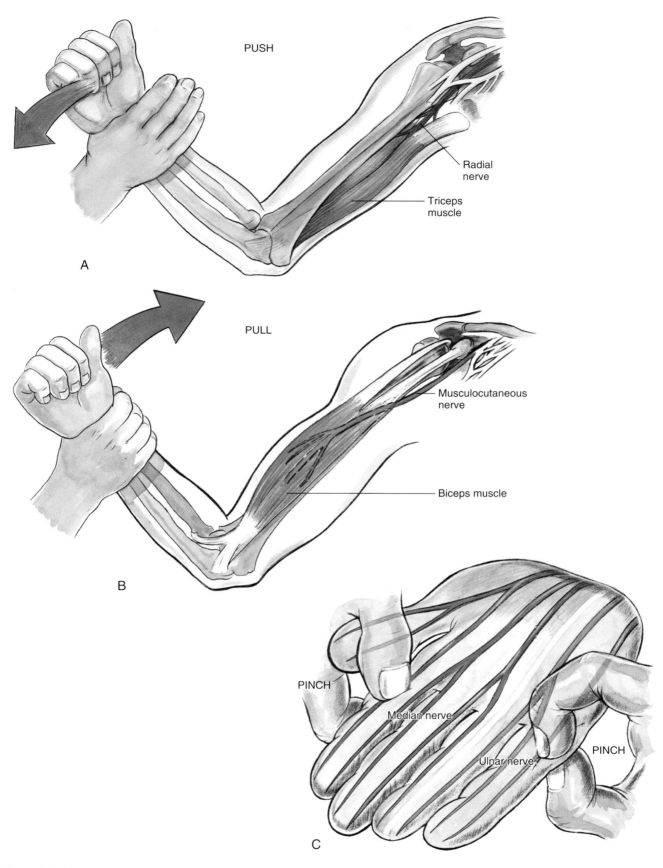

Figure 3-8. Upper extremity peripheral nerve function mnemonic: "push (A), pull (B), pinch, pinch (C)."

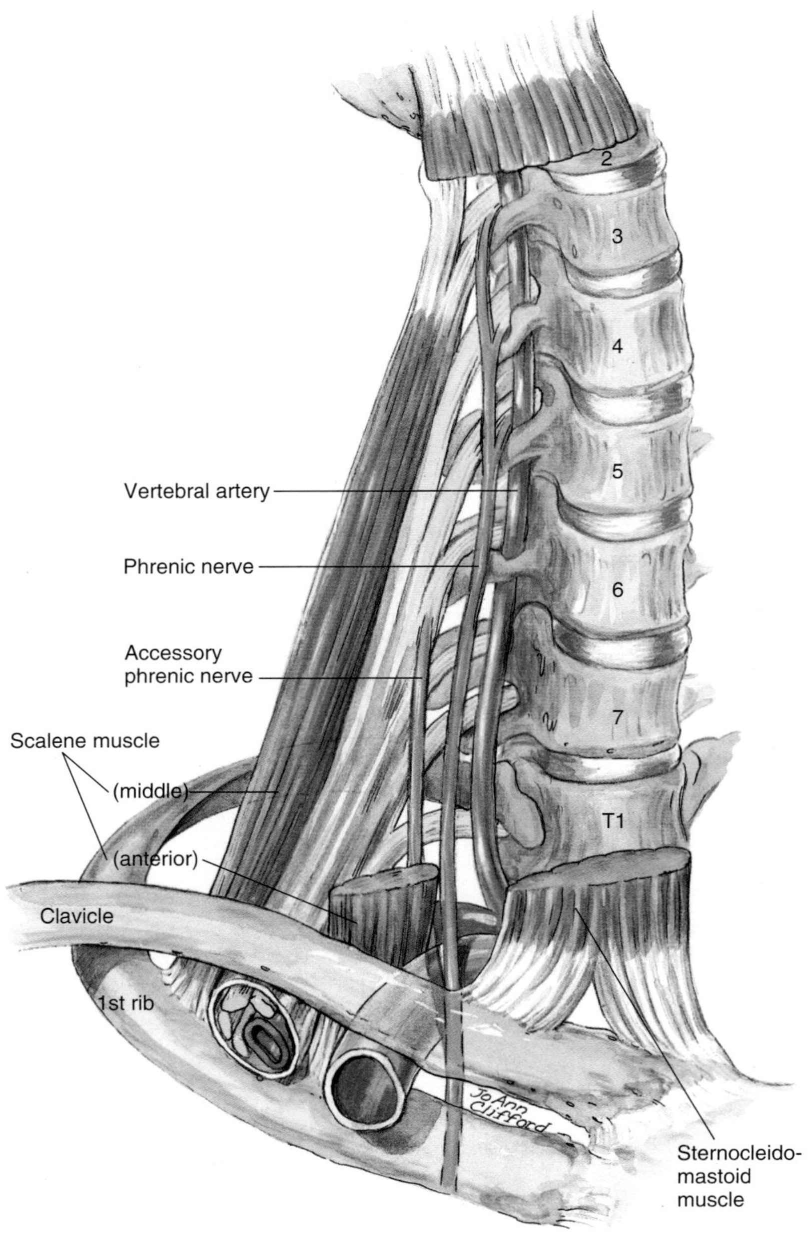

Figure 3-9. Supraclavicular regional block: functional anatomy.

depict the nerves in a stacked arrangement at this point. However, radiologic, clinical, ultrasonographic, and anatomic investigations demonstrate that the nerves are not discretely "stacked" at this point, but rather assume a posterior and cranial relationship to the subclavian artery (Fig. 3-10). This is important when one is carrying out supraclavicular nerve block and is using the rib as an anatomic landmark. The relationship of the nerves to the artery means that if one simply walks the needle tip closely along the first rib, one may not as easily elicit paresthesias because the nerves are more cranial in relationship to the first rib.

Another anatomic detail that needs highlighting is the proximal axillary anatomy at a parasagittal section through the coracoid process. At this transition site, the brachial plexus is changing from the brachial plexus cords to the peripheral nerves as it surrounds the subclavian and axillary arteries (Fig. 3-11). At the site of this parasagittal section, the borders of the proximal axilla are formed by the following anatomic structures:

Anterior: posterior border of the pectoralis minor muscle and brachial head of the biceps

Posterior: scapula and subscapularis, latissimus dorsi, and teres major muscles

Medial: lateral aspect of chest wall, including the ribs and intercostal and serratus anterior muscles

Lateral: medial aspect of upper arm

These anatomic relationships are important during continuous techniques of infraclavicular block.

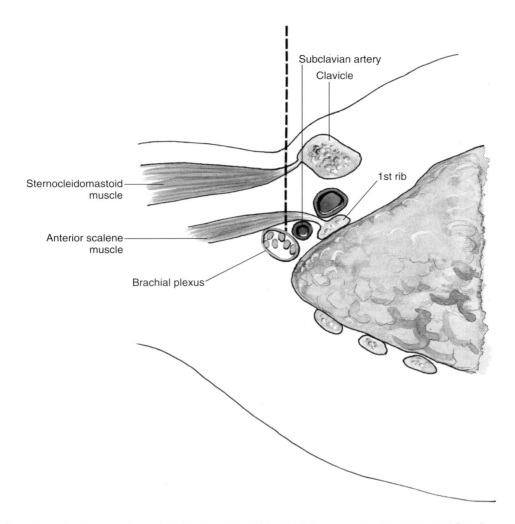

Figure 3-10. Supraclavicular block anatomy: functional anatomy of brachial plexus, subclavian artery, and first rib.

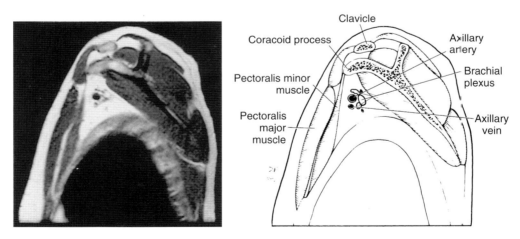

Figure 3-11. Parasagittal magnetic resonance image and line drawing of the important anatomy in the infraclavicular block.
(Reproduced with permission of the Mayo Foundation, Rochester, Minn.)

Interscalene Block

4

Ehab Farag with David L. Brown

PERSPECTIVE

Interscalene block (classic anterior approach) is especially effective for surgery of the shoulder or upper arm because the roots of the brachial plexus are most easily blocked with this technique. Frequently the ulnar nerve and its more peripheral distribution in the hand can be spared, unless one makes a special effort to inject local anesthetic caudad to the site of the initial paresthesia. This block is ideal for reduction of a dislocated shoulder and often can be achieved with as little as 10 to 15 mL of local anesthetic. This block also can be performed with the arm in almost any position and thus can be useful when brachial plexus block needs to be repeated during a prolonged upper extremity procedure.

Patient Selection. Interscalene block is applicable to nearly all patients because even obese patients usually have identifiable scalene and vertebral body anatomy. However, interscalene block should be avoided in patients with significantly impaired pulmonary function. This point may be moot if one is planning to use a combined regional and general anesthetic technique, which allows intraoperative control of ventilation. Even when a long-acting local anesthetic is chosen for the interscalene technique, usually phrenic nerve, and thus pulmonary, function has returned to a level that patients can tolerate by the time the average-length surgical procedure is completed.

Pharmacologic Choice. Useful agents for interscalene block are primarily the amino amides. Lidocaine and mepivacaine provide surgical anesthesia for 2 to 3 hours without epinephrine and for 3 to 5 hours when epinephrine is added. These drugs can be useful for less complex or outpatient surgical procedures. For more extensive surgical procedures requiring hospital admission, longer-acting agents such as bupivacaine or ropivacaine can be chosen. The more complex surgical procedures on the shoulder often require muscle relaxation; thus bupivacaine concentrations of at least 0.5% are needed. Plain bupivacaine produces surgical anesthesia lasting from 4 to 6 hours; the addition of epinephrine may prolong this to 8 to 12 hours. Ropivacaine's effects are slightly shorter in duration.

TRADITIONAL BLOCK TECHNIQUE

PLACEMENT

Anatomy. Surface anatomy of importance to anesthesiologists includes the larynx, sternocleidomastoid muscle, and external jugular vein. Interscalene block is most often performed at the level of the C6 vertebral body, which is at the level of the cricoid cartilage. Thus by projecting a line laterally from the cricoid cartilage, one can identify the level at which one should roll the fingers off the sternocleidomastoid muscle onto the belly of the anterior scalene and then into the interscalene groove. When firm pressure is applied, in most individuals it is possible to feel the transverse process of C6, and in some people it is possible to elicit a paresthesia by deep palpation. The external jugular vein often overlies the interscalene groove at the level of C6, although this should not be relied on (Fig. 4-1).

It is important to visualize what lies under the palpating fingers; again, the key to carrying out successful interscalene block is the identification of the interscalene groove. Figure 4-2 allows us to look beneath surface anatomy and develop a sense of how closely the lateral border of the anterior scalene muscle deviates from the border of the sternocleidomastoid muscle. This feature should be constantly kept in mind. The anterior scalene muscle and the interscalene groove are oriented at an oblique angle to the long axis of the sternocleidomastoid muscle. Figure 4-3 removes the anterior scalene and highlights the fact that at the level of C6, the vertebral artery begins its route to the base of the brain by traveling through the root of the transverse process in each of the more cephalad cervical vertebrae.

Position. The patient lies supine with the neck in the neutral position and the head turned slightly opposite the site to be blocked. The anesthesiologist then asks the patient to lift the head off the table to tense the sternocleidomastoid muscle and allow identification of its lateral border. The fingers then roll onto the belly of the anterior scalene and subsequently into the interscalene groove. This maneuver should be carried out in the horizontal plane through the cricoid cartilage—thus at the level of C6. To roll the

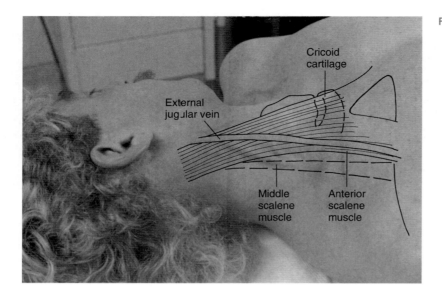

Figure 4-1. Interscalene block: surface anatomy.

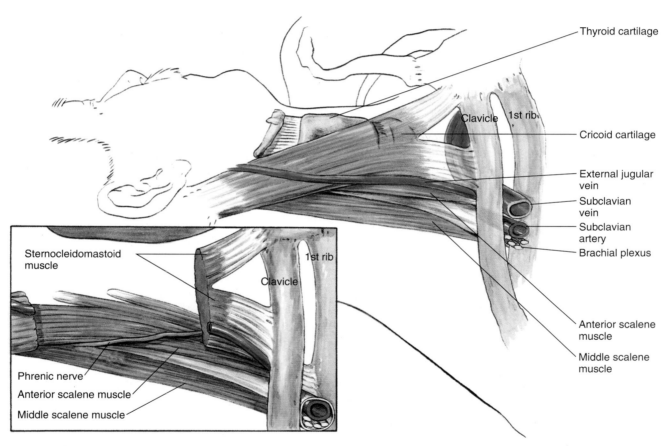

Figure 4-2. Interscalene block: functional anatomy of scalene muscles.

fingers effectively (Fig. 4-4), the operator should stand at the patient's side.

Needle Puncture. When the interscalene groove has been identified and the operator's fingers are firmly pressing in it, the needle is inserted, as shown in Figure 4-5, in a slightly caudal and slightly posterior direction. As a further directional help, if the needle for this block is imagined to be long and inserted deeply enough, it would exit the neck posteriorly in approximately the midline at the level of the C7 or T1 spinous process. If a paresthesia or motor response is not elicited on insertion, the needle is "walked" while maintaining the same needle angulation as shown in Figure

4-4 in a plane joining the cricoid cartilage to the C6 transverse process. Because the brachial plexus traverses the neck at virtually a right angle to this plane, a paresthesia or motor response is almost guaranteed if small enough steps of needle reinsertion are carried out. When undertaking the block for shoulder surgery, this is probably the one brachial plexus block in which a large volume of local anesthetic coupled with a single needle position allows effective anesthesia. For shoulder surgery, 25 to 35 mL of lidocaine, mepivacaine, bupivacaine, or ropivacaine can be used. If the interscalene block is being carried out for forearm or hand surgery, a second, more caudal needle

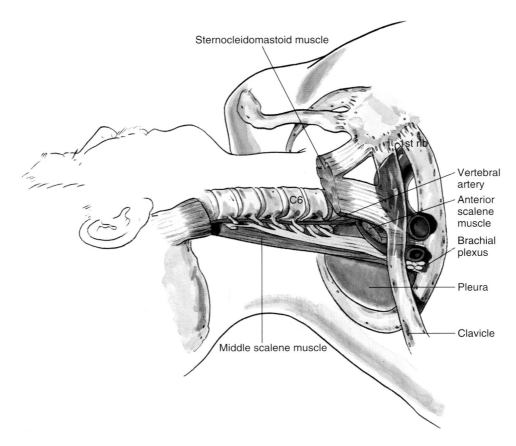

Figure 4-3. Interscalene block: functional anatomy of vertebral artery.

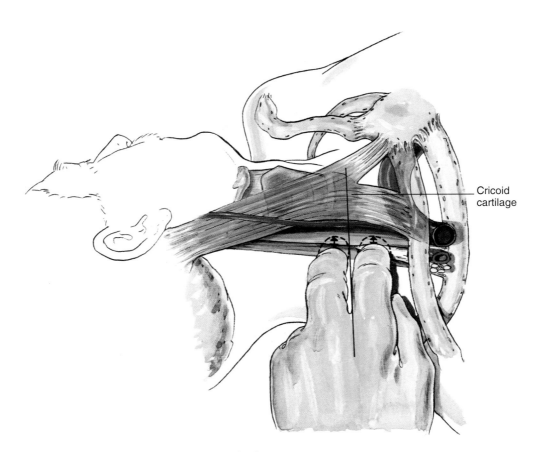

Figure 4-4. Interscalene block technique: palpation.

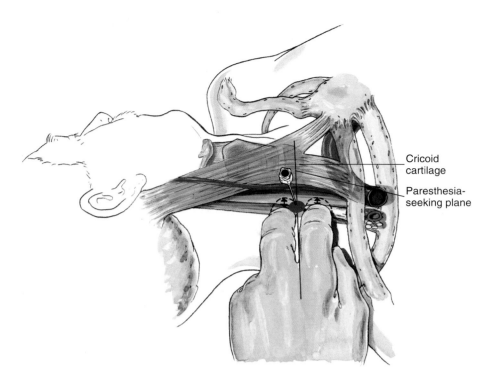

Cricoid
cartilage

Paresthesia-
seeking plane

Figure 4-5. Interscalene block technique: "paresthesia-seeking" plane.

position is desirable, in which 10 to 15 mL of additional local anesthetic is injected to allow spread along more caudal roots.

POTENTIAL PROBLEMS

Problems that can arise from interscalene block include subarachnoid injection, epidural block, intravascular injection (especially in the vertebral artery), pneumothorax, and phrenic block.

PEARLS

This block is most applicable to shoulder procedures, as opposed to forearm and hand surgical procedures, although some practitioners combine interscalene and axillary blocks to produce an approximation of a supraclavicular block. For shoulder surgery block that requires muscle relaxation, a local anesthetic concentration that provides adequate motor block should be chosen (i.e., mepivacaine and lidocaine at 1.5%, bupivacaine at 0.5%, and ropivacaine at 0.75% concentrations). Because this block is most often carried out through a single injection site and the operator relies on the spread of local anesthetic solution, one must allow sufficient "soak time" after the injection. This often means from 20 to 35 minutes.

If there is difficulty in identifying the anterior scalene muscle, one maneuver is to have the patient maximally inhale while the anesthesiologist palpates the neck. During this maneuver the scalene muscles should contract before the sternocleidomastoid muscle contracts, and this may allow clarification of the anterior scalene muscle in the difficult-to-palpate neck. Further, if the operator is finding it difficult to elicit a paresthesia or produce a motor

response during nerve stimulation with this block, it is almost always because the needle entry site has been placed too far posteriorly. For example, Figure 4-6 shows that if the right side of the neck is divided into a 180-degree arc, the needle entry site should be approximately at 60 degrees from the sagittal plane to optimize production of the block.

Most of the injection difficulties that result in complications can be avoided if one remembers that this should be a very "superficial" block; if the palpating fingers apply sufficient pressure, no more than 1 to 1.5 cm of the needle should be necessary to reach the plexus. It is when the needle is inserted deeply that one must be cautious about subarachnoid, epidural, and intravascular injection. For an operation that requires ulnar nerve block, I would not choose the interscalene block. The ulnar nerve is difficult to block with the interscalene approach because it is derived from the eighth cervical nerve (this nerve is difficult to block after injection at a more cephalic injection site). Finally, one should be cautious about using this block in a patient with significant pulmonary impairment because phrenic block is almost guaranteed with the interscalene block.

ULTRASOUND FOR INTERSCALENE BLOCK

KEY POINTS

- A small linear (20- to 25-mm) footprint is preferred for this block.
- The most successful way to perform this block is to visualize the brachial plexus in the supraclavicular region and then scan cephalad to identify the roots

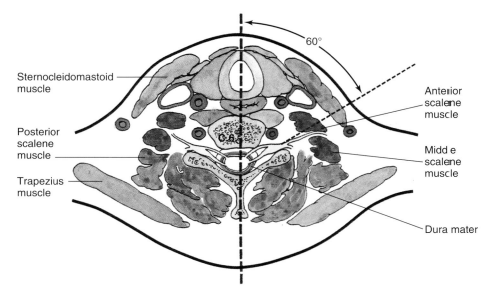

Figure 4-6. Interscalene block anatomy: an angle of approximately 60 degrees from the sagittal plane is the optimal needle angle for the block.

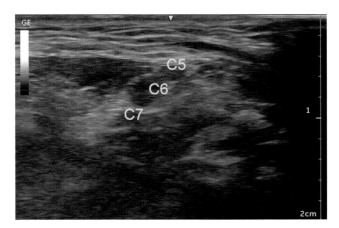

Figure 4-7. Interscalene ultrasound.

that are sandwiched between the anterior scalene and middle scalene muscles.

• Insertion of the needle and the catheter between C5 and C6 or C6 and C7 will help to properly anchor the catheter and ensure good analgesia after shoulder surgery.

SONOANATOMY

The interscalene block is performed in the posterior triangle (Figs 4-7 through 4-9), which lies between the posterior border of the sternocleidomastoid muscle and the trapezius muscle, next to the sixth and seventh cervical vertebra. In the interscalene block, the brachial plexus is made of nerve roots (C5, C6, C7) or trunks. The brachial plexus in the interscalene block appears as hypoechogenic nodules (due to the high ratio of neural/nonneural tissue in this region) located between the anterior and middle scalene muscles under the prevertebral fascia. The dorsal scapular and long thoracic nerves of the brachial plexus are

frequently located in the middle scalene muscle at less than 1 cm posterior to the plexus. The nerves appear as hyperechoic structures containing a hypoechoic center.

INDICATIONS

• The principal indication for interscalene block is surgery of the shoulder. Local anesthetic spread after the block includes the supraclavicular (nonbrachial plexus) nerve (C3 to C4), which supplies sensory innervation to the cape of the shoulder.
• The interscalene block can be used for surgery on the humerus neck; however, it is not sufficient for hand surgeries, as it misses the lower roots and the trunk of the plexus.

TECHNIQUE

The patient position is usually either supine with the head turned to the opposite side to be blocked or in the lateral decubitus position. We prefer to insert the block in the lateral decubitus position, especially during the catheter insertion. The supraclavicular region is usually scanned to identify the brachial plexus superficial and lateral to the subclavian artery. The brachial plexus is then followed cephalad to identify the roots of the brachial plexus in the interscalene region sandwiched between the anterior scalene and middle scalene muscles. In the transverse short-axis view of the plexus, the in-plane needle passes from the lateral into the medial direction in the supine position or from the posterior into the anterior direction in the lateral decubitus direction. The needle should be positioned between C5 and C6 or C6 and C7 in order to achieve a proper block for the shoulder surgery. In the case of catheter insertion, we prefer to pass the Tuohy needle through the middle scalene muscle below the dorsal scapular and long thoracic nerves to give the catheter better

Myotome innervation of the upper limb

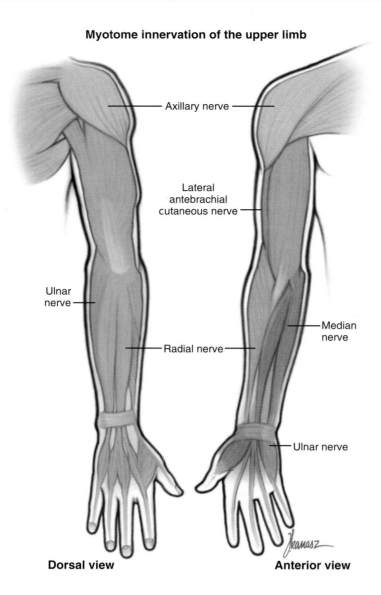

Figure 4-8. The myotome innervation of the upper limb.

Axillary nerve

Lateral antebrachial cutaneous nerve

Ulnar nerve

Median nerve

Radial nerve

Ulnar nerve

Dorsal view   **Anterior view**

anchoring into the plexus. A fascial click is often felt when the needle penetrates the middle scalene fascia in order to reach the interscalene space (Figs 4-10 through 4-17).

PEARLS

- The phrenic nerve and brachial plexus are within 2 mm of each other at the cricoid cartilage level, with additional 3 mm separation for every cm more caudal in the neck. Therefore puncture localization 1 to 2 cm caudal to the cricoid cartilage can be helpful in reducing phrenic nerve palsy after interscalene block.

- The transverse cervical artery or dorsal scapular artery is sometimes visible at the targeted site of injection. Therefore color Doppler can be useful to identify those vessels, as they might be misidentified as nerve structures.

- The needle insertion in the middle scalene muscle should be at a lower level to the dorsal scapular and long thoracic nerves. Injury to the dorsal scapular nerve is characterized by a dull ache along the medial border of the scapula and weakness and hypotrophy of the rhomboid and/or the levator scapulae muscles. Injury to the long thoracic nerve will result in chronic pain syndrome of the shoulder and different degree of serratus muscle weakness.

Figure 4-9. Sclerotome innervation of the upper limb.

Sclerotome innervation of the upper limb

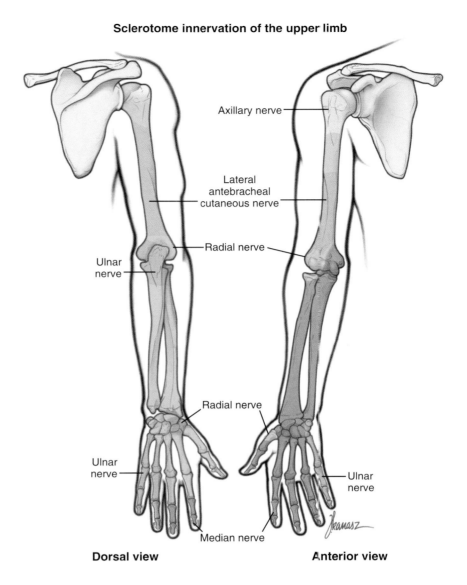

Axillary nerve

Lateral antebracheal cutaneous nerve

Radial nerve

Ulnar nerve

Radial nerve

Ulnar nerve

Ulnar nerve

Median nerve

Dorsal view   **Anterior view**

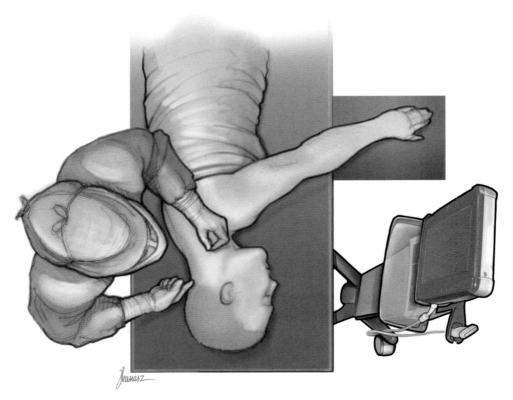

Figure 4-10. Lateral decubitus position (posterior approach) for the interscalene block.

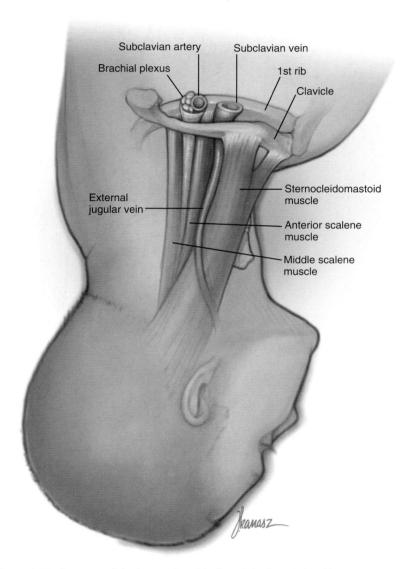

Figure 4-11. Anatomy of the interscalene block and the lateral decubitus position.

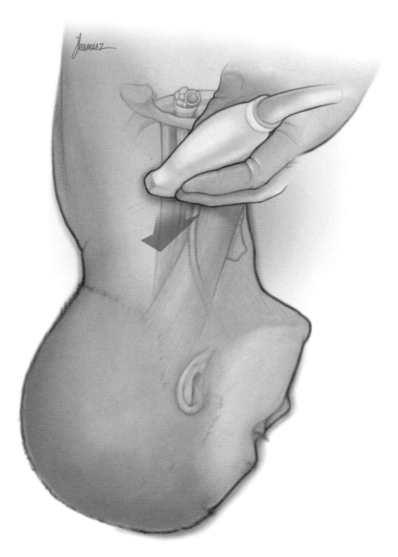

Figure 4-12. The brachial plexus is scanned in the chephlad direction from supraclavicular region to identify the roots of brachial plexus in the interscalene region between anterior and middle scalene muscle.

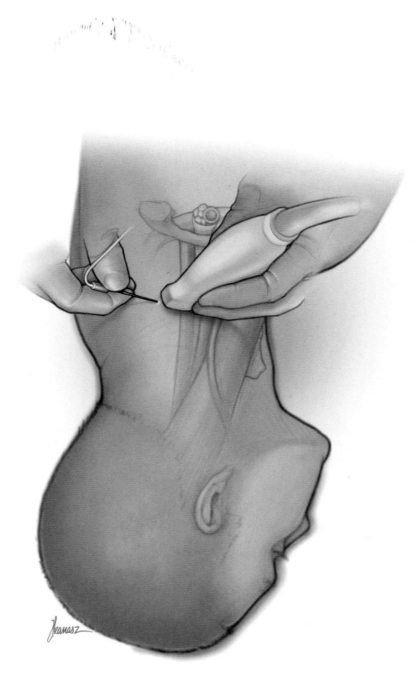

Figure 4-13. In-plane technique for interscalene block with the needle direction from posterior to anterior in the lateral decubitus position.

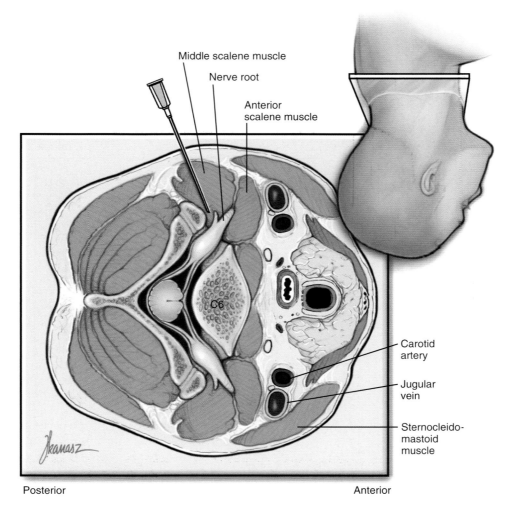

Middle scalene muscle

Nerve root

Anterior
scalene muscle

C6

Carotid
artery

Jugular
vein

Sternocleido-
mastoid
muscle

Posterior   Anterior

Figure 4-14. Interscalene block. Notice the needle has to pass through middle scalene muscle to reach the roots of the brachial plexus in the interscalene groove.

Figure 4-15. The needle position between C5 and C6 roots of the brachial plexus.

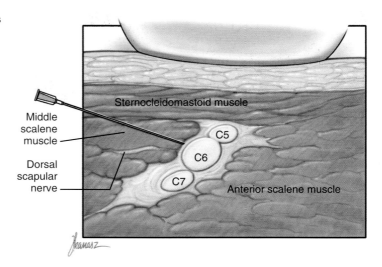

Sternocleidomastoid muscle

Middle
scalene
muscle

Dorsal
scapular
nerve

C5

C6

C7

Anterior scalene muscle

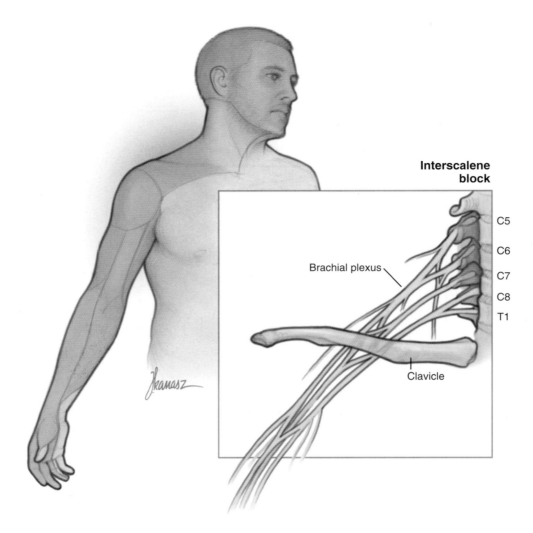

Interscalene block

Brachial plexus

Clavicle

C5
C6
C7
C8
T1

Figure 4-16. The anatomy of the interscalene block. Notice the roots are blocked in this technique.

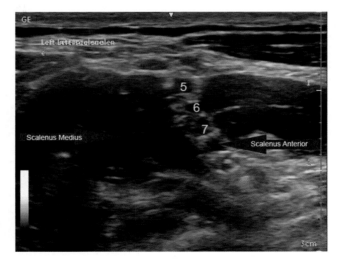

GE

Left Interscalene

5
6
7

Scalenus Medius

Scalenus Anterior

3cm

Figure 4-17. Ultrasound of interscalene. Note the roots of the brachial plexus are sandwiched between the scalenus anterior and the scalenus medius.

Supraclavicular Block 5

Ehab Farag and David L. Brown

PERSPECTIVE

Supraclavicular block provides anesthesia of the entire upper extremity in the most consistent, efficient manner of any brachial plexus technique. It is the most effective block for all portions of the upper extremity and is carried out at the division level of the brachial plexus; perhaps this is why there is often little or no sparing of peripheral nerves if an adequate paresthesia is obtained. If this block is to be used for shoulder surgery, it should be supplemented with a superficial cervical plexus block to anesthetize the skin overlying the shoulder.

Patient Selection. Almost all patients are candidates for this block, with the exception of those who are uncooperative. In addition, in less experienced hands it may be inappropriate for outpatients. Although pneumothorax is an infrequent complication of the block, such an event often becomes apparent only after a delay of several hours, when an outpatient may already be at home. Also, because the supraclavicular block relies principally on bony and muscular landmarks, very obese patients are not good candidates because they often have supraclavicular fat pads that interfere with easy application of this technique.

Pharmacologic Choice. As with other brachial plexus blocks, the prime consideration in drug selection should be the length of the procedure and the degree of motor blockade desired. Mepivacaine (1% to 1.5%), lidocaine (1% to 1.5%), bupivacaine (0.5%), and ropivacaine (0.5% to 0.75%) are all applicable to brachial plexus block. Lidocaine and mepivacaine will produce 2 to 3 hours of surgical anesthesia without epinephrine and 3 to 5 hours when epinephrine is added. These drugs can be useful for less involved or outpatient surgical procedures. For extensive surgical procedures requiring hospital admission, a longer-acting agent like bupivacaine can be chosen. Plain bupivacaine produces surgical anesthesia lasting from 4 to 6 hours, and the addition of epinephrine may prolong this time to 8 to 12 hours, whereas ropivacaine is slightly shorter acting.

TRADITIONAL BLOCK TECHNIQUE

PLACEMENT

Anatomy. The anatomy of interest for this block is the relationship between the brachial plexus and the first rib, the subclavian artery, and the cupola of the lung (Fig. 5-1). Our experience suggests that this block is more difficult to teach than many of the other regional blocks, and for that reason two approaches to the supraclavicular block are illustrated: the classic Kulenkampff approach and the vertical ("plumb bob") approach. The vertical approach has been developed in an attempt to overcome the difficulty and time necessary to become skilled in the classic supraclavicular block approach. Both techniques are clinically useful once mastered. As the subclavian artery and brachial plexus pass over the first rib, they do so between the insertion of the anterior and middle scalene muscles onto the first rib (Fig. 5-2). The nerves lie in a cephaloposterior relationship to the artery; thus a paresthesia may be elicited before the needle contacts the first rib. At the point where the artery and plexus cross the first rib, the rib is broad and flat, sloping caudad as it moves from posterior to anterior, and although the rib is a curved structure, there is a distance of 1 to 2 cm on which a needle can be "walked" in a parasagittal anteroposterior direction. Remember that immediately medial to the first rib is the cupola of the lung; when the needle angle is too medial, pneumothorax may result.

Position: Classic Supraclavicular Block. The patient lies supine without a pillow, with the head turned opposite the side to be blocked. The arms are at the sides, and the anesthesiologist can stand either at the head of the table or at the side of the patient, near the arm to be blocked.

Needle Puncture: Classic Supraclavicular Block. In the classic approach, the needle insertion site is approximately 1 cm superior to the clavicle at the clavicular midpoint (Fig. 5-3). This entry site is closer to the middle of the clavicle than to the junction of the middle and medial thirds (as often described in other regional anesthesia texts). In addition, if the artery is palpable in the supraclavicular fossa, it can be used as a landmark. From this point, the needle and syringe are inserted in a plane approximately parallel to the patient's neck and head, taking care that the axis of the syringe and needle does not aim medially toward the cupola of the lung. A 22-gauge, 5-cm needle typically will contact the rib at a depth of 3 to 4 cm, although in a very large patient it is sometimes necessary to insert it to a depth of 6 cm. The initial needle insertion should not be carried out past 3 to 4 cm until a careful search in an anteroposterior plane does not identify the first rib. During the insertion of the needle and syringe, the assembly should be controlled with the hand, as illustrated in Figure 5-4. The hand can rest lightly against the patient's

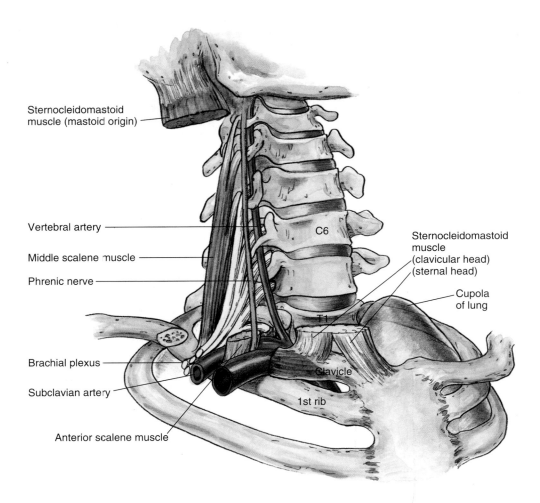

Sternocleidomastoid
muscle (mastoid origin)

Vertebral artery

Middle scalene muscle

Phrenic nerve

C6

Sternocleidomastoid
muscle
(clavicular head)
(sternal head)

Cupola
of lung

T1

Brachial plexus

Subclavian artery

Clavicle

1st rib

Anterior scalene muscle

Figure 5-1. Supraclavicular block: anatomy.

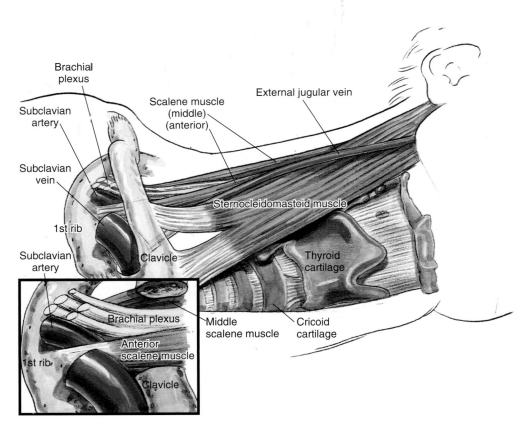

Brachial
plexus

Subclavian
artery

Subclavian
vein

1st rib

Subclavian
artery

Scalene muscle
(middle)
(anterior)

External jugular vein

Sternocleidomastoid muscle

Clavicle

Thyroid
cartilage

Brachial plexus

Middle
scalene muscle

Cricoid
cartilage

Anterior
scalene muscle

1st rib

Clavicle

Figure 5-2. Supraclavicular block: functional anatomy (with detail).

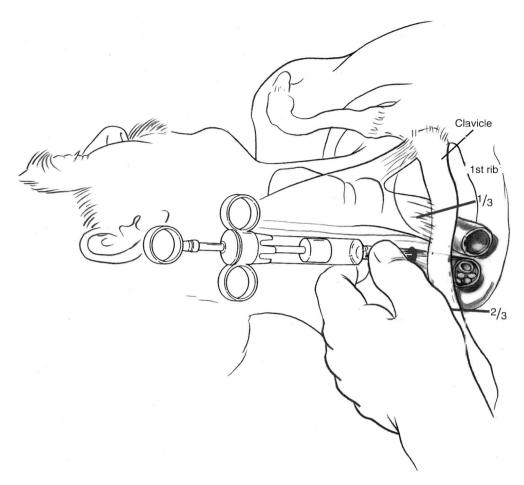

Figure 5-3. Supraclavicular block (classic approach): insertion site.

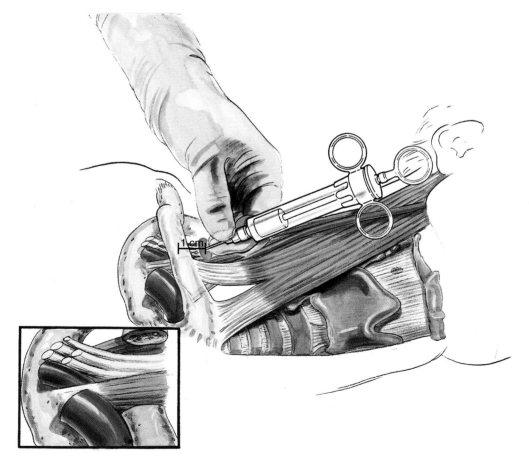

Figure 5-4. Supraclavicular block (classic approach): hand and syringe assembly positioning.

supraclavicular fossa because patients often move the shoulder with elicitation of a paresthesia.

Position: Vertical (Plumb Bob) Supraclavicular Block. The vertical approach to the supraclavicular block was developed to simplify the anatomic projection necessary for the block. The patient should be positioned in a manner similar to that used for the classic approach, lying supine without a pillow, with the head turned slightly away from the side to be blocked. The anesthesiologist should stand lateral to the patient at the level of the patient's upper arm. This block involves inserting the needle and syringe assembly at approximately a 90-degree angle to that used in the classic approach.

Needle Puncture: Vertical (Plumb Bob) Supraclavicular Block. Patients are asked to raise the head slightly off the block table so that the lateral border of the sternocleidomastoid muscle can be marked as it inserts onto the clavicle. From that point, a plane is visualized running parasagittally through that site (Fig. 5-5). The name "plumb bob" was chosen for this block concept because if one were to suspend a plumb bob vertically over the entry site (Fig. 5-6), needle insertion through that point, along the continuation of the vertical line defined by the plumb bob, would result in contact with the brachial plexus in most patients. Figure 5-6 also illustrates a parasagittal section obtained by magnetic resonance imaging in the sagittal plane necessary to carry out this block. As illustrated, the brachial plexus at the level of the first rib lies posterior and cephalad to the subclavian artery. Once this skin mark has been placed immediately superior to the clavicle at the lateral border of the sternocleidomastoid muscle as it inserts into the clavicle, the needle is inserted in the parasagittal plane at a 90-degree angle to the tabletop. If a paresthesia is not elicited on the first pass, the needle and syringe are redirected cephalad in small steps through an arc of approximately 20 degrees. If a paresthesia still has not been obtained, needle and syringe are reinserted at the starting position and then moved in small steps through an arc of approximately 20 degrees caudad (Fig. 5-7).

Because the brachial plexus lies cephaloposterior to the artery as it crosses the first rib, often a paresthesia can be elicited before either the artery or the first rib is contacted. If that occurs, approximately 30 mL of local anesthetic is inserted at this single site.

If a paresthesia is not elicited with the maneuvers described but the first rib is contacted, the block is carried out just as it is in the classic approach—by "walking" along the first rib until a paresthesia is elicited. As in the classic

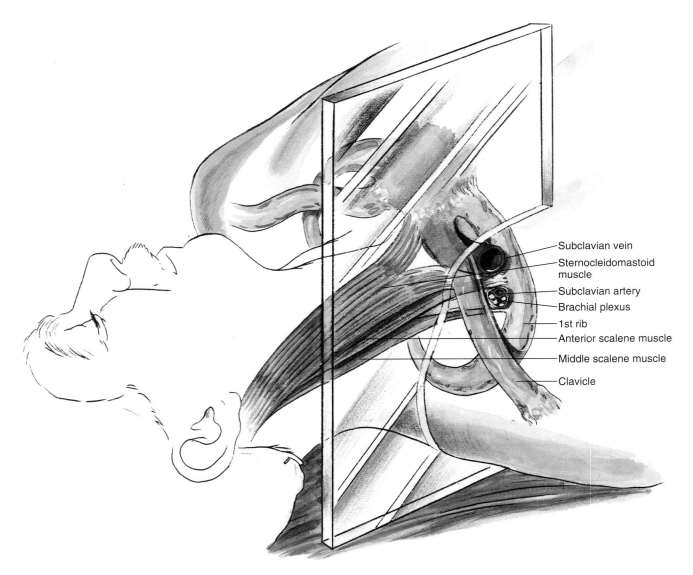

Subclavian vein
Sternocleidomastoid muscle
Subclavian artery
Brachial plexus
1st rib
Anterior scalene muscle
Middle scalene muscle
Clavicle

Figure 5-5. Supraclavicular block (plumb bob): functional anatomy.

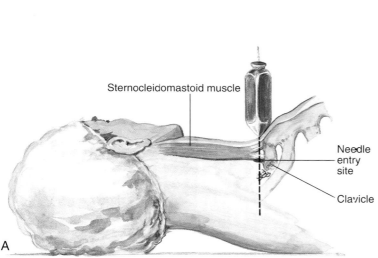

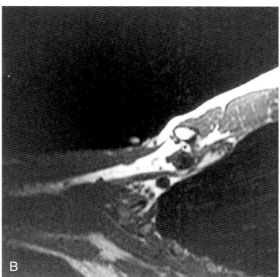

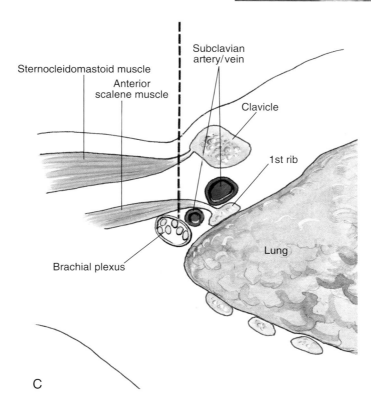

Figure 5-6. Supraclavicular block (plumb bob): parasagittal anatomy. A, Schematic, showing plumb bob and needle path. B, Magnetic resonance image. C, Needle path.

approach, care should be taken not to allow the syringe and needle assembly to aim medially toward the cupola of the lung.

POTENTIAL PROBLEMS

The most feared complication of this block is pneumothorax, the principal cause of which is a needle/syringe angle that aims toward the cupola of the lung. Special attention should be directed to "walking" the needle in a strict anteroposterior direction. Pneumothorax incidence is between 0.5% and 5% and becomes less frequent as an anesthesiologist becomes skilled. The cupola of the lung rises proportionally higher in the neck in thin, asthenic individuals, and perhaps in these individuals the incidence

of pneumothorax is higher. Pneumothorax most often develops over a number of hours as the result of impingement of the needle on the lung, rather than due to immediate entrance of air into the pleural space as the needle is inserted. Phrenic nerve block occurs probably in the range of 30% to 50% of patients, and the block's use in patients with significantly impaired pulmonary function must be weighed. The development of hematoma after supraclavicular block as a result of puncture of the subclavian artery usually simply requires observation.

PEARLS

The predictability and rapid onset of this block allow the anesthesiologist to keep up with a fast orthopedic surgeon.

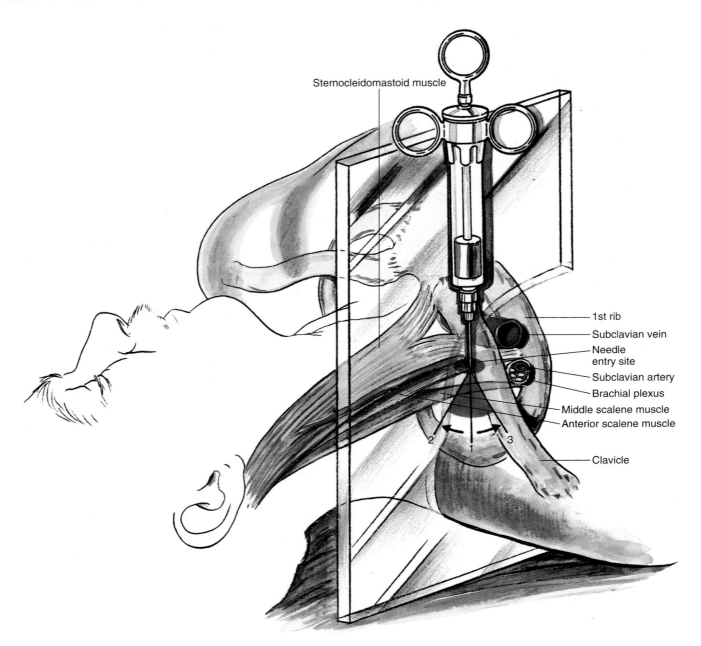

Figure 5-7. Supraclavicular block (plumb bob): paresthesia-seeking approach.

Use of this block allows regional anesthesia to be used for hand surgery, even in a busy practice. Because this block requires a longer time for the anesthesiologist to attain proficiency than most other regional blocks, the anesthesiologist should develop a system for its use. "Wishful" probing at the root of the neck without a system is not the way to approach this block. Likewise, one should choose either the classic or the vertical approach and give each a fair trial before abandoning either.

If a pneumothorax occurs after supraclavicular block, it most often can be observed while the patient is reassured. If the pneumothorax is large enough to cause dyspnea or patient discomfort, aspiration of the pneumothorax through a small-gauge catheter is often all that is necessary for treatment. The patient should be admitted for observation; however, it is the exceptional patient who needs formal, large-bore chest tube placement for reexpansion of the lung. Obviously, difficult patients should not be chosen as subjects while the anesthesiologist is developing expertise with this block.

Some anesthesiologists combine the axillary and interscalene blocks (in the so-called AXIS block) to approximate the results achieved from a more typical supraclavicular block. An AXIS block requires that the total doses of local anesthetic be increased; one must be willing to use almost 60 mL of whichever drug is injected. Time will tell whether this combined approach offers any advantages over the supraclavicular block. In the AXIS block, the axillary portion should be blocked first, with the interscalene block performed second to minimize the risk of injecting into an area already blocked by local anesthetic.

ULTRASONOGRAPHY-GUIDED TECHNIQUE

SONOANATOMY

The brachial plexus in the supraclavicular region is composed mainly of three trunks: superior, middle, and

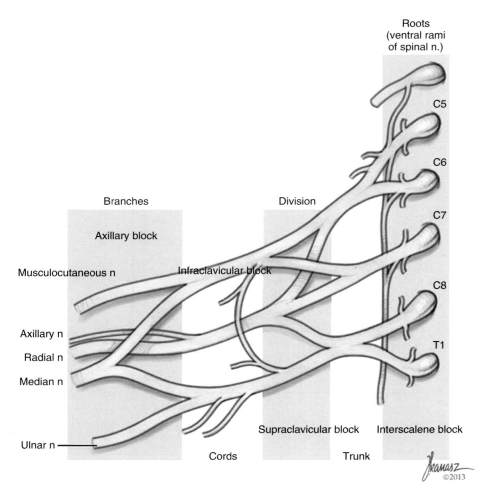

Figure 5-8. Comparing the different block positions for the different techniques of brachial plexus block.

inferior. These trunks pass across the upper surface of the first rib, where they lie posterior and superior to the subclavian artery. The trunks then divide into anterior and posterior divisions behind the clavicle. With ultrasonography, the six divisions can be seen compactly arranged and located superior and posterior to the subclavian artery as the artery passes over the first rib. Practically, in the supraclavicular approach for the brachial plexus, the trunks and the divisions appear as a compact group of nerves (like a bunch of grapes) lying superior and posterior to the artery (Figs. 5-8 through 5-10).

INDICATIONS

- The supraclavicular block is very efficient for upper limb and hand surgeries.
- This block can be used for shoulder surgery; however, it can miss the suprascapular nerve, which supplies the sensory innervation to the glenohumeral joint. Therefore the block could fail to provide appropriate analgesia after shoulder surgery.

TECHNIQUE

The patient could be in either a semisitting position (beach-chair position) by elevating the head of the bed 45 degrees or a supine position with the patient's head turned to the opposite side to be blocked. The first position is preferable in obese patients. The usual probe position is in the coronal oblique plane behind the midpoint of the clavicle to obtain the short-axis view. Scan the supraclavicular fossa to identify the subclavian artery and brachial plexus in the short-axis view. The first rib and the cervical pleura should be identified in this view as well. We prefer to use the in-plane approach for this technique, and the needle will be inserted from the posterior to anterior direction (Figs. 5-11 through 5-14).

KEY POINTS

- A small linear (20- to 25-mm footprint) transducer is preferred for this block.
- Try to identify the cervical pleura and keep the needle direction in a parallel position to the first rib to avoid injuring the pleura and prevent the development of pneumothorax.
- For catheter insertion, the Tuohy needle is usually used. The catheter is typically inserted superior to the subclavian artery in the case of shoulder surgery or in the corner pocket between the artery and the first rib in the case of hand surgery. The correct position of the catheter can be confirmed under ultrasound by either injecting local anesthetic or 1 mL of air via the catheter and observing its distribution in relation to the plexus.

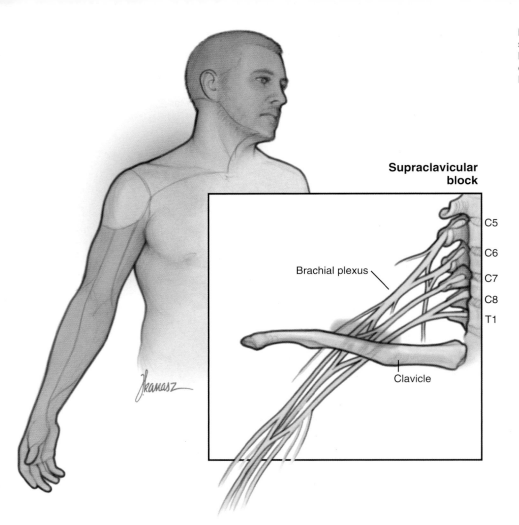

Figure 5-9. Anatomy of supraclavicular block. Note the block is performed at the level of trunks and divisions of brachial plexus.

Supraclavicular block

Brachial plexus

Clavicle

C5
C6
C7
C8
T1

Cutaneous innervation of the upper limb

Figure 5-10. Anatomy of the supraclavicular.

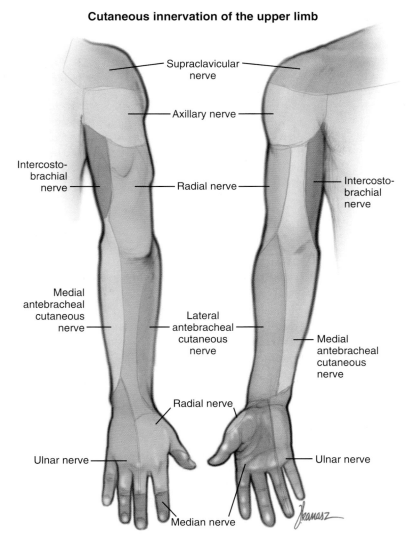

Supraclavicular nerve

Axillary nerve

Intercosto-brachial nerve

Radial nerve

Intercosto-brachial nerve

Medial antebracheal cutaneous nerve

Lateral antebracheal cutaneous nerve

Medial antebracheal cutaneous nerve

Radial nerve

Ulnar nerve

Ulnar nerve

Median nerve

Dorsal view

Anterior view

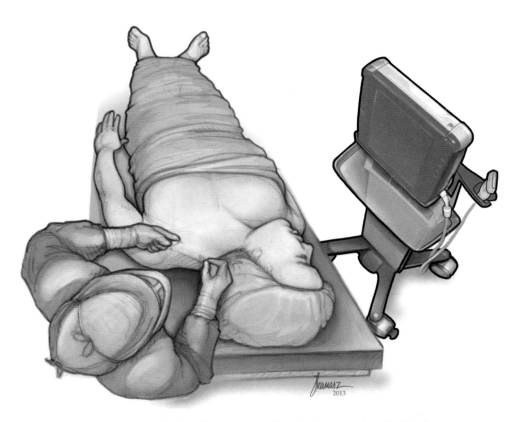

Figure 5-11. Patient position with the ultrasound machine for the supraclavicular block.

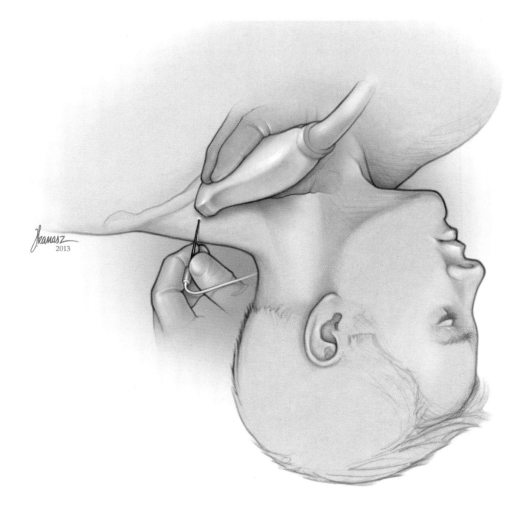

Figure 5-12. The probe is in the coronal oblique plane. Note the in-plane position of the needle with the direction of the needle from posterior to anterior.

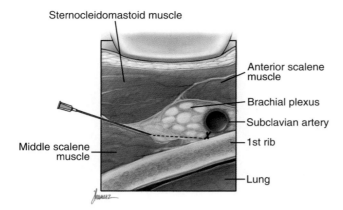

Figure 5-13. The needle position beneath the brachial plexus parallel to the first rib.

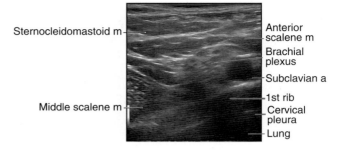

Figure 5-14. Ultrasound image of Figure 5-13.

PEARLS

- For hand surgery, the local anesthetic should be inserted in the corner pocket between the subclavian artery and the first rib to avoid missing the lower trunk/divisions and therefore the ulnar nerve.
- For shoulder surgeries, try to visualize the suprascapular nerve by scanning more proximal away from the artery.
- If the patient developed chest pain and cough during the procedure, he or she might have developed pneumothorax. The procedure should be abandoned and chest x-ray should be ordered to confirm the diagnosis.

- Try to examine the anterior chest wall by ultrasound after every supraclavicular block to confirm the absence of pneumothorax by visualizing the intact pleura (sliding sign).
- Injury to the suprascapular nerve following supraclavicular block is usually presented by severe shoulder pain followed by weakness in the supraspinatus and infraspinatus muscles. To avoid this complication, try not to inject above the plexus to avoid exposing the nerve to toxic high concentrations of local anesthetics. In addition, avoiding injection above the plexus might decrease the incidence of phrenic nerve palsy after the block.
- Parsonage-Turner syndrome has the same physical presentations as suprascapular nerve injury. However, Parsonage-Turner syndrome is often idiopathic in its etiology, although its onset has been associated with physical stressors, including surgery.

Suprascapular Block 6

Wael Ali Sakr Esa

SONOANATOMY

The suprascapular nerve (SSN) arises from the C5 and C6 nerve roots, emerges from the superior trunk of the brachial plexus, and then enters the supraspinatus fossa via the suprascapular notch underneath the superior transverse scapular ligament. With application of color Doppler, the SSN can be visualized medial to the pulsation of the suprascapular artery as an oval or round, slightly hyperechoic structure. In the supraspinous fossa, the nerve is in direct contact with bone and exits the suprascapular fossa lateral to the infrascapular fossa lateral to the spinoglenoid notch (Fig. 6-1).

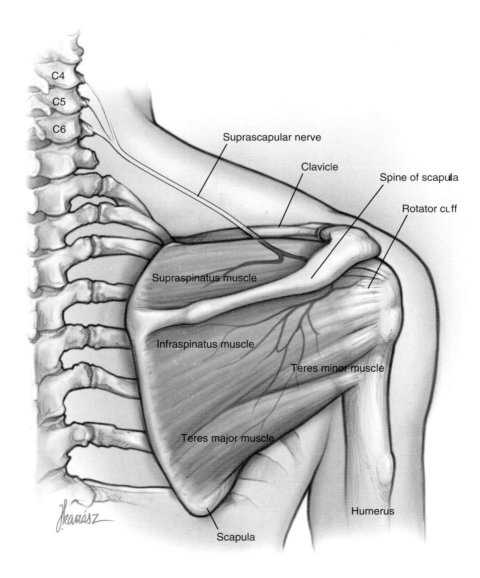

Figure 6-1. Anatomy of the suprascapular nerve.

INDICATIONS

- Shoulder arthroscopic surgeries that approach the joint from its posterior aspect. The SSN innervates up to 70% of the superior and posterior part of the shoulder. The superior articular branch from the SSN supplies the coracohumeral ligament, subacromial bursa, and posterior aspect of the acromioclavicular joint capsule, whereas the inferior articular branch from the SSN supplies the posterior joint capsule. The SSN has no innervation to the anterior and inferior shoulder regions.
- Frozen shoulder, dislocated shoulder, rotator cuff syndrome, and scapular fracture.
- Supplementation to the supraclavicular block for shoulder replacement surgeries if the patient has pain on the posterior part of the shoulder joint postoperatively.

TECHNIQUE

The patient ideally should be placed in a sitting position, and the operator should be behind the patient with the ultrasound machine in front of the patient and facing the operator. This will allow an uninterrupted field of view of the ultrasound screen. The ultrasound transducer should be placed parallel to the scapular spine. A transverse plane

of imaging is optimum for the ultrasound-guided SSN block. By moving the transducer cephalad, the suprascapular fossa can be identified. While imaging the supraspinatus muscle and the bony fossa underneath, the ultrasound transducer should be slowly moved laterally to locate the suprascapular notch. The SSN should be seen as a round, hyperechoic structure beneath the transverse scapular ligament in the scapular notch. Also, with application of color Doppler, the SSN can be visualized medial to the pulsation of the suprascapular artery as an oval or round, slightly hyperechoic structure. We prefer to use the in-plane approach for this technique. The echoic needle should be advanced using the in-plane approach medial to lateral to visualize the whole length of the needle (Fig. 6-2). The endpoint for injection is an ultrasound image demonstrating the needle tip in proximity to the SSN in the suprascapular notch below the transverse scapular ligament and the spread of the local anesthetic confirmed as a separation between the supraspinatus muscle and the spine of the scapula (Figs 6-3 and 6-4).

KEY POINTS

- High-frequency, 38-mm broadband linear array transducer is preferred for this block.
- For catheter insertion, the Tuohy needle is usually used. The catheter is placed beneath the transverse scapular ligament around the SSN. The correct

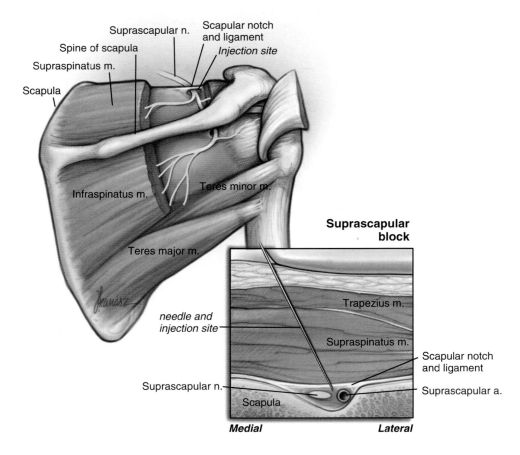

Figure 6-2. In-plane technique for suprascapular block. The needle direction is from medial to lateral.

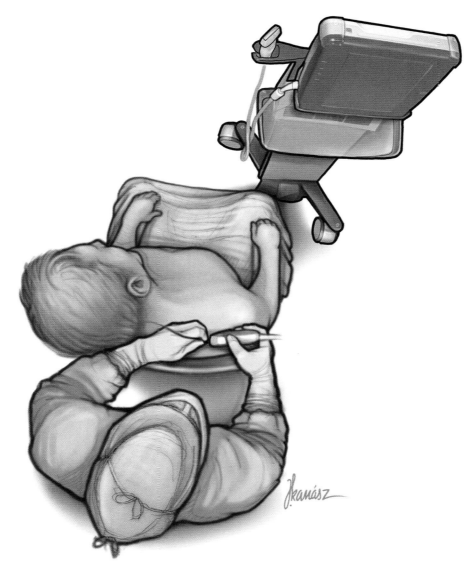

Figure 6-3. Position of the patient and ultrasound machine.

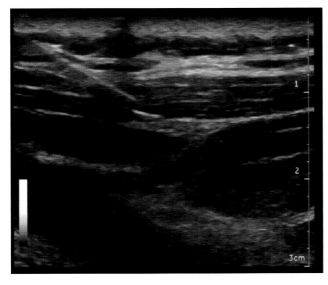

Figure 6-4. Ultrasound image of a 22 G needle directed toward the supra scapular nerve.

position of the catheter can be confirmed under ultrasound by injecting either local anesthetic or 1 mL of air via the catheter and observing its distribution in relation to the SSN and the transverse scapular ligament.

- The incidence of pneumothorax associated with SSN block is reported as less than 1%. The use of ultrasound and the in-plane approach will decrease this risk markedly.

PEARLS

- Adjust the focal point to the suprascapular notch to get a better image.
- If possible, ask the patient to adduct the arm and move it forward, thus bringing the nerve more superficially.
- Using color Doppler can be very helpful, as the SSN usually lies medial to the suprascapular artery.

- The block is painful, as the needle will pass through muscles, so prepare your patient with local anesthesia, midazolam, and fentanyl.
- Always use echogenic needles, as visualization of the needle is difficult due to the steep angle used in performing this block. Also, you can reduce the needle angle by using an insertion point as far as possible from the ultrasound probe while still maintaining an in-line approach and visualization of the entire needle during the block.

Infraclavicular Block 7

Kenneth C. Cummings III and David L. Brown

PERSPECTIVE

Infraclavicular brachial plexus block is often used for patients requiring prolonged brachial plexus analgesia and is increasingly used for surgical anesthesia by modifying it into a single-injection technique. Anesthesia or analgesia with this technique results in a "high" axillary block. Thus it is most useful for patients undergoing procedures on the elbow, forearm, or hand. Like the axillary block, this technique is carried out distant from both the neuraxial structures and the lung, thus minimizing complications associated with those areas.

Patient Selection. To undergo an infraclavicular block, the patient need not abduct the arm at the shoulder, as is required for the axillary block, and thus the technique can substitute for an axillary block in patients who cannot abduct their arms. Nevertheless, abduction of the arm at the shoulder may make identification of the axillary artery easier and can provide an enhanced sense of three-dimensional anatomy during the technique.

Pharmacologic Choice. Because prolonged brachial plexus analgesia requires less motor blockade than is needed for surgical anesthesia, the concentration of local anesthetic can be decreased during postoperative analgesia regimens. An appropriate drug is bupivacaine 0.25% or ropivacaine 0.2%, both administered at initial rates of approximately 8 to 12 mL/hr. If a single-injection technique is used, appropriate drugs are lidocaine (1% to 1.5%), mepivacaine (1% to 1.5%), bupivacaine (0.5%), or ropivacaine (0.5% to 0.75%). Lidocaine and mepivacaine produce 2 to 3 hours of surgical anesthesia without epinephrine and 3 to 5 hours with the addition of epinephrine. These drugs are useful for less involved procedures or outpatient surgical procedures. For more extensive surgical procedures requiring hospital admission, longer-acting agents such as bupivacaine or ropivacaine are appropriate. Plain bupivacaine and ropivacaine produce surgical anesthesia lasting 4 to 6 hours; the addition of epinephrine may prolong this period to 8 to 12 hours. The local anesthetic timeline must be considered when prescribing a drug for outpatient infraclavicular block because blocks lasting as long as 18 to 24 hours can result from higher concentrations of bupivacaine with added epinephrine.

TRADITIONAL BLOCK TECHNIQUE

PLACEMENT

Anatomy. At the level of the proximal axilla, where the infraclavicular block is performed, the axilla is a pyramid-shaped space with an apex, a base, and four sides (Fig. 7-1A). The base is the concave armpit, and the anterior wall is composed of the pectoralis major and minor muscles and their accompanying fasciae. The posterior wall of the axilla is formed by the scapula and the scapular musculature, the subscapularis, and the teres major. The latissimus dorsi muscle abuts the teres major muscle to form the inferior aspect of the posterior wall of the axilla (Fig. 7-1B). The medial wall of the axilla is composed of the serratus anterior muscle and its fascia, and the lateral wall is formed by the converging muscle and tendons of the anterior and posterior walls as they insert into the humerus (see Fig. 7-1B). The apex of the axilla is triangular and is formed by the convergence of the clavicle, the scapula, and the first rib. The neurovascular structures of the limb pass into the pyramid-shaped axilla through its apex (Fig. 7-2A).

The contents of the axilla are blood vessels and nerves—the axillary artery and vein and the brachial plexus, respectively—and lymph nodes and loose areolar tissue. The neurovascular elements are enclosed within the anatomically variable, multipartitioned axillary sheath, a fascial extension of the prevertebral layer of cervical fascia covering the scalene muscles. The axillary sheath adheres to the clavipectoral fascia behind the pectoralis minor muscle and continues along the neurovascular structures until it enters the medial intramuscular septum of the arm (Fig. 7-2B).

The brachial plexus divisions become cords as they enter the axilla. The posterior divisions of all three trunks unite to form the posterior cord; the anterior divisions of the superior and middle trunks form the lateral cord; and the nonunited anterior division of the inferior trunk forms the medial cord. These cords are named according to their relationship to the second part of the axillary artery (Fig. 7-3). From these cords, nerves to the subscapularis, pectoralis major and minor, and latissimus dorsi muscles leave the brachial plexus. The medial brachial cutaneous, medial antebrachial cutaneous, and axillary nerves also leave the brachial plexus from the level of the cords.

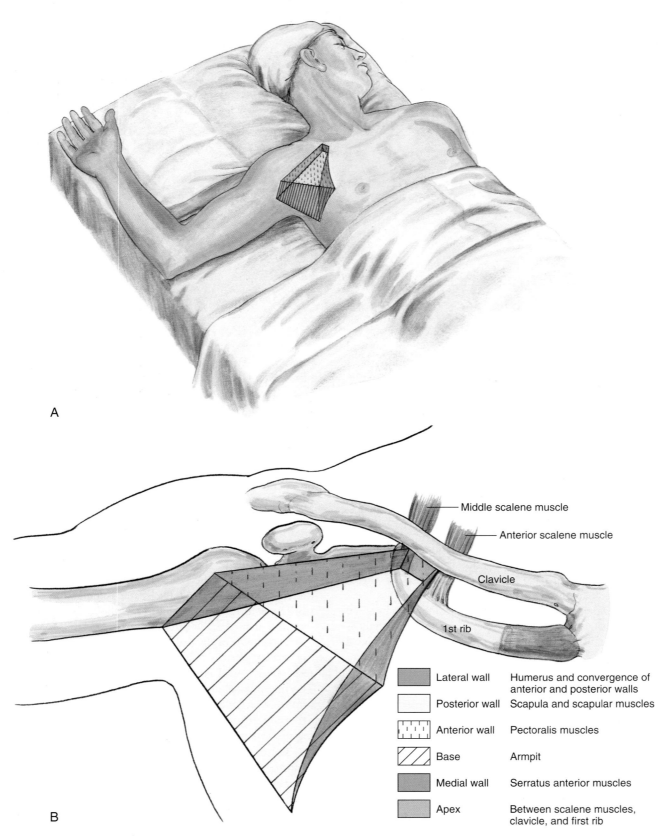

Figure 7-1. A, Surface anatomy of infraclavicular block. B, The concept of the pyramid-shaped axilla is important for infraclavicular block.

At the lateral border of the pectoralis minor muscle (which inserts onto the coracoid process), the three cords reorganize to give rise to the peripheral nerves of the upper extremity. In a simplified scheme, the branches of the lateral and medial cords are all "ventral" nerves to the upper extremity. The posterior cord, in contrast, provides all "dorsal" innervation to the upper extremity. Thus the radial nerve supplies all the dorsal muscles in the upper extremity below the shoulder. The musculocutaneous nerve supplies muscular innervation in the arm and provides cutaneous innervation to the forearm. In contrast, the median and ulnar nerves are nerves of passage in the arm,

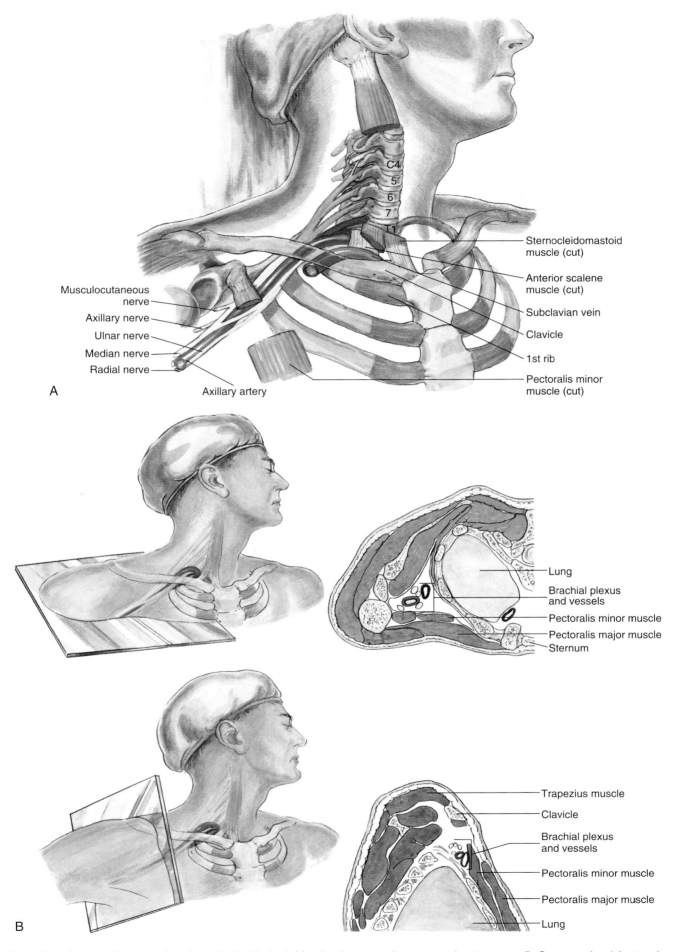

C4
5
6
7
T1

Musculocutaneous nerve

Axillary nerve

Ulnar nerve

Median nerve

Radial nerve

Axillary artery

Sternocleidomastoid muscle (cut)

Anterior scalene muscle (cut)

Subclavian vein

Clavicle

1st rib

Pectoralis minor muscle (cut)

A

Lung

Brachial plexus and vessels

Pectoralis minor muscle

Pectoralis major muscle

Sternum

Trapezius muscle

Clavicle

Brachial plexus and vessels

Pectoralis minor muscle

Pectoralis major muscle

Lung

B

Figure 7-2. Anatomy important for infraclavicular block. A, Muscles, bones, and neurovascular structures. B, Cross-sectional *(top)* and parasagittal *(bottom)* anatomy.

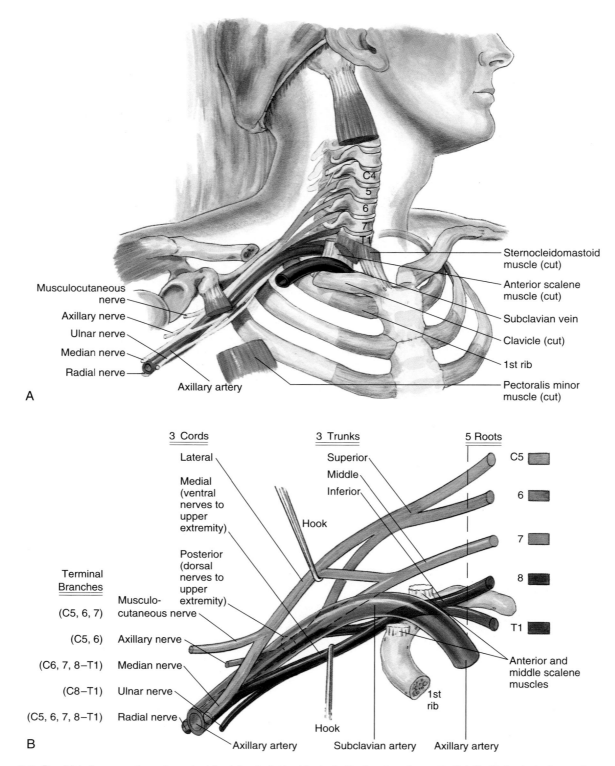

Figure 7-3. Brachial plexus anatomy important for infraclavicular block. **A,** Regional anatomy. **B,** Detailed infraclavicular anatomy.

but in the forearm and hand they provide the ventral musculature with motor innervation. These nerves can be further categorized: the median nerve innervates more heavily in the forearm, whereas the ulnar nerve innervates more heavily in the hand.

Position. The patient is placed supine, with the arm to be blocked abducted at the shoulder to a 90-degree angle if possible. If pain prevents this, the arm can be left at the patient's side and adjustments can be made with skin markings. The anesthesiologist can stand on the ipsilateral

or the contralateral side of the patient, depending on his or her preference and the patient's body habitus. We prefer to stand on the ipsilateral side of the patient.

Needle Puncture. With the arm abducted at the shoulder, the coracoid process is identified by palpation and a skin mark placed at its most prominent portion. The skin entry mark is then made at a point 2 cm medial and 2 cm caudad to the previously marked coracoid process (Fig. 7-4A). Deeper infiltration is then performed with a 25-gauge, 5-cm needle while the needle is directed from the insertion

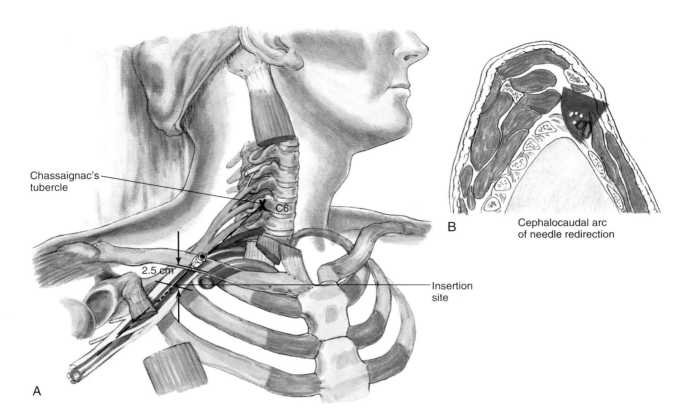

Figure 7-4. Technique of infraclavicular block. A, Surface markings for block. B, Parasagittal view showing arc of needle redirection.

site in a vertical parasagittal plane. Then a 7- to 9.5-cm, 20- to 22-gauge needle is inserted in a direction similar to that taken by the infiltration needle. If a paresthesia technique is used, a distal upper extremity paresthesia is sought; if a nerve stimulator technique is used, a distal upper extremity motor response is sought. If needle redirection is needed to achieve either a paresthesia or a motor response, the needle should be redirected in a cephalocaudad arc (Fig. 7-4B). The depth of contact with the brachial plexus depends on body habitus and needle angulation; it ranges from 2.5 to 3 cm in slender patients and from 8 to 10 cm in larger individuals.

Once adequate needle position has been achieved, either the single-injection dose of local anesthetic is administered incrementally or 20 mL of preservative-free normal saline solution is injected before threading the continuous brachial plexus catheter. For a single-injection technique, the block can be administered in a manner similar to that used in either a supraclavicular or an axillary block. For a continuous technique, we currently use a stimulating catheter device to optimize catheter placement.

POTENTIAL PROBLEMS

An infraclavicular block should not cause neuraxial or pulmonary complications. Although vascular compromise (puncture of the axillary artery or vein) is theoretically possible, in our experience this occurs infrequently. If a continuous catheter technique is chosen, there is the possibility that despite adequate initial needle position, the catheter may be threaded too far away from the plexus to result in an effective block. However, the use of stimulating catheters has decreased this concern.

ULTRASONOGRAPHY-GUIDED TECHNIQUE

SONOANATOMY

The brachial plexus in the infraclavicular region consists of three cords, each named for its classical position relative to the axillary artery: medial, lateral, and posterior. There is, however, significant anatomic variation. The cords and axillary vessels lie deep to the pectoralis major and minor muscles, just below the fascia of the pectoralis minor. The ultrasound transducer should be placed in a parasagittal orientation caudal to the coracoid process, roughly perpendicular to the clavicle, so that the plane of the ultrasound beam cuts the brachial plexus cords and axillary vessels in the short-axis view. The axillary artery is seen in cross-section as a hypoechoic, noncompressible pulsatile structure, whereas the axillary vein usually lies inferior and/or superficial to the artery. With the left side of the screen oriented cephalad, the lateral, posterior, and medial cords are often found at 9 to 10 o'clock, 6 to 7 o'clock, and 4 to 5 o'clock relative to the artery, respectively. The cords are often difficult to distinctly identify, emphasizing the importance of placing the local anesthetic deep to the pectoral fascia (Fig. 7-5). Depending on how medially the transducer is placed, ribs and/or pleura may be identified in the inferior part of the image.

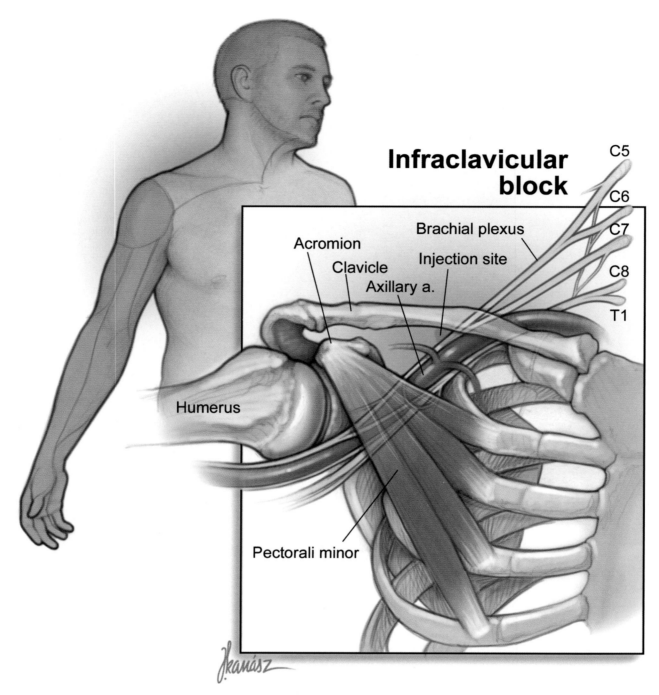

Figure 7-5. Anatomy of infraclavicular block

INDICATIONS

- Infraclavicular blocks are very effective for arm, elbow, forearm, and hand surgeries.
- Both single-shot and continuous techniques are possible. Continuous infraclavicular nerve blocks may provide superior analgesia compared with other techniques.[1]

[1]Mariano ER, Sandhu NS, Loland VJ, Bishop ML, Madison SJ, Abrams RA, et al. A randomized comparison of infraclavicular and supraclavicular continuous peripheral nerve blocks for postoperative analgesia. *Reg Anesth Pain Med.* 2011 Jan-Feb;36(1):26-31.

TECHNIQUE

The patient may be placed either supine or semisitting. The patient's head should be turned away from the side to be blocked. In the classic technique for the infraclavicular block, the arm is adducted to the side; therefore it is called the lateral infraclavicular technique. However, to improve visualization of the cords, we prefer to use the medial infraclavicular approach in which the arm is abducted 110 degrees, externally rotated, and the elbow is flexed 90 degrees. This will bring the cords closer together, superior to the axillary artery, and they may lie closer to the skin. The puncture site is made at the apex of the deltopectoral groove in the parasagittal plane. An in-plane approach is

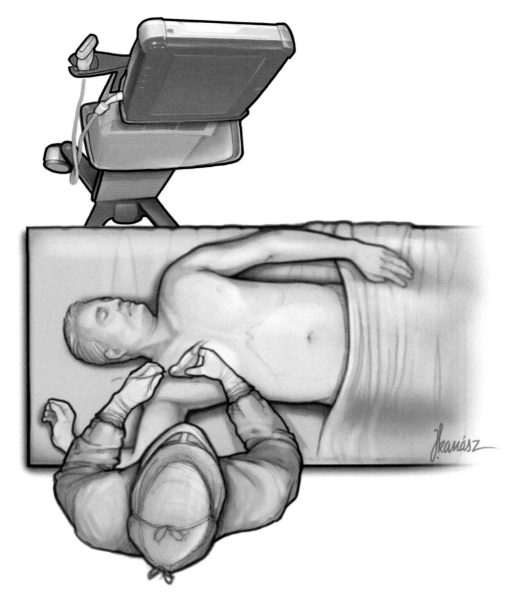

Figure 7-6. Medial approach for infraclavicular block. Note the arm is abducted.

recommended from the cephalad end of the probe along its long axis. In the case of catheter insertion, we prefer to use a 22-gauge needle to inject the local anesthetics around the three cords separately first; then we use Touhy needle to place the catheter beneath the posterior cord (Figs. 7-6 through 7-8).

KEY POINTS

- A linear or small curved transducer is preferred for this block to minimize the transducer footprint.
- The axillary artery is usually 4 to 5 cm below the skin in a typical patient.
- Because of the steep angle of needle insertion relative to the ultrasound beam, direct visualization of the needle may be difficult.
- Approximately 15 to 30 mL of local anesthetic is typically sufficient to provide complete block of the plexus. A single injection at the 6 o'clock position commonly suffices, but multiple injections may be required to ensure spread around the three cords.

- Unlike an axillary block, the medial brachial and antebrachial cutaneous nerves are blocked with this technique. The intercostobrachial nerve (arising from T2) may be separately blocked under the arm if desired.
- For catheter insertion, a Touhy needle is usually used. The catheter is usually inserted posterior to the axillary artery and advanced 2 to 3 cm past the needle tip. The correct position of the catheter can be confirmed under ultrasound by injecting either local anesthetic or 1 mL of air via the catheter and observing its distribution relative to the plexus.
- Catheters are typically coiled on the skin over the insertion site and covered with a transparent sterile dressing.

PEARLS

- If visualization of all three cords is not possible, it is typically sufficient to ensure that local anesthetic spreads in a "U" shape surrounding the axillary

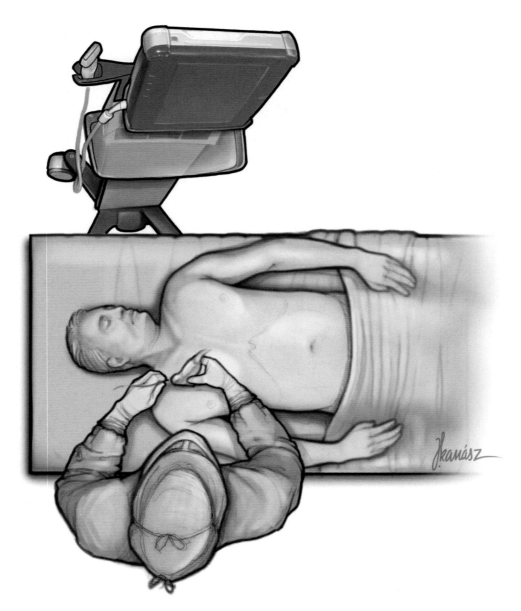

Figure 7-7. Lateral approach for infraclavicular block. Note the arm is adducted. In both, the in-plane technique is used with the needle direction from proximal to distal.

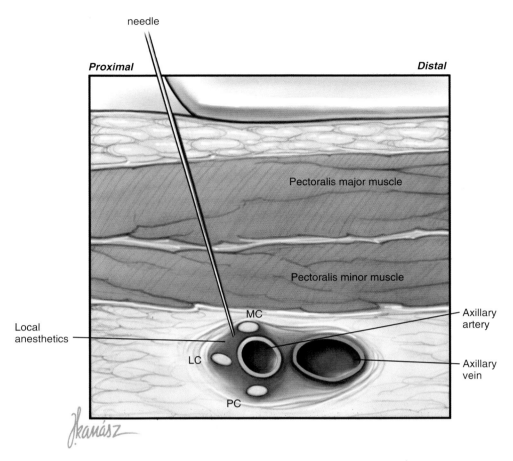

Figure 7-8. In-plane technique of infraclavicular block. The needle direction is from proximal to distal. Lateral cord (LC), Medial cord (MC), Posterior cord (PC).

artery. The contrast provided by the local anesthetic commonly improves visualization of the cords during the block.

- A reverberation artifact from the axillary artery may lead to the incorrect impression of a nerve structure deep to the artery.
- Because of the acute needle-to-transducer angle, it may be necessary to rely on indirect signs of needle location such as hydrodissection with normal saline or tissue movement while jiggling the needle.
- Excessive transducer pressure may occlude veins and increase the chance of inadvertent intravenous injection or hematoma formation.
- Placing the transducer as laterally as possible (but still medial to the coracoid process) increases the distance to the pleura and provides a larger margin of safety.

- Because of the increased distance between the plexus structures at this level, a larger volume of local anesthetic is commonly needed compared with more proximal brachial plexus blocks. Larger patient-controlled boluses (8 to 12 mL once per hour in our practice) via an indwelling catheter are also often needed to provide adequate analgesia.
- The infraclavicular location is particularly appealing for continuous blocks because the insertion site is away from the patient's head and neck, and passing through the pectoral muscles stabilizes the catheter.
- The infraclavicular approach does not produce phrenic nerve paralysis in contrast to the interscalene or supraclavicular approaches for brachial plexus blocks, which makes this technique very appealing in patients with compromised pulmonary function.

Axillary Block 8

Wael Ali Sakr Esa and David L. Brown

PERSPECTIVE

Axillary brachial plexus block is most effective for surgical procedures distal to the elbow. Some patients can undergo procedures on the elbow or lower humerus with an axillary technique, but strong consideration should be given to a supraclavicular block for those requiring more proximal procedures. It is discouraging to carry out a "successful" axillary block only to find that the surgical procedure extends outside the area of the block. This block is appropriate for hand and forearm surgery; thus it is often the most appropriate technique for outpatients in a busy hand surgery practice. Some anesthesiologists find the axillary block suitable for elbow surgical procedures, and continuous axillary catheter techniques may be indicated for postoperative analgesia in these patients. Because this block is carried out distant from both the neuraxial structures and the lung, complications associated with those areas are avoided.

Patient Selection.   To undergo an axillary block, patients must be able to abduct the arm at the shoulder. As the experience of the operator increases, the need for abduction decreases, but this block cannot be carried out with the arm at the side. Because the block is most appropriate for forearm and hand surgery, it is a rare patient with a surgical condition at those sites who cannot abduct the arm as needed.

Pharmacologic Choice.   Because hand and wrist procedures often require less motor blockade than procedures on the shoulder, the concentration of local anesthetic needed for axillary block can usually be slightly less than that needed for supraclavicular or interscalene block. Appropriate drugs are lidocaine (1% to 1.5%), mepivacaine (1% to 1.5%), bupivacaine (0.5%), and ropivacaine (0.5% to 0.75%). Lidocaine and mepivacaine produce 2 to 3 hours of surgical anesthesia without epinephrine and 3 to 5 hours with the addition of epinephrine. These drugs can be useful for less involved procedures or outpatient surgical procedures. For more extensive surgical procedures requiring hospital admission, a longer-acting agent such as bupivacaine can be chosen. Plain bupivacaine and ropivacaine produce surgical anesthesia that lasts from 4 to 6 hours; the addition of epinephrine may prolong this period to 8 to 12 hours. The local anesthetic timeline must be considered when prescribing a drug for outpatient axillary block because blocks lasting as long as 18 to 24 hours can result from higher concentrations of bupivacaine with added epinephrine. With continuous catheter techniques used for postoperative analgesia or chronic pain syndromes, 0.25% bupivacaine or 0.2% ropivacaine may be used, and even lower concentrations of these drugs may be used after a trial.

TRADITIONAL BLOCK TECHNIQUE

PLACEMENT

Anatomy.   At the level of the distal axilla, where the axillary block is undertaken (Fig. 8-1), the axillary artery can be visualized as the center of a four-quadrant neurovascular bundle. We conceptualize these nerves in quadrants like a clock face because multiple injections during axillary block result in more acceptable clinical anesthesia than does injection at a single site. The musculocutaneous nerve is found in the 9 to 12 o'clock quadrant in the substance of the coracobrachialis muscle. The median nerve is most often found in the 12 to 3 o'clock quadrant; the ulnar nerve is "inferior" to the median nerve in the 3 to 6 o'clock quadrant; and the radial nerve is located in the 6 to 9 o'clock quadrant. The block does not need to be performed in the axilla; in fact, needle insertion in the middle to lower portion of the axillary hair patch or even more distal to this is effective. It is clear from radiographic and anatomic study of the brachial plexus and the axilla that separate and distinct sheaths are associated with the plexus at this point. Keeping this concept in mind will help decrease the number of unacceptable blocks performed. Also, this more distal approach to axillary block is similar to the midhumeral brachial plexus block.

Position.   The patient is placed supine, with the arm forming a 90-degree angle with the trunk, and the forearm forming a 90-degree angle with the upper arm (Fig. 8-2). This position allows the anesthesiologist to stand at the level of the patient's upper arm and palpate the axillary artery, as illustrated in Figure 8-2. A line should be drawn tracing the course of the artery from the midaxilla to the lower axilla; overlying this line, the index and third fingers of the anesthesiologist's left hand are used to identify the artery and minimize the amount of subcutaneous tissue overlying the neurovascular bundle. In this manner, the anesthesiologist can develop a sense of the longitudinal course of the artery, which is essential for performing an axillary block.

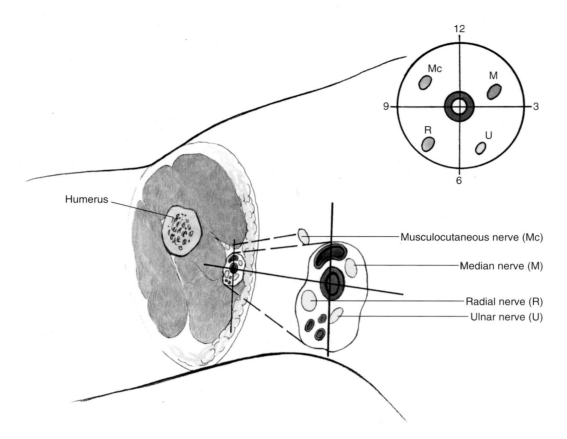

Figure 8-1. Axillary block: functional quadrant anatomy of distal axilla.

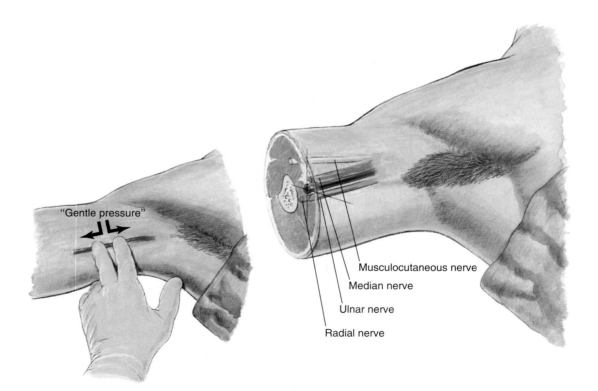

Figure 8-2. Axillary block: position of patient arm and clinician's fingers for palpation of axillary artery.

Needle Puncture. While the axillary artery is identified with two fingers, the needle and syringe are inserted as shown in Figure 8-3. Some local anesthetic should be deposited in each of the quadrants surrounding the axillary artery. If paresthesia is obtained, it is beneficial, although undue time should not be expended or patient discomfort incurred from an attempt to elicit a paresthesia. As illustrated in Figure 8-4, effective axillary block is produced by using the axillary artery as an anatomic landmark and infiltrating in a fanlike manner around the artery. Anesthesia of the musculocutaneous nerve is best achieved by infiltrating into the mass of the coracobrachialis muscle. This

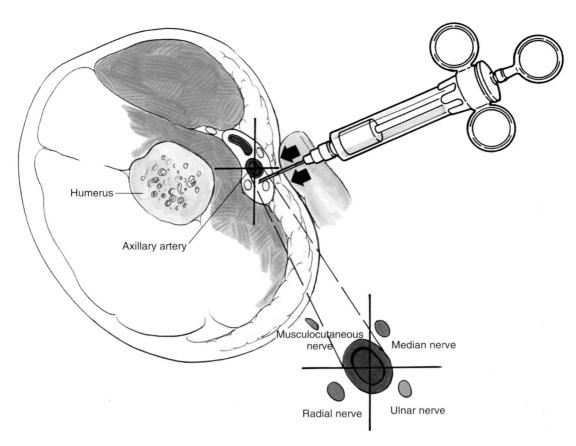

Figure 8-3. Axillary block: needle and syringe insertion.

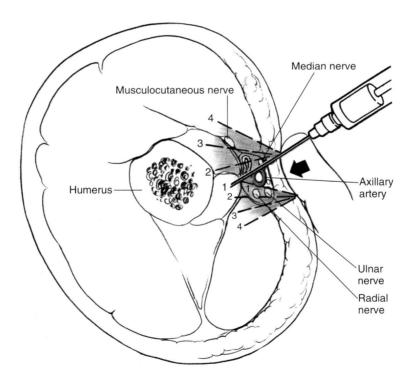

Figure 8-4. Axillary block: fanlike injection pattern using axillary artery as guide.

maneuver can be carried out by identifying the coracobrachialis and injecting anesthetic into its substance, or by inserting a longer needle until it contacts the humerus and injecting in a fanlike manner near the humerus (see Fig. 8-4).

When using a continuous catheter technique for an axillary block, stimulating or nonstimulating catheter kits may be used; we prefer the stimulating catheter (Fig. 8-5). With the nonstimulating catheter, the epidural needle is positioned either with the assistance of a nerve stimulator or with elicitation of paresthesia as an endpoint. After the needle is positioned, 20 mL of preservative-free normal saline solution is injected through the needle, and then the appropriate-size catheter is inserted approximately 10 cm

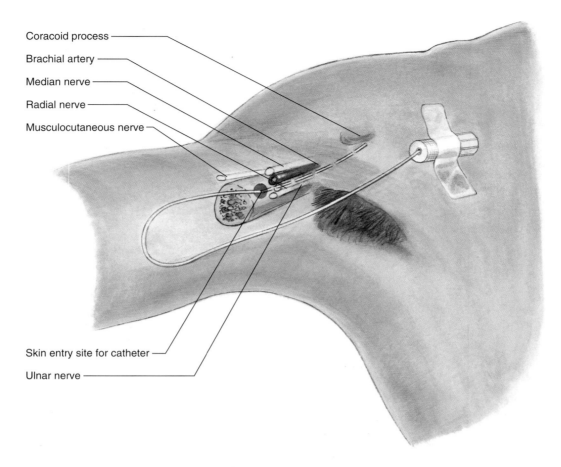

Coracoid process

Brachial artery

Median nerve

Radial nerve

Musculocutaneous nerve

Skin entry site for catheter

Ulnar nerve

Figure 8-5. Axillary block: continuous catheter technique after threading 10 cm of catheter proximally.

past the needle tip. Once the catheter has been secured with a plastic occlusive dressing, the initial bolus of drug is injected and the infusion is started.

POTENTIAL PROBLEMS

Problems with axillary block are infrequent because of the distance of this block from neuraxial structures and the lung. One occasional complication, which can be minimized by using multiple injections rather than a fixed needle, is systemic toxicity. Use of a single immobile needle to inject large volumes of a local anesthetic increases the potential for systemic toxicity relative to the use of smaller volumes of local anesthetic injected at multiple sites. Another potential problem with axillary block is the development of postoperative neuropathy, but one should not assume that axillary block is the cause of all neuropathy after upper extremity surgery. One must follow a logical and systematic approach when seeking the cause of a neuropathy if we are to understand the true incidence and causes of this condition after brachial plexus block and upper extremity surgery.

SONOANATOMY

The lateral cord of the brachial plexus divides into the musculocutaneous nerve and the lateral portion of the median

nerve, the medial cord divides into the ulnar nerve and medial portion of the median nerve, and the posterior cord divides into the radial nerve and the axillary nerve. In the axilla, the median, ulnar, and radial nerves travel in a neurovascular bundle with the axillary artery medial to the humerus. The musculocutaneous nerve travels separately and usually lies in the plane between the biceps and coracobrachialis muscles or in the body of the coracobrachialis.

The target nerves for the axillary block are the radial, median, ulnar, and musculocutaneous nerves. The structures of interest, including the axillary artery and surrounding nerves, are superficial (1 to 3 cm) from the skin surface of the anteromedial aspect of the proximal arm. The median nerve is located superficial and lateral to the artery, whereas the ulnar nerve is superficial and medial to the artery, and the radial nerve is posterior and lateral or medial to the artery.

Under ultrasound, the median, ulnar, and radial nerves have a honeycomb appearance or can be seen as round hyperechoic structures. The musculocutaneous nerve is usually seen under ultrasound as a hypoechoic, flattened oval with a bright hyperechoic border (Fig. 8-6).

INDICATIONS

- Surgeries from midarm down to elbow (brachiobasilic fistula, elbow fixation)
- Surgeries on the hand and wrist

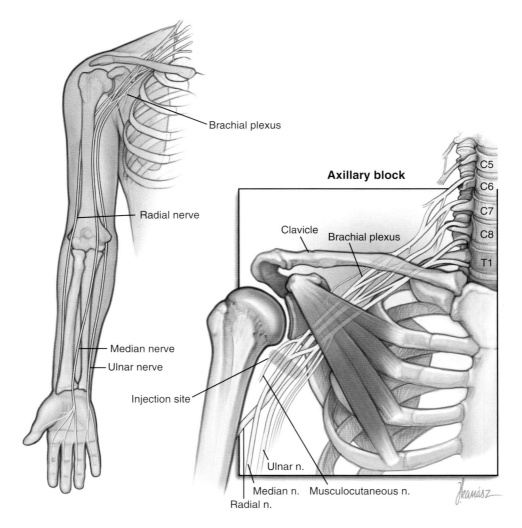

Figure 8-6. Anatomy of axillary approach of brachial plexus block.

TECHNIQUE

The patient ideally should be placed in the supine position, with the arm abducted 90 degrees and externally rotated so the dorsum of the hand rests on the bed, and the operator should be preferably behind the patient with the ultrasound machine in front of the patient and facing the operator. Injured extremities should be well supported during positioning. The ultrasound probe is placed transversely on the proximal medial upper aspect of the arm in order to view the axillary artery and surrounding nerves in short-axis view. This starting point should place the ultrasound transducer over both the biceps and triceps muscles. Then slide the ultrasound transducer across the axilla until the thick-walled pulsatile axillary artery and the hyperechoic surrounding nerves are visualized. Relative to the axillary artery, the median nerve usually lies around the 9 to 12 o'clock position, the ulnar nerve around 2 to 3 o'clock, and the radial nerve around 5 to 6 o'clock. We prefer to use the in-plane approach and a 2-inch, 22-gauge echogenic needle. The needle is inserted in plane from the cephalad aspect and directed to the location of the median, ulnar, and radial nerves using careful hydrodissection with a small amount of local anesthetic. Finally, the needle is withdrawn to the biceps muscle and redirected toward the hypoechoic flattened oval with a bright hyperechoic border musculocutaneous nerve (Figs. 8-7 and 8-8).

KEY POINTS

- High-frequency, 38-mm broadband linear array transducer is preferred for this block.
- Use between 20 and 25 mL of 0.5% ropivacaine or bupivacaine to inject the four nerves.
- We usually block the nerves around the axillary artery first—which are the median, ulnar, and radial nerves—and then the needle is withdrawn to the biceps muscle and redirected toward the hypoechoic, flattened oval musculocutaneous nerve.

PEARLS

- A reverberation artifact deep to the artery is often misinterpreted for the radial nerve. When you are in doubt, you can use nerve stimulation to confirm the location of the nerve.

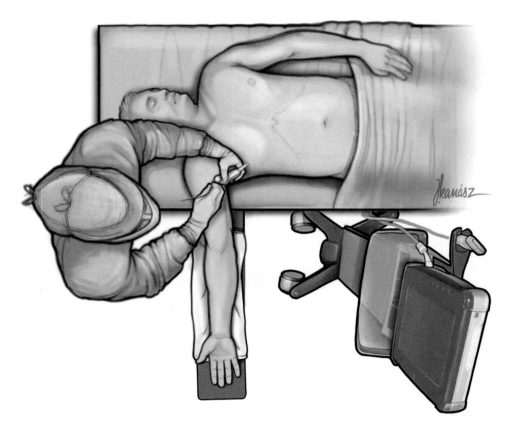

Figure 8-7. Patient position with the arm abducted 90 degrees and externally rotated.

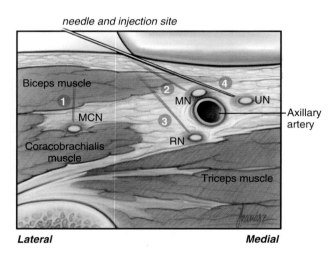

Figure 8-8. In-plane technique for axillary block. Note the multiple injections of local anesthetics around the musculocutaneous nerve (MCN), radial nerve (RN), and ulnar nerve (UN).

- The axillary nerve is not blocked because it departs from the posterior cord high up in the axilla; that's why the deltoid muscle is not anesthetized by the axillary block.
- Always aspirate before injection, and watch for the spread and the dose of the local anesthetic to avoid toxicity.
- When scanning, use minimal pressure with the ultrasound transducer to avoid obliteration of the veins, rendering the veins invisible and easily prone to being punctured with the needle if care is not taken.
- Unintentional multiple punctures of the veins surrounding the axillary artery can predispose the patient to local anesthetic toxicity.

ULNAR, MEDIAN, AND RADIAL BLOCK AT THE ELBOW

PERSPECTIVE

In general, distal upper extremity blocks—those at the elbow or wrist—are not frequently required if facility with more proximal blocks is gained. These more distal peripheral blocks are perceived to be associated with a slightly higher likelihood of nerve injury, perhaps because many of the peripheral branches are anatomically located in sites where the nerve is contained within bony and ligamentous surroundings. Although it is not difficult to localize the nerves at these peripheral sites, especially with ultrasonographic guidance, the "entrapment" of these nerves makes more proximal blocks, such as the axillary block, my preferred approach. Further, because a significant portion of hand and forearm surgery is carried out using an upper arm tourniquet, use of more distal blocks mandates significantly heavier sedation so that the patient can tolerate tourniquet inflation pressures.

Patient Selection. Few patients should require distal upper extremity block; an exception might be those needing supplementation after brachial plexus block. In any event, comprehensive anesthesia care should be possible without frequent use of these blocks.

Pharmacologic Choice. These peripheral blocks are usually considered for superficial surgery; thus lower concentrations of local anesthetic are appropriate because motor blockade should not be an issue. Therefore 0.75% to 1% mepivacaine or lidocaine, 0.25% bupivacaine, or 0.2% ropivacaine should be sufficient.

PLACEMENT

AT THE ELBOW

Anatomy. Of the three major nerves at the elbow—radial, median, and ulnar—the ulnar is most predictable in location. As illustrated in Figure 9-1, the ulnar nerve is located in the ulnar groove, which is a bony fascial canal between the medial epicondyle of the humerus and the olecranon process. This area is extremely well protected by fibrous

tissue, and, although it may seem at first like an easy site to carry out block, the nerve is well protected (and potentially vulnerable) in the ulnar groove. The median nerve at the elbow lies medial to the brachial artery, which lies just medial to the biceps muscle. Conversely, the radial nerve has a somewhat variable course; it pierces the lateral intramuscular septum on its way to the forearm and lies between the brachialis muscle and the brachioradialis muscle in the distal aspect of the upper arm. It is more effectively blocked in the axilla than at the elbow.

Position. All three of these nerves are blocked with the patient in the supine position and the arm supinated and abducted at the shoulder at a 90-degree angle. In addition, when the ulnar nerve block is performed, the forearm is flexed on the upper arm to more easily identify the ulnar groove (as illustrated in Fig. 9-3).

Needle Puncture: Median Nerve Block. A line should be drawn between the medial and lateral epicondyles of the humerus (at the level of the "pane of glass" shown in Fig. 9-1). Immediately medial to the brachial artery, the needle is inserted in the plane of the pane of glass, and paresthesia is sought or a nerve stimulator or ultrasonographic guidance is used to direct the needle (Fig. 9-2). After the needle is positioned, 3 to 5 mL of solution is injected medial to the brachial artery.

Needle Puncture: Radial Nerve Block. The radial nerve is likewise blocked at the level of the pane of glass in Figure 9-1. The biceps tendon at that level should be identified, and then a mark is made 1 to 2 cm lateral to the tendon. Again, a small-gauge, 3-cm needle is inserted through the mark in the plane of the pane of glass, and paresthesia is sought or a nerve stimulator or ultrasonographic guidance is used to direct the needle, and 3 to 5 mL of solution is injected at that site (see Fig. 9-2).

Needle Puncture: Ulnar Nerve Block. As illustrated in Figure 9-3, the forearm is flexed on the upper arm and the ulnar groove is palpated. At a point approximately 1 cm proximal to a line drawn between the olecranon process and the medial epicondyle, a small-gauge, 2-cm needle is inserted. Paresthesia should be easily obtainable, and once it is, the needle is withdrawn 1 mm, and 3 to 5 mL of local anesthetic is injected through the needle. A larger volume of solution should not be injected directly into the ulnar groove because high pressure in this tightly contained fascial space may increase the risk of nerve injury.

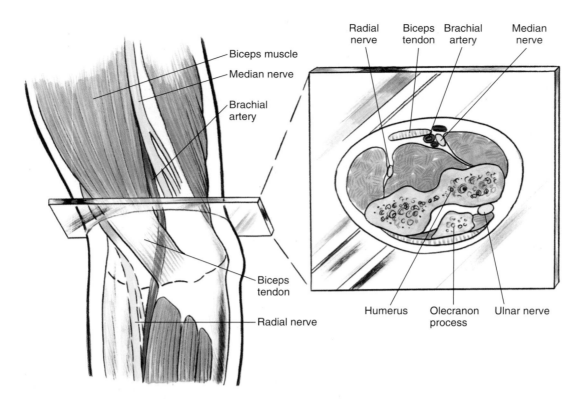

Figure 9-1. Elbow nerve blocks: functional anatomy.

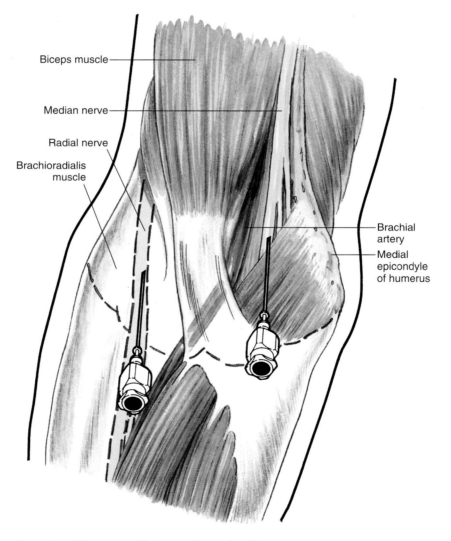

Figure 9-2. Elbow nerve blocks: median and radial nerves.

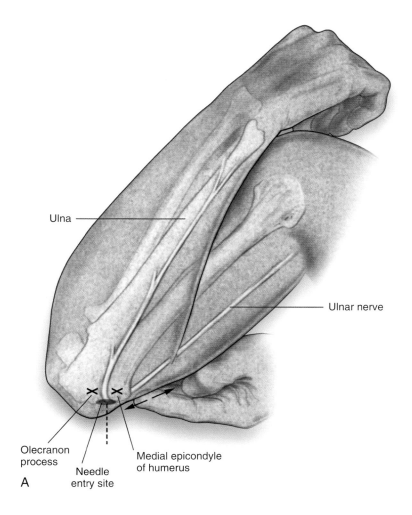

Ulna

Ulnar nerve

Olecranon
process

Needle
entry site

Medial epicondyle
of humerus

A

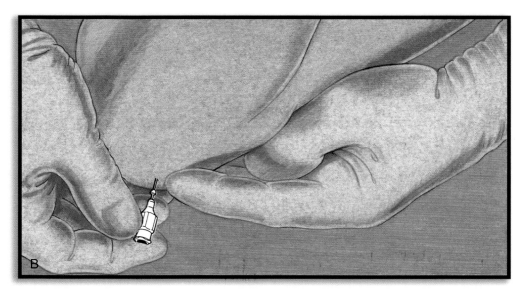

B

Figure 9-3. Ulnar nerve block: positioning. A, Palpation of the ulnar groove. B, Needle insertion.

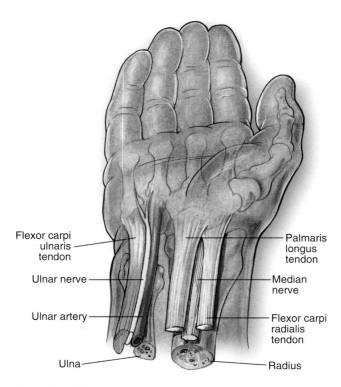

Flexor carpi ulnaris tendon

Ulnar nerve

Ulnar artery

Ulna

Palmaris longus tendon

Median nerve

Flexor carpi radialis tendon

Radius

Figure 9-4. Wrist nerve blocks: functional anatomy.

AT THE WRIST

Anatomy. The ulnar nerve lies immediately lateral to the tendon of the flexor carpi ulnaris muscle and immediately medial to the ulnar artery (Fig. 9-4). The median nerve lies between the tendon of the palmaris longus muscle and the tendon of the flexor carpi radialis muscle. That places the median nerve in the long axis of the radius. The radial nerve at the wrist has already divided into a number of its peripheral branches, and effective radial block requires a field block along the radial aspect of the wrist.

Position. For a peripheral block at the wrist, the patient rests supine while the arm is extended at the shoulder and supported on an arm board (Fig. 9-5). The wrist is flexed over a small support, and the most effective position for the anesthesiologist is to stand in the long axis of the arm board. Thus while performing the block, the anesthesiologist may observe the patient's face.

Needle Puncture: Ulnar Nerve Block. It should be easy to palpate the tendon of the flexor carpi ulnaris and the ulnar artery immediately proximal to the ulnar styloid process. A small-gauge, short-bevel needle can be inserted perpendicular to the wrist at this site, and paresthesia should be easy to elicit. Three to 5 mL of solution can be injected at this site; if no paresthesia is obtained, a similar amount can be injected in a fanlike manner between those two structures with near certainty of block.

Needle Puncture: Median Nerve Block. On a line between the styloid process of the ulna and the prominence of the distal radius, the palmaris longus tendon and the tendon of the flexor carpi radialis are identified. These tendons can be accentuated by having the patient flex the wrist while making a fist. The median nerve lies deep and between those structures, so a blunt-beveled, small-gauge, short

needle is inserted between the tendons. If paresthesia is obtained, 3 to 5 mL of solution is injected; if none is obtained, a similar amount is injected in a fanlike manner between the two tendons.

Needle Puncture: Radial Nerve Block. Blocking the radial nerve at the wrist requires infiltration of its multiple peripheral branches, which descend along the dorsal and radial aspects of the wrist. A field block is performed at the subcutaneous level in and around the anatomic snuffbox. The injection should be carried out superficial to the extensor pollicis longus tendon, which is easily identified by having the patient extend the thumb. This block may require from 5 to 6 mL of local anesthetic and is used infrequently.

POTENTIAL PROBLEMS

As outlined, problems with peripheral blocks primarily involve the potential for compression nerve injury and possibly a slightly increased incidence of neuropathy. Theoretically, this occurs because of the tight fascial compartments in which these nerves run through the distal arm, forearm, and wrist. Likewise, blocking these distal nerves does not allow for tourniquet use, which is often the clinically limiting factor.

PEARLS

Suggestions for the successful use of these blocks involve avoiding them when possible. Understanding the concepts outlined for the axillary nerve block (see Chapter 8, Axillary Block) should make the necessity of these blocks infrequent.

DIGITAL NERVE BLOCK

PERSPECTIVE

Digital nerve block is commonly used in emergency departments, but is not frequently used by anesthesiologists. It can be used for any surgery that requires a digital operation. However, its widest use is in repair of lacerations.

Patient Selection. The most common use for this block is in emergency departments, although its use may be appropriate in an occasional elective surgical patient with a single-digit surgical problem.

Pharmacologic Choice. As with any of the more peripheral upper extremity blocks, lower concentrations of any of the amide local anesthetics are appropriate for digital block, with the strong recommendation to avoid epinephrine-containing solutions.

PLACEMENT

Anatomy. As illustrated in Figure 9-6, the digital nerves can be conceptualized as running at the "corners" of the proximal phalanx. The nerves run near arteries and veins and are the distal continuations of both the median and ulnar nerves.

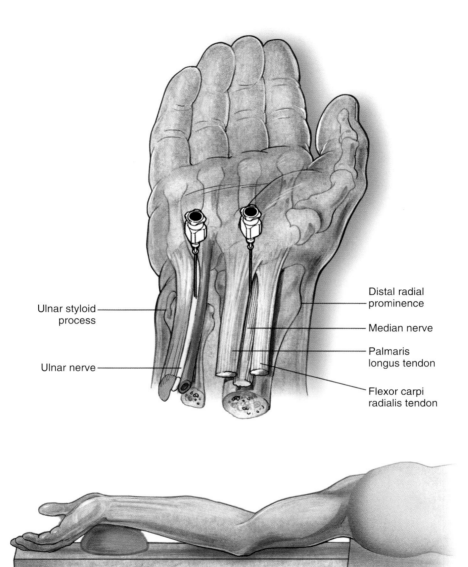

Ulnar styloid
process

Ulnar nerve

Distal radial
prominence

Median nerve

Palmaris
longus tendon

Flexor carpi
radialis tendon

Figure 9-5. Wrist nerve blocks: needle insertion and arm positioning.

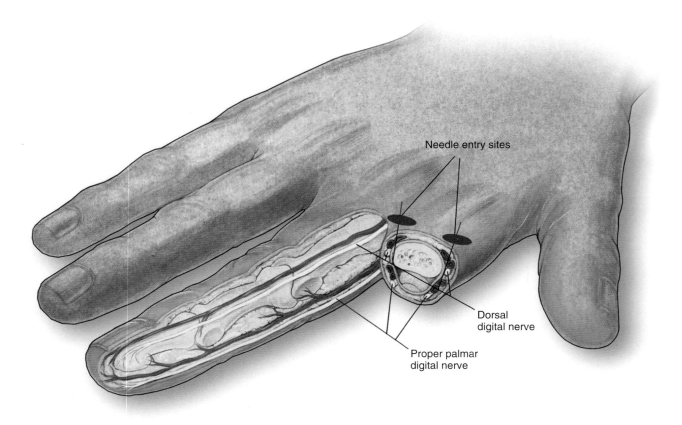

Figure 9-6. Digital nerve block: anatomy and needle insertion.

Position. Digital nerve block is most effectively carried out with the hand pronated. The skin over the dorsum of the finger is less tightly fixed to the underlying structures than it is on the ventral surface.

Needle Puncture. Skin wheals are raised at the dorsolateral borders of the proximal phalanx, and a blunt-beveled, small-gauge, short needle is inserted at the dorsal surface of the lateral border of the phalanx. Infiltration of both the dorsal and the ventral branches of the digital nerve is carried out bilaterally, and a total of 1 to 2 mL at each site should be sufficient for block.

POTENTIAL PROBLEMS

Epinephrine-containing solutions should not be used for digital nerve block.

PEARLS

These blocks should be used principally for emergency department procedures, and comprehensive anesthesia care requires at least familiarity with the technique.

Intravenous Regional Block 10

David L Brown

PERSPECTIVE

Intravenous (IV) regional anesthesia was introduced by Bier in 1908. As illustrated in Figure 10-1, in the initial description a surgical procedure was required to cannulate a vein, and both proximal and distal tourniquets were used to contain the local anesthetic in the venous system. After its introduction, the technique fell into disuse until the less toxic amino amides became available in the midtwentieth century. This technique can be used for a variety of upper extremity operations, including both soft tissue and orthopedic procedures, primarily in the hand and forearm. The technique has also been used for foot procedures with a calf tourniquet.

Patient Selection. The technique is best suited for patients in whom there is no disruption of the venous system of the involved upper extremity, because the technique relies on an intact venous system. It can be used for distal orthopedic fractures and soft tissue operations. Intravenous regional block may not be appropriate for patients in whom movement of the upper extremity causes significant pain, because movement of the upper extremity is required to exsanguinate blood from the venous system adequately.

Pharmacologic Choice. The most commonly used agent for IV regional anesthesia is a dilute concentration of lidocaine; however, prilocaine has also been successfully used. Lidocaine is used in a 0.5% concentration; approximately 50 mL is used for an upper extremity IV regional block.

PLACEMENT

Anatomy. The only anatomic detail necessary for clinical use of the IV regional block is identification of a peripheral vein; one must be cannulated in the involved extremity.

Position. The patient should be resting supine on the operating table with an IV tube already established in the nonsurgical arm. The involved arm should be extended on an arm board near available supplies (Fig. 10-2).

Needle Puncture. Before placement of the IV catheter in the operative extremity, a tourniquet, either double or single, should be placed around the upper arm of the patient. An IV cannula is then inserted in the operative extremity as distally as possible, most commonly in the dorsum of the hand (Fig. 10-3). There are two methods for exsanguinating the venous blood from the operative extremity. The traditional technique requires wrapping an Esmarch bandage from distal to proximal (Fig. 10-4). When the Esmarch bandage is not available or the patient is in too much pain to allow its placement, another method is to raise the arm for 3 to 4 minutes to allow gravity to exsanguinate the operative upper extremity (Fig. 10-5). After the blood has been exsanguinated from the upper extremity, the tourniquet is inflated. If a double tourniquet is used, only the upper tourniquet is inflated. Recommendations for tourniquet inflation pressures range from 50 mm Hg above systolic blood pressure with a wide cuff, to a cuff pressure double the systolic blood pressure, to 300 mm Hg regardless of blood pressure. Until more information is available, I caution against using pressures greater than 300 mm Hg during upper extremity block.

If an Esmarch bandage has been used, the elastic bandage is then unwrapped, and in the average adult 50 mL of 0.5% lidocaine without a vasoconstrictor is injected. Onset of the block usually occurs within 5 minutes, and the block is effective for procedures lasting as long as 90 to 120 minutes. This time limit is due to tourniquet time constraints rather than to diminution of the local anesthetic effect. The IV cannula is removed before preparation for operation. The block persists as long as the cuff is inflated and disappears shortly after deflation.

POTENTIAL PROBLEMS

The principal disadvantage of IV regional anesthesia is that physicians unfamiliar with treating local anesthetic toxicity may use the technique when appropriate resuscitation measures are not available. Although some workers report successful use of IV regional anesthesia for lower extremity surgery, especially if a calf tourniquet is used for foot surgery, its use is not widespread. During upper extremity use, a considerable number of patients complain about tourniquet pressure even when a double tourniquet is used, and this is often the clinically limiting feature of this technique. Appropriate use of IV sedatives is important for patient comfort.

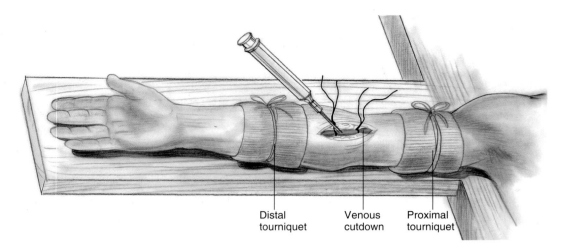

Distal tourniquet   Venous cutdown   Proximal tourniquet

Figure 10-1. Early Bier block: surgical technique.

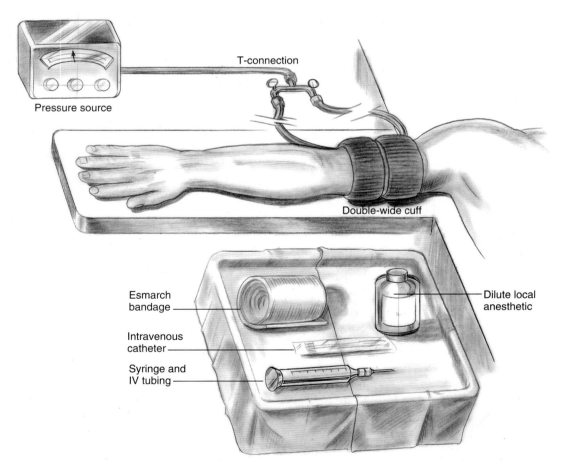

T-connection

Pressure source

Double-wide cuff

Esmarch bandage

Intravenous catheter

Syringe and IV tubing

Dilute local anesthetic

Figure 10-2. Intravenous regional block: equipment.

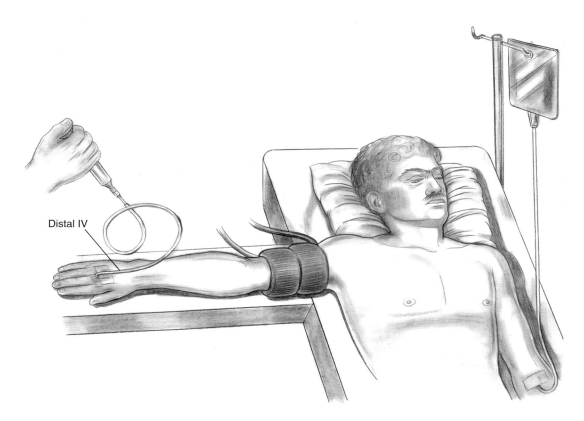

Distal IV

Figure 10-3. Intravenous regional block: distal IV site.

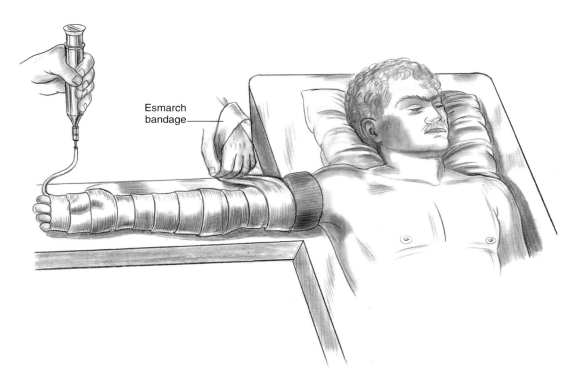

Esmarch bandage

Figure 10-4. Intravenous regional block: venous exsanguination with Esmarch bandage.

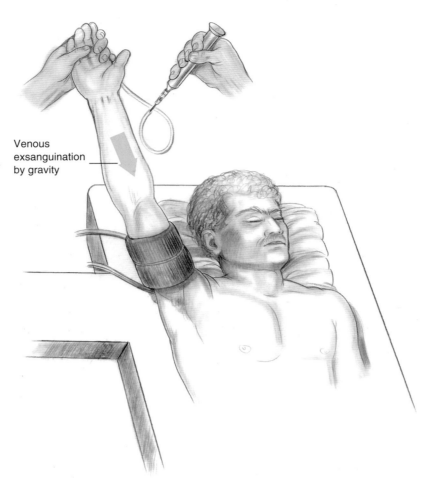

Venous
exsanguination
by gravity

Figure 10-5. Intravenous regional block: venous exsanguination by gravity.

PEARLS

Figure 10-6 illustrates the two complementary theories of how IV regional anesthesia produces block. The figure conceptualizes local anesthetic entering the venous system and producing block by blocking the peripheral nerves running with the venous structures. It also outlines a theory that may be complementary—that is, the local anesthetic leaves the veins and blocks small distal branches of peripheral nerves. It is likely that both of these theories are operative. If IV regional anesthesia is to be used successfully, all members of the operating team should understand the importance of tourniquet integrity because the most significant problems with the technique involve unintentional deflation of the tourniquet.

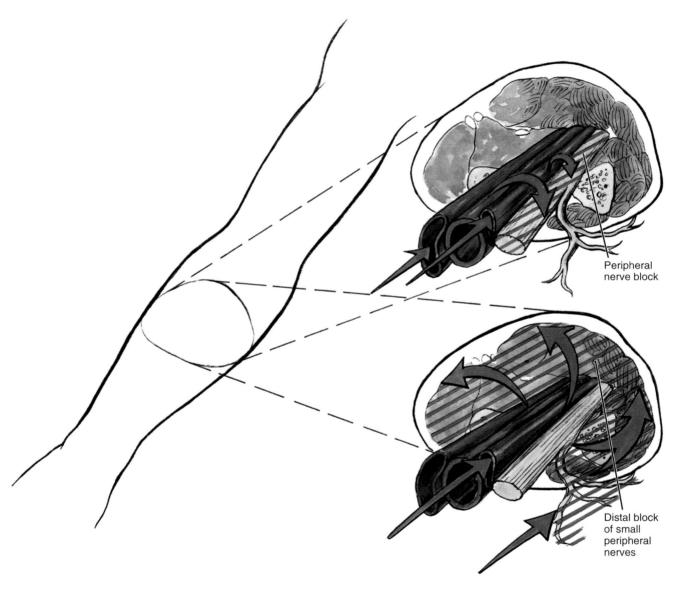

Peripheral
nerve block

Distal block
of small
peripheral
nerves

Figure 10-6. Intravenous regional block: potential mechanism(s) of action.

SECTION III
Lower Extremity Blocks

Lower Extremity Block Anatomy

11

David L Brown

Anesthesiologists are more comfortable carrying out lower extremity regional block than upper extremity regional block because of the ease and simplicity of blocking the lower extremities with neuraxial techniques. Also, in no anatomic site outside the neuraxis are the lower extremity plexuses as compactly packaged as are the nerves to the upper extremity in the brachial plexus. If one compares the path of lower extremity nerves over the pelvic brim with the path of the brachial plexus over the first rib, it is clear that the four major nerves to the lower extremity exit from four widely differing sites (Figs 11-1 and 11-2). Thus regional block of the lower extremity focuses on block of individual peripheral nerves, and my approach to anatomy will follow that concept.

Two major nerve plexuses innervate the lower extremity: the lumbar plexus and the lumbosacral plexus. The lumbar plexus primarily innervates the ventral aspect, whereas the lumbosacral plexus primarily innervates the dorsal aspect of the lower extremity (see Fig. 11-2).

The lumbar plexus is formed from the ventral rami of the first three lumbar nerves and part of the fourth lumbar nerve. In approximately half of patients, a small branch from the twelfth thoracic nerve joins the first lumbar nerve. The lumbar plexus forms from the ventral rami of these nerves anterior to the transverse processes of the lumbar vertebrae deeply within the psoas muscle (Fig. 11-3). The cephalad portion of the lumbar plexus (i.e., the first lumbar nerve, and often a portion of the twelfth thoracic nerve) splits into superior and inferior branches. The superior branch redivides into the iliohypogastric and ilioinguinal nerves, and the smaller inferior branch unites with a small superior branch of the second lumbar nerve to form the genitofemoral nerve (see Fig. 11-1).

The iliohypogastric nerve penetrates the transversus abdominis muscle near the crest of the ilium and supplies motor fibers to the abdominal musculature. It ends in an anterior cutaneous branch to the skin of the suprapubic region and a lateral cutaneous branch in the hip region (Fig. 11-4).

The ilioinguinal nerve courses slightly inferior to the iliohypogastric nerve. It then traverses the inguinal canal and ends cutaneously in branches to the upper and medial parts of the thigh and near the anterior scrotal nerves, which supply the skin at the root of the penis and the anterior part of the scrotum in males (see Fig. 11-4). In females, the comparable anterior labial nerves supply the skin of the mons pubis and labia majora.

The genitofemoral nerve divides at a variable level into genital and femoral branches. The genital branch is small; it enters the inguinal canal at the deep inguinal ring and supplies the cremaster muscle, small branches to the skin and fascia of the scrotum, and adjacent parts of the thigh. The femoral branch is the more medial of the two branches and continues under the inguinal ligament on the anterior surface of the external iliac artery. Below the inguinal ligament, it pierces the femoral sheath and passes through the saphenous opening to supply the skin over the femoral triangle lateral to that supplied by the ilioinguinal nerve (see Fig. 11-4). These three nerves are clinically important during regional block for inguinal herniorrhaphy or other groin procedures carried out under regional block.

Caudal to these three nerves are three major nerves of the lumbar plexus that exit from the pelvis anteriorly and innervate the lower extremity. These are the lateral femoral cutaneous, femoral, and obturator nerves (see Figs. 11-1 and 11-2).

The lateral femoral cutaneous nerve passes under the lateral end of the inguinal ligament. It may be superficial or deep to the sartorius muscle, and it descends at first deep to the fascia lata. It provides cutaneous innervation to the lateral portion of the buttock distal to the greater trochanter and to the proximal two-thirds of the lateral aspect of the thigh.

The obturator nerve descends along the medial posterior aspect of the psoas muscle and through the pelvis to the obturator canal into the thigh. This nerve supplies the adductor group of muscles, the hip and knee joints, and often the skin on the medial aspect of the thigh proximal to the knee.

The femoral nerve is the largest branch of the lumbar plexus. It emerges through the fibers of the psoas muscle at the muscle's lower lateral border and descends in the groove between the psoas and the iliacus muscles. It passes under the inguinal ligament within this groove. Slightly before or on entering the femoral triangle of the upper thigh, the femoral nerve breaks into numerous branches supplying the muscles and skin of the anterior thigh, knee, and hip joints.

The lumbosacral plexus is formed by the ventral rami of the lumbar fourth and fifth and the sacral first, second, and third nerves. Occasionally, a portion of the fourth sacral nerve contributes to the sacral plexus. The nerve from the plexus that is of primary interest to anesthesiologists during lower extremity block is the sciatic nerve. The posterior

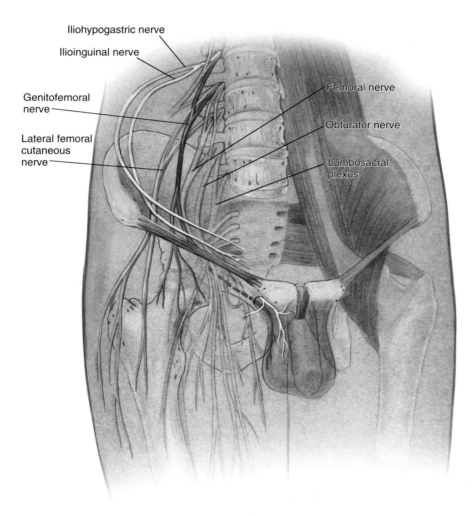

Iliohypogastric nerve

Ilioinguinal nerve

Genitofemoral nerve

Lateral femoral cutaneous nerve

Femoral nerve

Obturator nerve

Lumbosacral plexus

Figure 11-1. Lower extremity anatomy: major nerves, anterior oblique view.

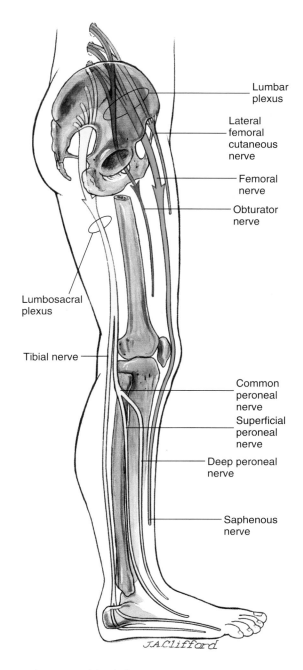

Figure 11-2. Lower extremity anatomy: major nerves, lateral view.

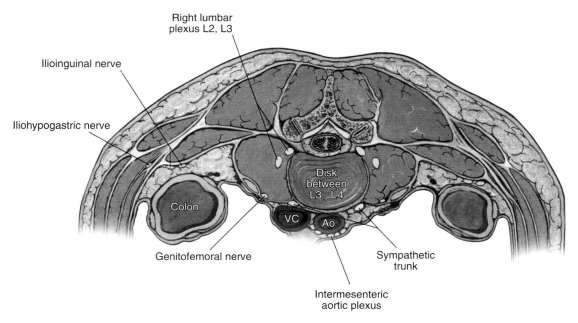

Figure 11-3. Lumbar plexus anatomy: cross-sectional view. Ao, aorta; VC, vena cava.

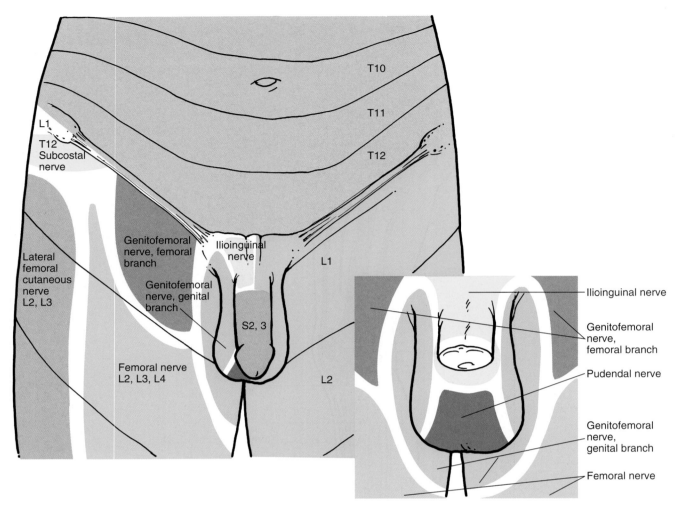

Figure 11-4. Lower extremity anatomy: proximal innervation (peripheral nerves labeled on right side of the body, dermatomes on the left).

femoral cutaneous nerve is sometimes listed as an additional branch important to anesthesiologists. In reality, the sciatic nerve is the combination of two major nerve trunks: the first is the tibial nerve, derived from the anterior branches of the ventral rami of the fourth and fifth lumbar and the first, second, and third sacral nerves, whereas the second is the common peroneal nerve, derived from the dorsal branches of the ventral rami of the same five nerves. These two major nerve trunks pass as the sciatic nerve through the upper leg to the popliteal fossa, where they divide into their terminal branches: the tibial and common peroneal nerves.

Figures 11-5 and 11-6 illustrate the cutaneous innervation of the peripheral nerves of the lower extremity. This subject is illustrated with the patient's lower extremity in both the anatomic and the lithotomy positions for greatest clinical utility. Figure 11-7 illustrates the dermatomal innervation of the lower extremities in a similar manner. Figure 11-8 illustrates the osteotome pattern of lower extremity innervation and will be most useful to anesthesiologists who are providing anesthesia for orthopedic procedures. Figure 11-9 helps clarify the cross-sectional anatomy pertinent to regional block of the lower extremity.

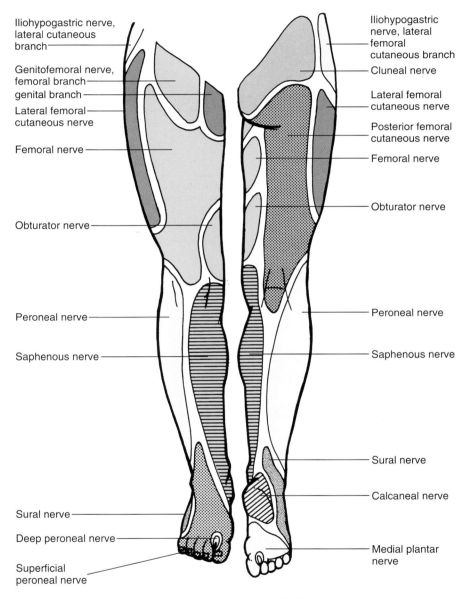

Iliohypogastric nerve, lateral cutaneous branch

Genitofemoral nerve, femoral branch genital branch

Lateral femoral cutaneous nerve

Femoral nerve

Obturator nerve

Peroneal nerve

Saphenous nerve

Sural nerve

Deep peroneal nerve

Superficial peroneal nerve

Iliohypogastric nerve, lateral femoral cutaneous branch

Cluneal nerve

Lateral femoral cutaneous nerve

Posterior femoral cutaneous nerve

Femoral nerve

Obturator nerve

Peroneal nerve

Saphenous nerve

Sural nerve

Calcaneal nerve

Medial plantar nerve

Figure 11-5. Lower extremity anatomy: proximal and distal innervation.

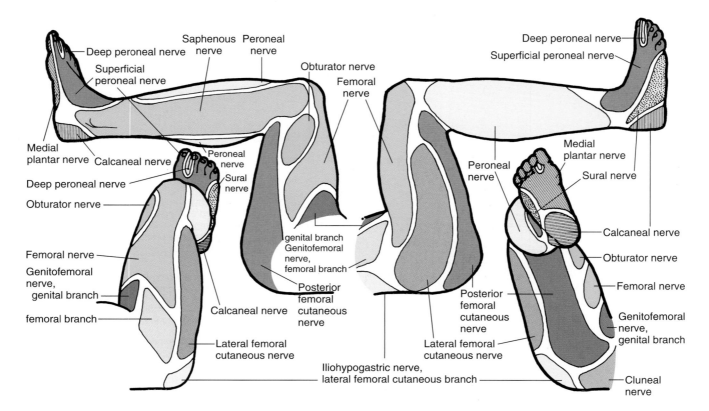

Figure 11-6. Lower extremity anatomy in lithotomy position: proximal and distal peripheral nerves.

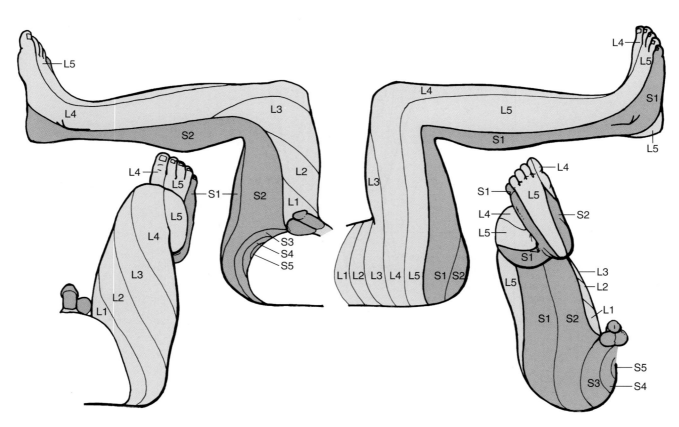

Figure 11-7. Lower extremity anatomy in lithotomy position: dermatomes.

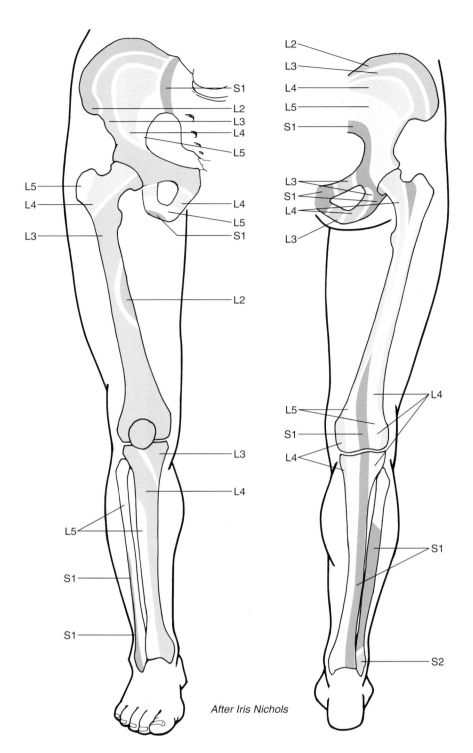

Figure 11-8. Lower extremity anatomy: osteotomes.

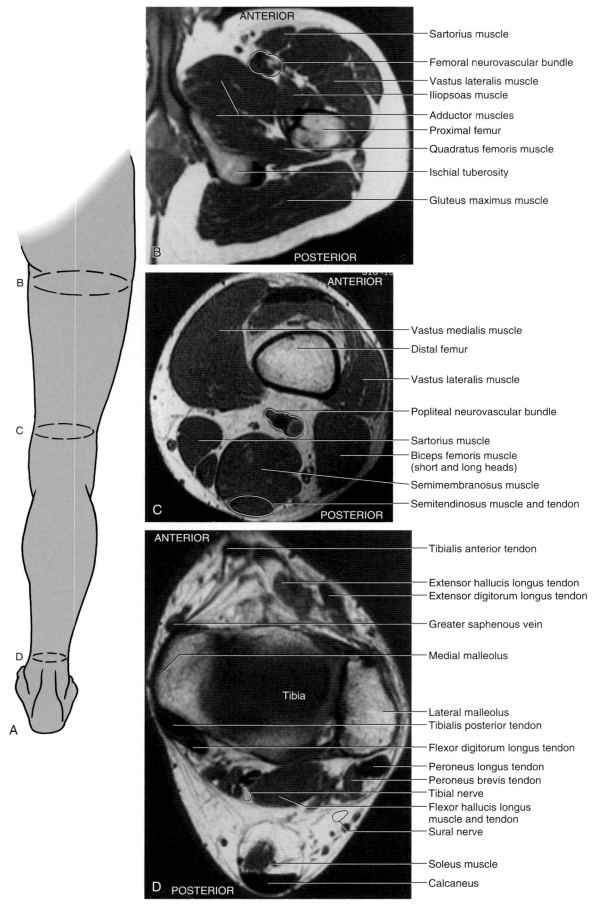

Figure 11-9. Lower extremity anatomy: cross-sectional magnetic resonance images. A, Location of sections. B, Upper leg (below the hip). C, Middle leg (above the knee). D, Lower leg (above the ankle).

Lumbar Plexus Block 12

Loran Mounir-Soliman and David L Brown

INGUINAL PERIVASCULAR BLOCK (THREE-IN-ONE BLOCK)

PERSPECTIVE

The inguinal perivascular block is based on the concept of injecting local anesthetic near the femoral nerve in an amount sufficient to track proximally along fascial planes to anesthetize the lumbar plexus. The three principal nerves of the lumbar plexus pass from the pelvis anteriorly: the lateral femoral cutaneous, the femoral, and the obturator nerves. As illustrated in Figure 12-1, the theory behind this block presumes that the local anesthetic will track in the fascial plane between the iliacus and the psoas muscles to reach the region of the lumbar plexus roots.

Patient Selection. As outlined, lower extremity block is often most effectively and efficiently performed with neuraxial blocks. Nevertheless, in some patients avoidance of bilateral block or sympathectomy may make an alternative approach necessary.

Pharmacologic Choice. Local anesthetics should be selected by deciding whether a primarily sensory or a sensory and motor block is needed. Any of the amino amides can be used. It has been suggested that the volume of local anesthetic needed for adequate lumbar plexus block from this approach can be estimated by dividing the patient's height, in inches, by three. That number is the volume of local anesthetic in milliliters that theoretically will provide lumbar plexus block.

PLACEMENT

Anatomy. The concept behind this block is that the only anatomy one needs to visualize is the extension of sheath-like fascial planes that surround the femoral nerve.

Position. The patient should be placed supine on the operating table with the anesthesiologist standing at the patient's side in position to palpate the ipsilateral femoral artery.

Needle Puncture. A short-beveled, 22-gauge, 5-cm needle is inserted immediately lateral to the femoral artery, caudal to the inguinal ligament in the lower extremity to be blocked. It is advanced with cephalad angulation until femoral paresthesia occurs; alternatively, nerve stimulation or ultrasonographic guidance is used to identify the correct perineural location of the needle tip. At this point, the needle is firmly fixed, and while the distal femoral sheath is digitally compressed, the entire volume of local anesthetic is injected.

POTENTIAL PROBLEMS

Our clinical experience suggests that the principal problem with this technique is a lack of predictability. In addition, whenever a large volume of local anesthetic is injected through a fixed "immobile" needle, the risk of systemic toxicity is increased. If the technique is used, incremental injection of local anesthetic, accompanied by frequent aspiration for blood, should be carried out.

PEARLS

This block should be used when the goal is lower extremity analgesia, not anesthesia during an operation. We do not believe one needs to master this technique to provide comprehensive regional anesthesia care.

PSOAS COMPARTMENT BLOCK

PERSPECTIVE

In theory, the psoas compartment block produces block of all lumbar and some sacral nerves, thus providing anesthesia of the anterior thigh. This block is described in *Chapter 37*. It is best termed a *lumbar paravertebral block*.

LUMBAR PLEXUS BLOCK

RELEVANT ANATOMY OF THE LUMBAR PLEXUS

The lumbar plexus is formed by the ventral rami of the first three lumbar nerves and the greater part of the ventral ramus of the fourth nerve. The first lumbar nerve, frequently supplemented by the twelfth thoracic nerve, splits into an upper branch that divides into the iliohypogastric and ilioinguinal nerves. The lower branch unites with a branch from the second lumbar to form the genitofemoral nerve.

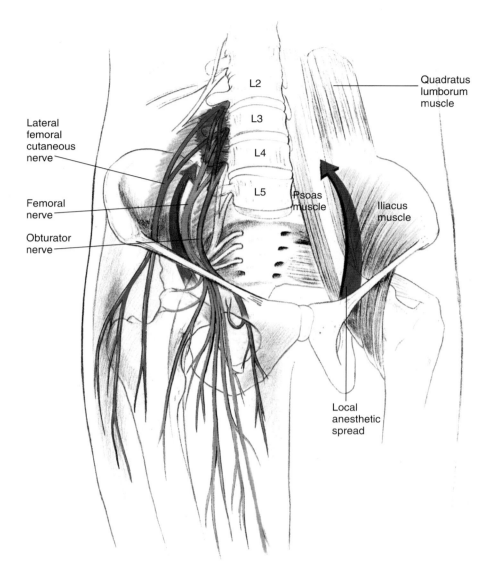

Figure 12-1. Lumbar plexus anatomy: proposed mechanism of proximal local anesthetic spread.

From the remains of the second lumbar nerve, the third and fourth nerves divide into ventral and dorsal divisions. The anterior divisions unite to form the obturator nerves, and the dorsal divisions form the lateral femoral cutaneous nerve and the larger femoral nerve.

The lumbar plexus and its branches are formed within the psoas major muscle in front of the transverse processes of the lumbar vertebrae. The anterior two-thirds of the psoas muscle originate from the anterolateral aspect of the vertebral body, and the posterior one-third of the muscle originates from the anterior aspect of the transverse processes, creating a fascial plane between both compartments of the muscle that hosts the lumbar plexus.

It is important to appreciate that the lumbar plexus is located anterior to the transverse processes of the lumbar vertebrae and posterior (embedded in the post wall) of the psoas muscle. The erector spinae muscle covers the lumbar spine posteriorly medially and the quadratus lumborum muscle laterally.

Appreciation of the relations between the different muscles and spine anatomy, as well as the sonographic characteristics of these structures, is crucial to perform the block.

TECHNIQUE

The lumbar plexus block is a deep block that requires a lower-frequency (2 to 5 MHz), curvilinear ultrasound probe. A 4- to 6-inch needle is used, depending on the body habitus. Two techniques are described to perform the block.

Paramedial Longitudinal Scanning Technique

With the patient in the prone position (this can also be performed in the lateral position with the side blocked upwards), the ultrasound probe is placed parallel to the long axis of the sacrum to identify its flat surface. The probe is moved cephalad to identify the intervertebral space between L5 and S1 as an interruption of the sacral line continuity. The probe is moved 3 to 4 cm laterally (keeping the same orientation) to identify the transverse process of L5. The transverse processes of the other lumbar vertebrae are identified by cephalad scan in ascending order. The acoustic shadow of the transverse processes has a characteristic appearance often referred to as a *trident sign*.

The psoas muscle is imaged through the acoustic windows between the hyperechoic shadows of the transverse processes. The lumbar plexus can be identified as hyperechoic striations in the posterior wall of the psoas muscle. However, appropriate identification of the plexus is confirmed by inducing quadriceps contraction or adduction when applying nerve stimulation to the insulated needle. The needle can be introduced using both the in-plane and out-of-place techniques in the middle of the probe or using the in-plane technique from the lower edge of the probe (Figs 12-2A and 12-2B).

Transverse Oblique Scanning Technique

This technique can be also used in the prone or lateral position with the side blocked up. The L3 to L4 transverse processes are identified by the same technique described earlier (scanning from the sacrum upwards). Once identified, the ultrasound probe is rotated horizontally parallel to the transverse processes. Next, it is directed slightly medially to scan the midline structures (transverse oblique orientation). The target structures of the ultrasound beam are:

- Quadratus lumborum (lateral) and erector spinae muscles (medial)
- Deeper to the muscles, the transverse processes of L3 to L4 and the anterolateral surface of the vertebral bodies can be scanned as hyperechoic structures with underlying drop-down shadows.
- The psoas muscle appears slightly hypoechoic with multiple hyperechoic striations deeper to the transverse processes.
- Slowly adjust the probe in the acoustic window between the transverse processes, allowing for visualization of the intervertebral foramen, and the articular process facet joint with the roots of the lumbar plexus as it emerges from the intervertebral foramen. The roots appear as hyperechoic structures adjacent to the posterior wall of the psoas muscle.

The lumbar plexus is approached with the needle in the plane with the ultrasound beam from the lateral side of the probe (the approach from the medial side is also described), targeting the posterior border of the psoas muscle at the level of the intervertebral foramen. Using nerve stimulation is very helpful to confirm the proximity of the needle to the lumbar plexus and avoid intramuscular injection where local psoas contraction is induced. Care should be taken to avoid advancing the needle too medially to reduce the risk of injury of the lumbar artery or its branches and to avoid spread of local anesthetic into the neuraxial space (Figs 12-3A and 12-3B).

INDICATION

- The lumbar plexus block is the most proximal approach to the lumbar plexus, providing the most reliable block of its major branches (femoral, obturator, and lateral femoral cutaneous nerves).
- The block is ideal for hip surgeries and surgeries above the knee.
- When combined with sciatic nerve block, it provides complete unilateral lower limb anesthesia suitable for lower extremity surgeries.
- Continuous catheterization can be used for prolonged analgesia (Fig. 12-4).

KEY POINTS

- The lumbar plexus block is a deep block that makes it difficult to appreciate the difference in the echogenicity of the anatomic structures, especially in obese and elderly patients.
- The use of nerve stimulation is necessary to identify the lumbar plexus.
- Identification of small lumbar arteries is hard to visualize at deeper scan, and the block should be avoided in patients with coagulation disorders or at risk of bleeding.
- The spread of local anesthetic at the posterior surface of the psoas muscle is satisfactory.

PEARLS

- The lumbar plexus block is a technically advanced procedure with major potential for complications. Experience with ultrasound anatomy, scanning skills, and needle manipulations is necessary before attempting ultrasound-guided lumbar plexus block.
- The lumbar plexus is embedded within the body of the psoas muscle; hence the name *psoas block* is synonymous with lumbar plexus block.
- The block can be performed in the prone and lateral positions. The advantage of the prone position is that it provides a more stable resting hand position, allowing more precise scanning and manipulations.
- At the level of L2 to L3, the kidney can be visualized as a hypoechoic structure that moves with respiration.
- Care should be taken to do frequent repeated aspiration and inject the local anesthetic in small increments to detect epidural or spinal spread early.
- The lumbar paravertebral space is a vascular and muscular space, which leads to significant systemic absorption of the local anesthetic and potentially high plasma levels.

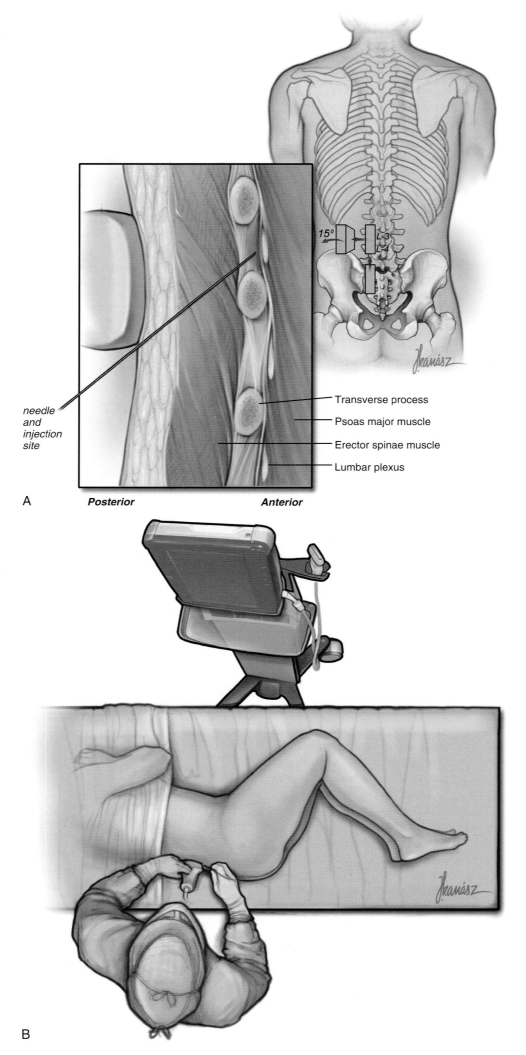

needle
and
injection
site

Transverse process

Psoas major muscle

Erector spinae muscle

Lumbar plexus

A   **Posterior**   **Anterior**

15º   L-3
      L-4

B

Figure 12-2. Paramedian longitudinal technique for lumbar plexus block.

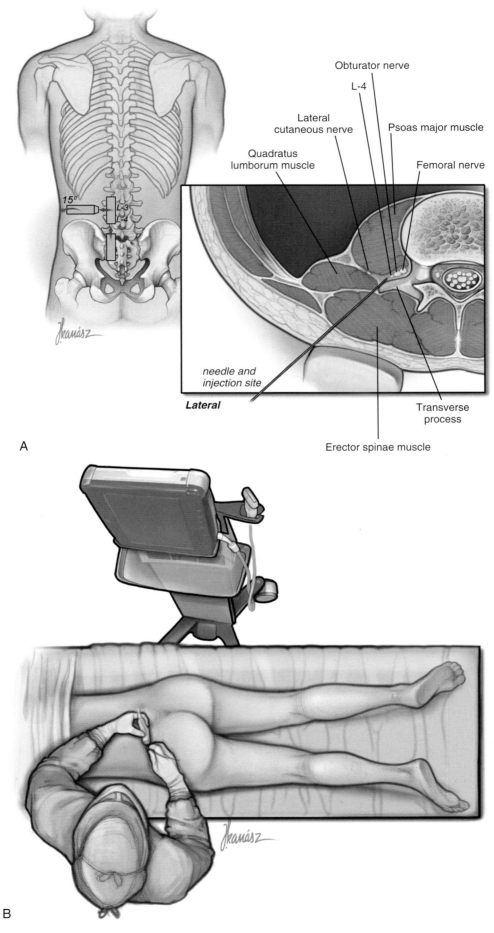

A

Obturator nerve

L-4

Lateral
cutaneous nerve

Psoas major muscle

Quadratus
lumborum muscle

Femoral nerve

15°

L-3
L-4

*needle and
injection site*

Lateral

Transverse
process

Erector spinae muscle

B

Figure 12-3. Transverse oblique technique for lumbar plexus block.

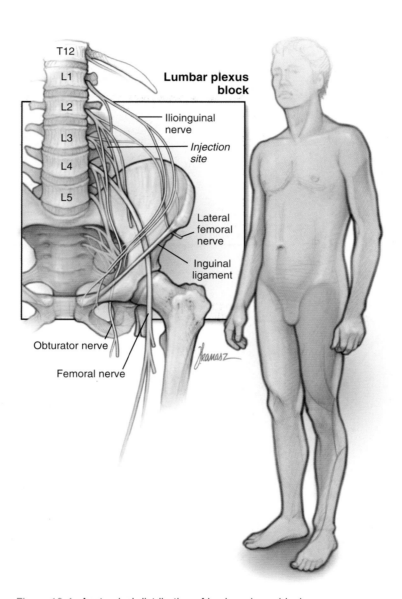

Figure 12-4. Anatomical distribution of lumbar plexus block.

Sciatic Block 13

Ehab Farag and David L Brown

PERSPECTIVE

The sciatic nerve is one of the largest nerve trunks in the body, yet few surgical procedures can be performed with sciatic block alone. It is most often combined with femoral, lateral femoral cutaneous, or an obturator nerve block. The block is also effective for analgesia of the lower leg and may provide pain relief from ankle fractures or tibial fractures before operative intervention.

Patient Selection.   This block may be indicated for patients needing analgesia before transport for definitive orthopedic surgical repair of lower leg or ankle fractures. For patients in whom it may be desirable to avoid the sympathectomy accompanying neuraxial block, sciatic block combined with femoral nerve block often allows ankle and foot procedures to be carried out. One group of patients in whom this block is often useful is those undergoing distal amputations of the lower extremity who have vascular compromise based on diabetes or peripheral vascular disease.

Pharmacologic Choice.   Sciatic nerve block requires from 20 to 25 mL of local anesthetic solution. When this volume is added to that required for other lower extremity peripheral blocks, the total may reach the upper end of an acceptable local anesthetic dose range. Conversely, uptake of local anesthetic from these lower extremity sites is not as rapid as with epidural or intercostal block; thus a larger mass of local anesthetic may be appropriate in this region. If motor blockade is desired with this block, 1.5% mepivacaine or lidocaine may be necessary, whereas 0.5% bupivacaine or 0.5% to 0.75% ropivacaine will be effective.

TRADITIONAL BLOCK TECHNIQUE

PLACEMENT

Anatomy.   The sciatic nerve is formed from the L4 through S3 roots. These roots of the sacral plexus form on the anterior surface of the lateral sacrum and are assembled into the sciatic nerve on the anterior surface of the piriformis muscle. The sciatic nerve results from the fusion of two major nerve trunks. The "medial" sciatic nerve is functionally the tibial nerve, which forms from the ventral branches of the ventral rami of L4 to L5 and S1 to S3; the posterior branches of the ventral rami of these same nerves form the "lateral" sciatic nerve, which is functionally the peroneal nerve. As the sciatic nerve exits the pelvis, it is anterior to the piriformis muscle and is joined by another nerve—the posterior cutaneous nerve of the thigh. At the inferior border of the piriformis, the sciatic and posterior cutaneous nerves of the thigh lie posterior to the obturator internus, the gemelli, and the quadratus femoris. At this point, these nerves are anterior to the gluteus maximus. Here, the nerve is approximately equidistant from the ischial tuberosity and the greater trochanter (Figs. 13-1 to 13-3). The nerve continues downward through the thigh to lie along the posteromedial aspect of the femur. At the cephalad portion of the popliteal fossa, the sciatic nerve usually divides to form the tibial and common peroneal nerves. Occasionally, this division occurs much higher, and sometimes the tibial and peroneal nerves are separate through their entire course. In the popliteal fossa, the tibial nerve continues downward into the lower leg, whereas the common peroneal nerve travels laterally along the medial aspect of the short head of the biceps femoris muscle.

CLASSIC APPROACH

Position.   The patient is positioned laterally, with the side to be blocked nondependent. The nondependent leg is flexed and its heel placed against the knee of the dependent leg (Fig. 13-4). The anesthesiologist is positioned to allow insertion of the needle, as shown in Figure 13-4.

Needle Puncture.   A line is drawn from the posterior superior iliac spine to the midpoint of the greater trochanter. Perpendicular to the midpoint of this line, another line is extended caudomedially for 5 cm. The needle is inserted through this point (Fig. 13-5). As a cross-check for proper placement, an additional line may be drawn from the sacral hiatus to the previously marked point on the greater trochanter. The intersection of this line with the 5-cm perpendicular line should coincide with the needle insertion site.

At this site, a 22-gauge, 10- to 13-cm needle is inserted, as illustrated in Figure 13-4. The needle should be directed through the entry site toward an imaginary point where the femoral vessels course under the inguinal ligament. The needle is inserted until paresthesia is elicited or until bone is contacted. If bone is encountered before paresthesia is elicited, the needle is redirected along the line joining the sacral hiatus and the greater trochanter until paresthesia or a motor response is elicited. During this redirection, the

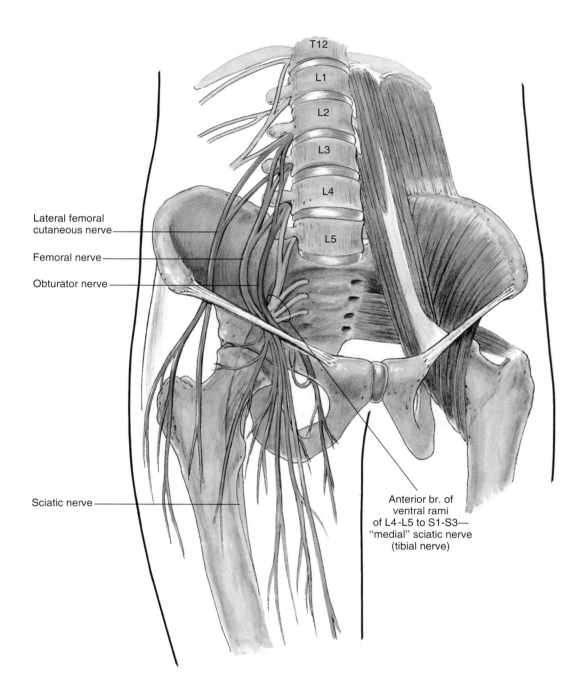

Figure 13-1. Sciatic nerve anatomy: anterior oblique view.

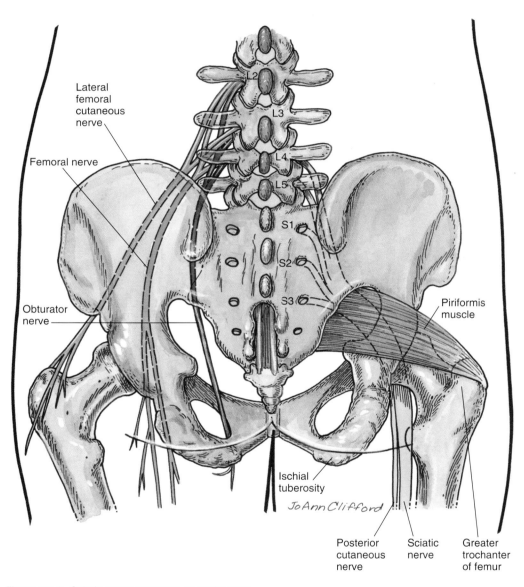

Figure 13-2. Sciatic nerve anatomy: posterior view.

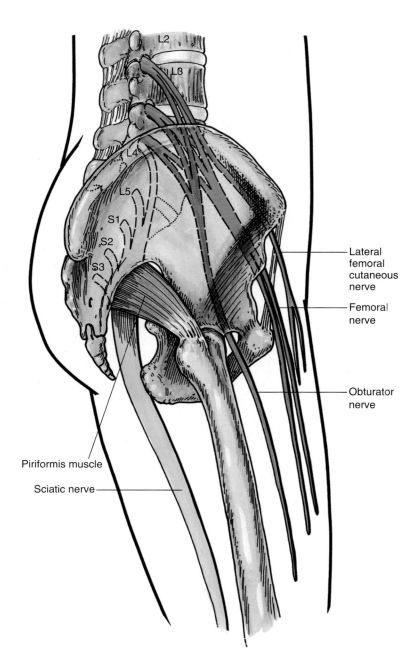

Figure 13-3. Sciatic nerve anatomy: lateral view.

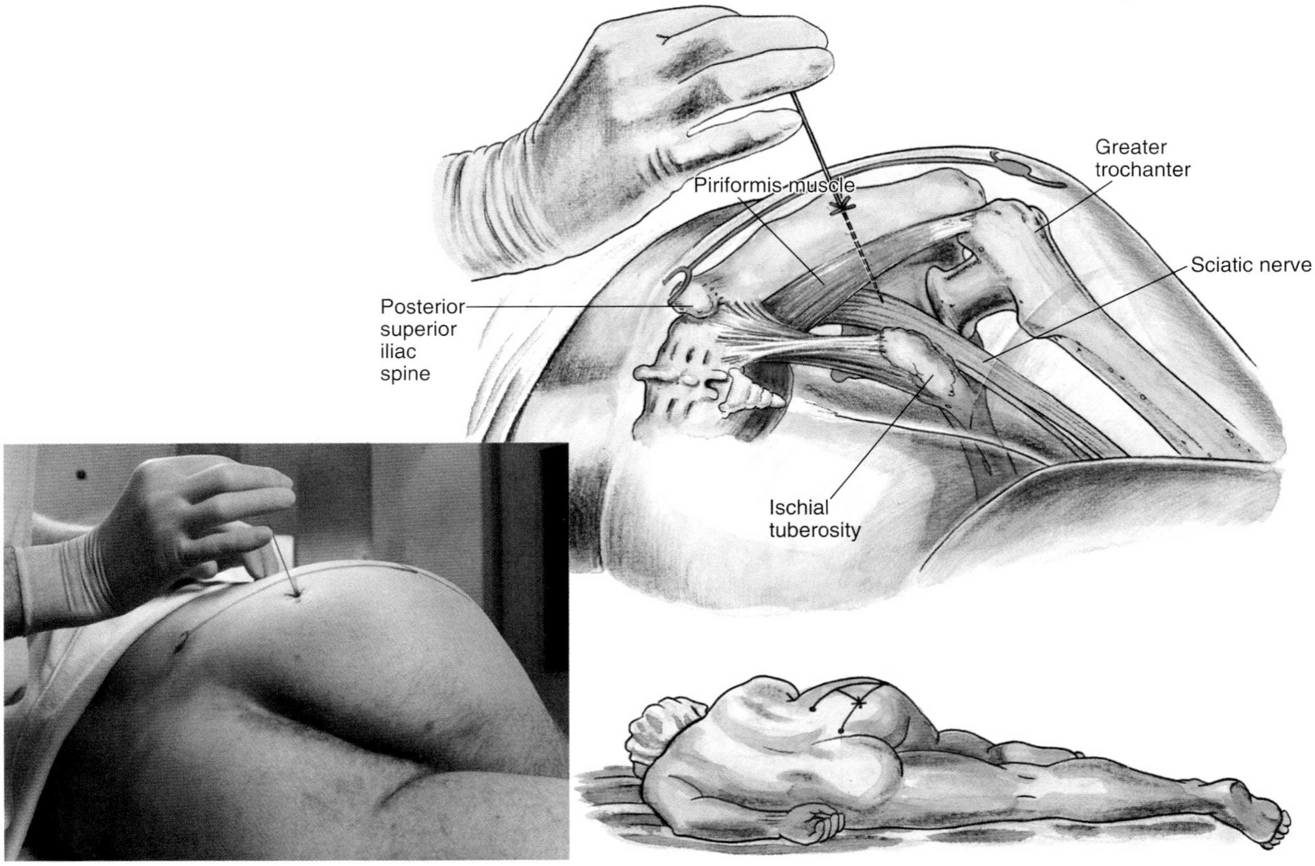

Figure 13-4. Sciatic nerve block: classic technique and positioning.

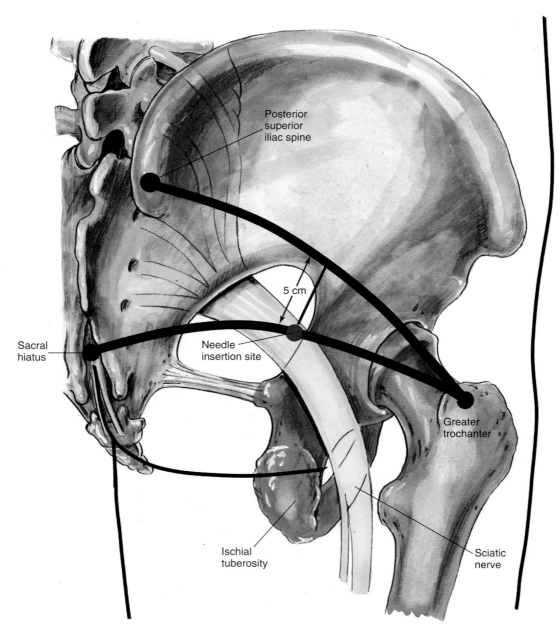

Figure 13-5. Sciatic nerve block: surface marking technique.

needle should not be inserted more than 2 cm past the depth at which bone was originally contacted, or the needle tip will be placed anterior to the site of the sciatic nerve. Once paresthesia or a motor response is elicited, 20 to 25 mL of local anesthetic is injected.

ANTERIOR APPROACH

Position.   The anterior block of the sciatic nerve can be carried out in the supine patient whose leg is in the neutral position. The anesthesiologist should be at the patient's side, similar to positioning during femoral nerve block.

Needle Puncture.   In the supine patient, a line should be drawn from the anterior superior iliac spine to the pubic tubercle. Another line should be drawn parallel to this line from the midpoint of the greater trochanter inferomedially, as illustrated in Figure 13-6. The first line is trisected, and

a perpendicular line is drawn caudolaterally from the juncture of the medial and middle thirds, as shown in Figure 13-6. At the point where the perpendicular line crosses the more caudal line, a 22-gauge, 13-cm needle is inserted so that it contacts the femur at its medial border. Once the needle has contacted the femur, it is redirected slightly medially to slide off the medial surface of the femur. At approximately 5 cm past the depth required to contact the femur, paresthesia or a motor response should be sought to ensure successful block (Fig. 13-7). Once paresthesia or a motor response is obtained, 20 to 25 mL of local anesthetic is injected.

POTENTIAL PROBLEMS

In patients in whom the block is being used for an injury to the lower extremity, the classic position is sometimes

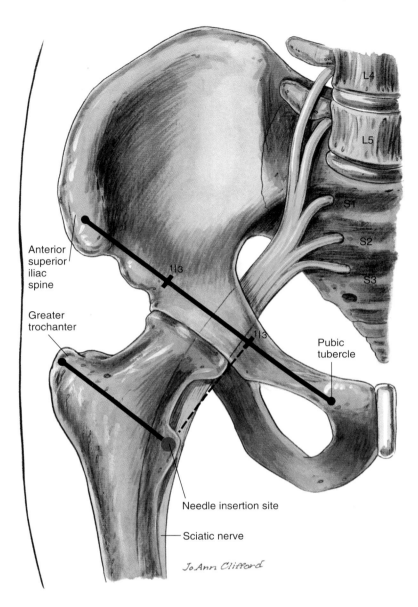

Figure 13-6. Sciatic nerve block: anterior technique.

difficult to use. This block can also be of long duration, and patients should be warned of this before surgery. Although it is unsubstantiated, some consider that dysesthesias may be more common after this block than after other peripheral blocks. The same problems pertaining to the classic approach should be considered with the anterior approach.

PEARLS

CLASSIC APPROACH

The keys to making this block work are adequate positioning of the patient and a systematic redirection of the needle until paresthesia is obtained.

ANTERIOR APPROACH

Although the anterior approach is conceptually simple, we are able to produce anesthesia using it slightly less often than when using the classic approach. Perhaps with additional experience, this difference would not be as apparent. One observation that may help to improve one's success rate with this block is to make sure that the lower extremity to be blocked is maintained in the neutral position and is not allowed to assume either a medially or a laterally rotated position. This block may be useful in supine patients who are in significant discomfort and cannot be positioned for the classic approach.

ULTRASONOGRAPHY-GUIDED TECHNIQUE

SONOANATOMY

The sciatic nerve in the subgluteal region lies in the middle between the greater trochanter laterally and the ischial tuberosity medially. Under ultrasound, the subgluteal sciatic nerve has a triangular shape defined by the long head of the biceps formis (posterolateral), the

ANTERIOR

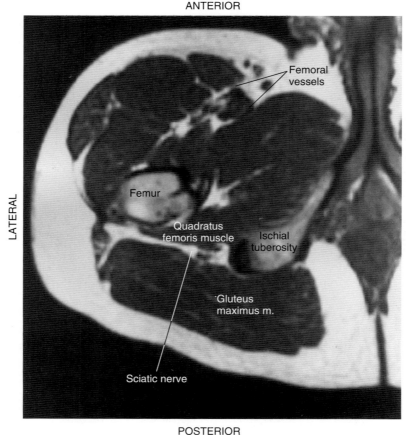

POSTERIOR

Figure 13-7. Magnetic resonance image (cross-sectional) at level of anterior sciatic nerve.

semitendinosus (posteromedial), and the adductor magnus (anterior). If it is difficult to identify the sciatic nerve in the subgluteal region, it can be identified in the midthigh region by tracing the nerve from the popliteal region (Fig. 13-8).

TECHNIQUE

The prone position is the preferred one to provide better imaging for the in-plane technique from the lateral aspect of the thigh. If the patient is not able to lie in the prone position, the lateral position with the hips and the knees flexed will be utilized. The curved array ultrasound probe is placed at the level of the inferior border of the gluteus maximus to visualize the sciatic nerve in the short axis as a hyperechoic structure between the greater trochanter and ischial tuberosity. The in-plane approach will be used with the needle direction from medial to lateral in the prone position; however, in the lateral position, the needle direction should preferably be from posterior to anterior. The use of nerve stimulation in addition to the ultrasound is preferred in this technique to confirm the nerve identification, especially in obese patients. The medium-frequency, linear, 50-mm footprint is used for the midthigh approach block for the sciatic nerve block. The continuous block can be performed using a catheter threaded through a Touhy needle. The catheter tip position can be identified by injecting local anesthetic and observing its distribution using ultrasound or by injecting 1 mL of air, which appears as a hyperechogenic artifact (Figs 13-9, 13-10 and 13-11).

CLINICAL PEARLS

- Continuous sciatic block is very helpful for managing phantom limb pain after either below-knee or above-knee amputations.
- Single-shot sciatic block using 0.1% ropivacaine is very helpful to manage posterior knee pain after total knee arthroplasty without affecting the motor power and/or neurological examination of the lower limb after total knee arthroplasty.
- Combined femoral and sciatic blocks are quite sufficient for lower limb procedures, especially in high-risk patients in whom general and/or neuroaxial anesthesia can disturb their hemodynamic stability, such as very tight aortic stenosis or heart failure.

KEY POINTS

- Subgluteal and midthigh approaches are the most commonly used techniques for sciatic nerve block using ultrasound.
- Short axis with in-plane approach with lateral to medial needle direction is the preferred ultrasound technique for both subgluteal and midthigh sciatic blocks.
- Using a nerve stimulator is very helpful to confirm the identification of the sciatic nerve in the subgluteal approach, especially in obese patients.

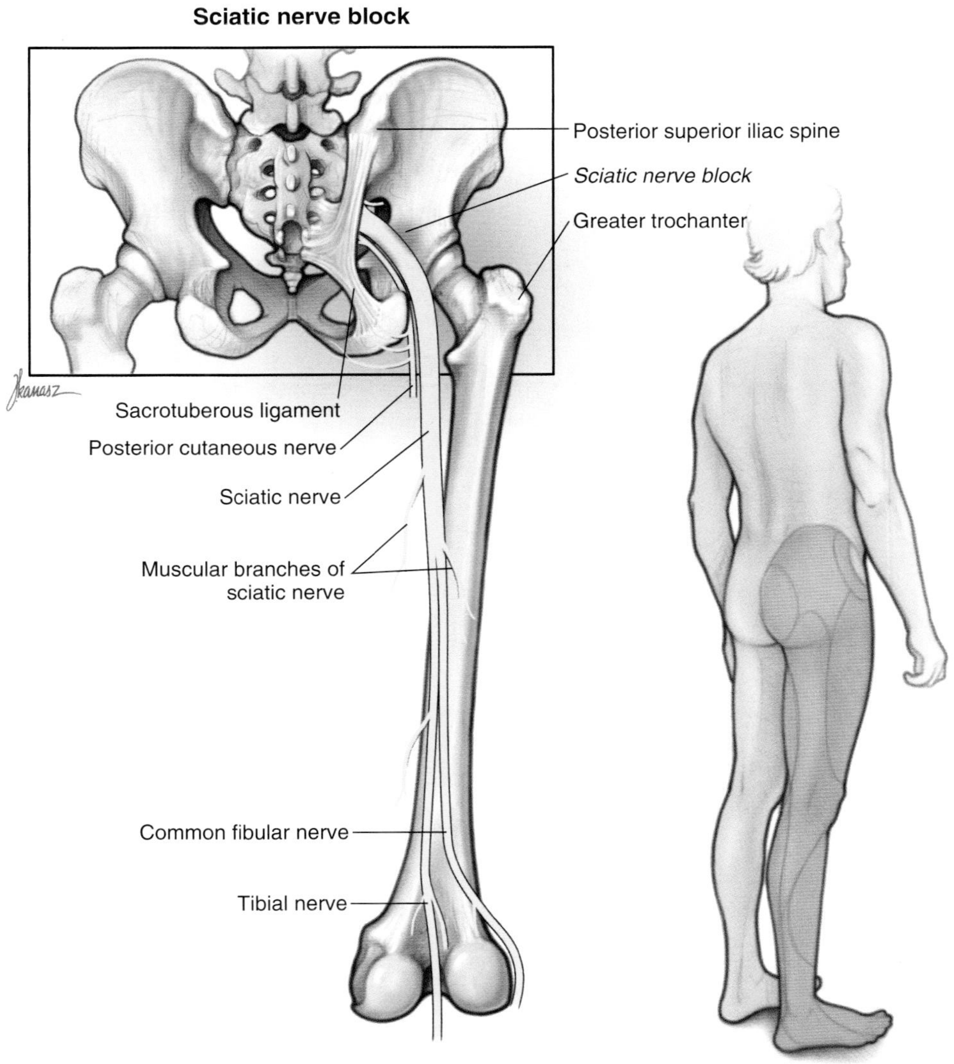

Sciatic nerve block

Posterior superior iliac spine

Sciatic nerve block

Greater trochanter

Sacrotuberous ligament

Posterior cutaneous nerve

Sciatic nerve

Muscular branches of
sciatic nerve

Common fibular nerve

Tibial nerve

Figure 13-8. Anatomy of the subgluteal sciatic nerve block.

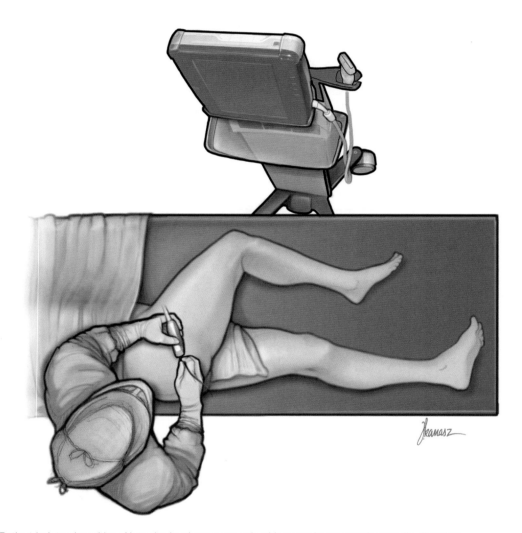

Figure 13-9. Patient in lateral position. Note the in-plane approach with posterior to anterior needle direction.

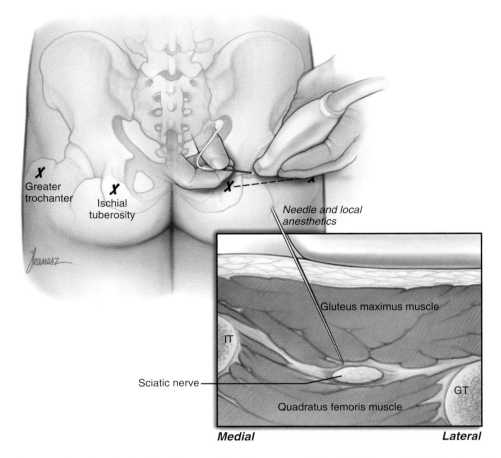

Figure 13-10. In-plane technique for subgluteal sciatic nerve block in prone position. Note the medial to lateral needle direction

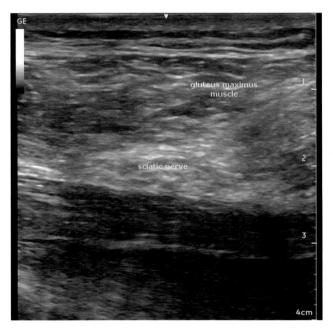

Figure 13-11. Ultrasound still of sciatic nerve block.

Femoral Block 14

Ehab Farag and David L. Brown

14

PERSPECTIVE

This block is useful for surgical procedures carried out on the anterior thigh, both superficial and deep. It is most frequently combined with other lower extremity peripheral blocks to provide anesthesia for operations on the lower leg and foot. As an analgesic technique, it is used for femoral fracture analgesia or for prolonged continuous catheter analgesia after surgery on the knee or femur.

Patient Selection. Because the patient is supine when this block is carried out, virtually any patient undergoing a surgical procedure of the lower extremity is a candidate. Because elicitation of paresthesia is not necessary to carry out femoral block, even anesthetized patients are candidates.

Pharmacologic Choice. As with all lower extremity blocks, a decision must be made about the extent of sensory and motor blockade desired. If motor blockade is necessary, higher concentrations of local anesthetic are needed. As with concerns about local anesthetic use in the sciatic block, the desire for motor blockade must be balanced against the volume of local anesthetic necessary if femoral, sciatic, lateral femoral cutaneous, and obturator blocks are combined. Approximately 20 mL of local anesthetic should be adequate to produce femoral block. With continuous catheter techniques used for postoperative analgesia, 0.25% bupivacaine or 0.2% ropivacaine may be used, and even lower concentrations of these drugs may be useful after a trial. With this technique, a rate of 8 to 10 mL per hour usually suffices.

TRADITIONAL BLOCK TECHNIQUE

PLACEMENT

Anatomy. The femoral nerve travels through the pelvis in the groove between the psoas and the iliacus muscles, as illustrated in Figure 14-1. It emerges beneath the inguinal ligament, posterolateral to the femoral vessels, as illustrated in Figure 14-2. It frequently divides into its branches at or above the level of the inguinal ligament.

Position. The patient is in a supine position, and the anesthesiologist should stand at the patient's side to allow easy palpation of the femoral artery.

Needle Puncture. A line is drawn connecting the antero-superior iliac spine and the pubic tubercle, as illustrated in Figure 14-3. The femoral artery is palpated on this line, and a 22-gauge, 4-cm needle is inserted, as illustrated in Figure 14-4. The initial insertion should abut the femoral artery in a perpendicular fashion, as shown in Figure 14-5 (*position 1*); a "wall" of local anesthetic is developed by redirecting the needle in a fanlike manner in progressive steps to *position 2*. (Ultrasonography highlights that the nerve is deep to the fascia iliaca, something difficult to appreciate without imaging guidance.) Approximately 20 mL of local anesthetic is injected incrementally in this fashion. It may also be useful to displace the needle entry site laterally 1 cm, direct the needle tip to lie immediately posterior to the femoral artery, and then inject an additional 2 to 5 mL of drug. This allows block of those fibers that may be in a more posterior relationship to the femoral artery. Elicitation of paresthesia is variable with this block; however, if one does occur, the mediolateral injection should still be carried out because the nerve often divides into branches cephalad to the inguinal ligament.

When using a continuous catheter technique, either stimulating catheter block kits or traditional epidural needles and matched catheters may be used in adults (Fig. 14-6). In the latter situation, the epidural needle is positioned either with the assistance of a nerve stimulator or with paresthesia elicitation as an endpoint. After the needle is positioned, 20 mL of preservative-free normal saline solution is injected through the needle, and then the appropriate-size catheter is inserted approximately 10 cm past the needle tip. Once the catheter has been secured with a plastic occlusive dressing, the initial bolus injection of drug is carried out and the infusion is started.

POTENTIAL PROBLEMS

Patients with peripheral vascular disease often require unilateral lower extremity block; thus a number of patients with prosthetic femoral arteries may be suitable candidates for this block. If lower extremity peripheral regional block has been chosen in a patient who has recently undergone placement of a prosthetic femoral artery, efforts should be made to avoid the prosthesis.

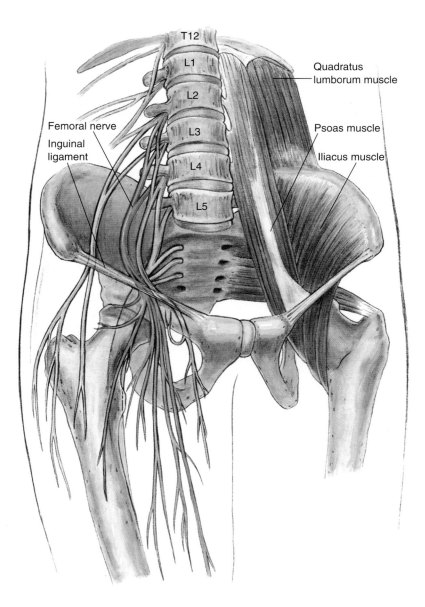

Figure 14-1. Femoral nerve anatomy: anterior oblique view.

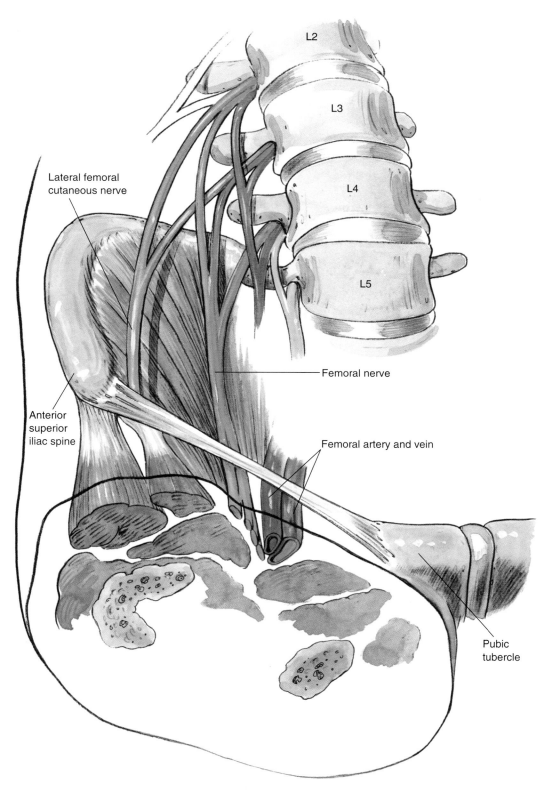

Figure 14-2. Femoral nerve anatomy: at inguinal ligament.

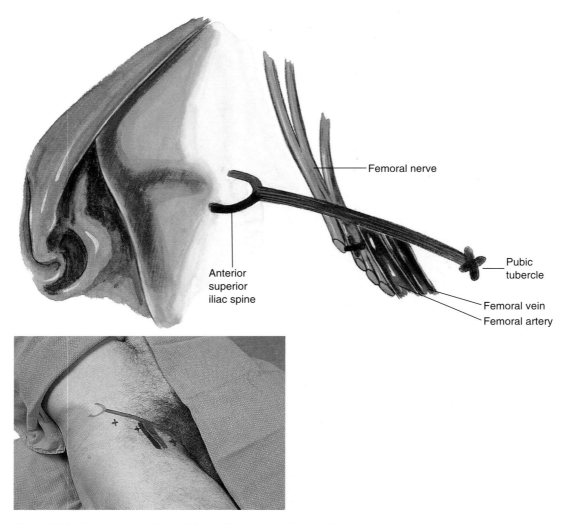

Femoral nerve

Pubic
tubercle

Femoral vein

Femoral artery

Anterior
superior
iliac spine

Figure 14-3. Femoral nerve block: skin markings for needle puncture.

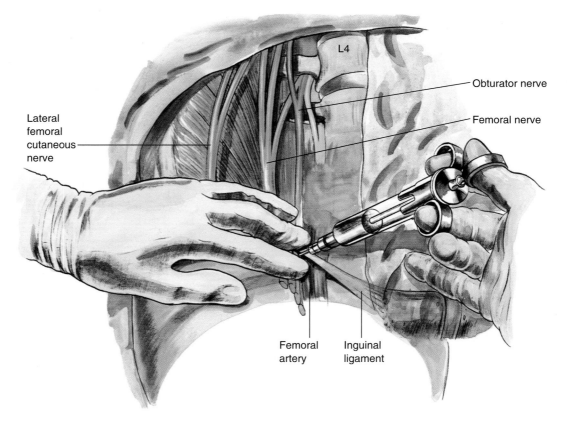

L4

Obturator nerve

Femoral nerve

Lateral
femoral
cutaneous
nerve

Femoral
artery

Inguinal
ligament

Figure 14-4. Femoral nerve block: needle puncture.

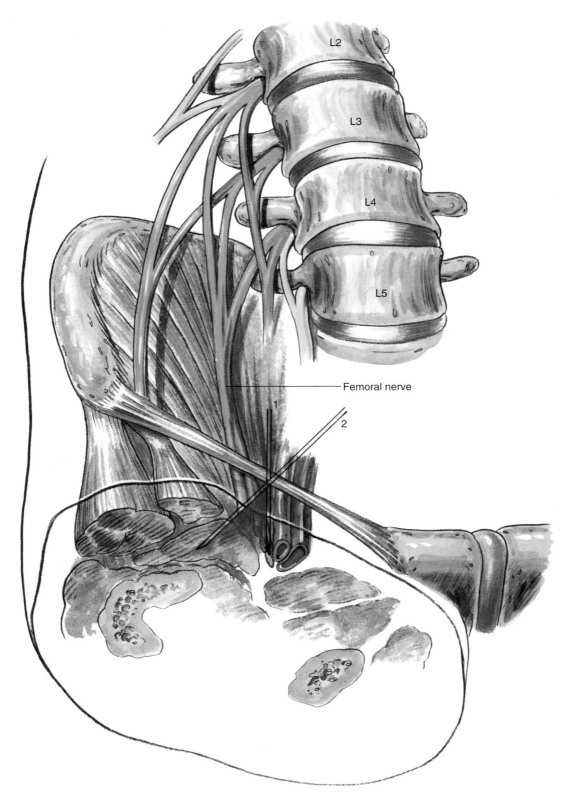

Figure 14-5. Femoral nerve block: local anesthetic injection.

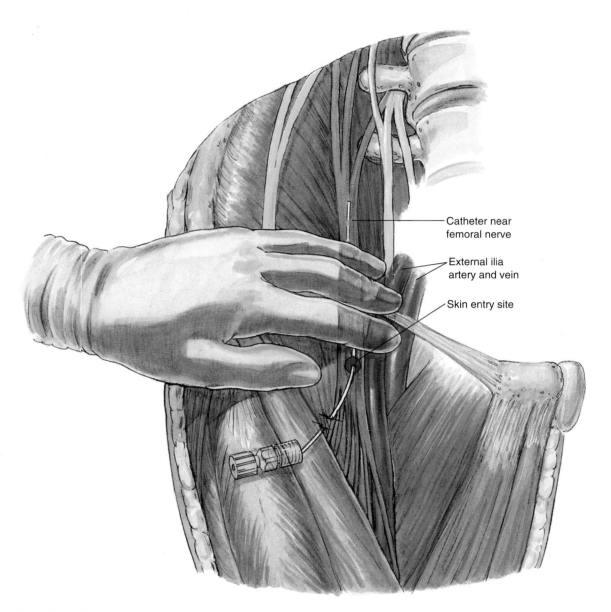

Figure 14-6. Femoral nerve block: use of continuous catheter.

Catheter near
femoral nerve

External ilia
artery and vein

Skin entry site

PEARLS

Because a traditional block is actually a field block, enough "soak time" must be allowed to produce satisfactory anesthesia. When sciatic and femoral blocks are combined, it is often helpful to place the femoral block before the sciatic block, thus allowing extra soak time. Increasingly, patients undergoing surgery on the knee are effectively being offered femoral block as part of the postoperative analgesia regimen. Most often, this is provided as a single-shot technique; however, some practitioners provide the analgesia using a continuous catheter method.

ULTRASONOGRAPHY-GUIDED TECHNIQUE

SONOANATOMY

The femoral nerve is the largest branch of the lumbar plexus and usually consists of the roots of segments L2 to L4. It runs distally to the inguinal region, typically positioned in the groove formed by the iliac and lateral psoas muscles posteriorly and covered by the iliac fascia anteriorly. At this level the iliac fascia, along with the internal aspect of the iliopsoas, thickens to form the iliopectineal band that separates the femoral vein and femoral artery from the nerve. The femoral nerve is often visualized distal to the inguinal ligament within a triangular hyperechoic region lateral to the femoral artery and superficial to the iliopsoas muscle. The nerve may be thin and flat in this region as it may divide into terminal branches. However, it can be visualized as a biconvex or oval hyperechoic structure. Therefore from superficial to deep, the fascia lata is first encountered, then the fascia iliaca, as a hyperechoic line (Figs 14-7 to 14-9).

INDICATIONS

- Analgesia for fractured neck/shaft of femur.
- Analgesia after hip joint replacement.

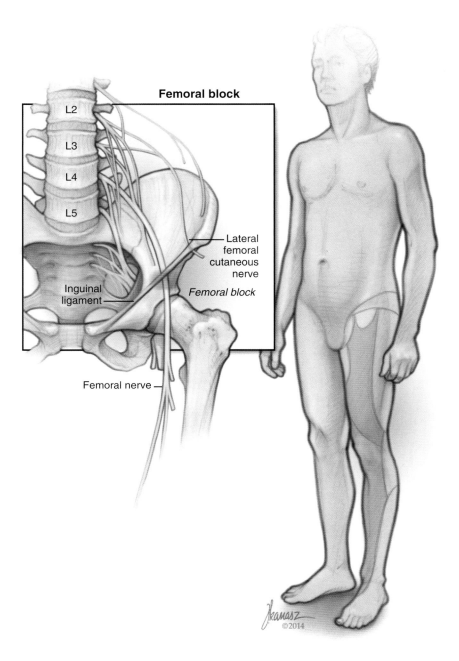

Femoral block

L2

L3

L4

L5

Lateral femoral cutaneous nerve

Femoral block

Inguinal ligament

Femoral nerve

©2014

Figure 14-7. Anatomy of femoral nerve.

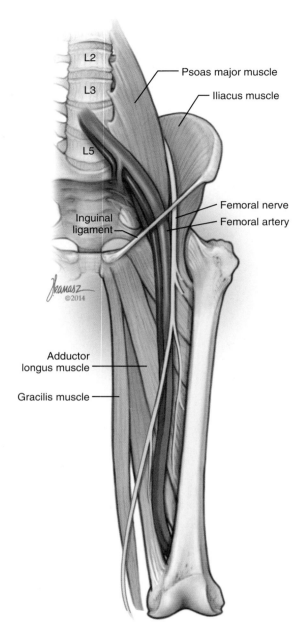

Figure 14-8. Anatomy of femoral nerve.

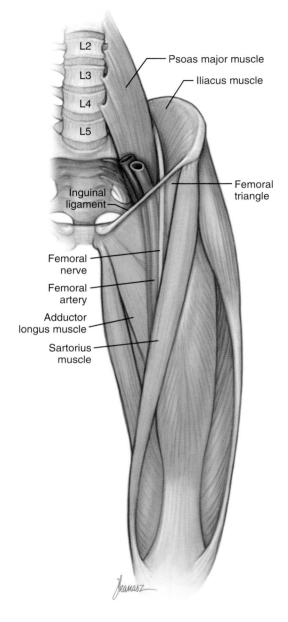

Figure 14-9. Anatomy of femoral nerve.

- Analgesia after knee joint surgeries, such as total knee arthroplasty or anterior cruciate ligament repair.
- It can be combined with popliteal block to provide anesthesia for lower leg or foot surgeries.

TECHNIQUE

While the patient is in a supine position the ultrasound probe will be parallel to the inguinal crease to obtain the short axis of the nerve within the triangular hypoechoic region. The in-plane technique is most commonly used for this block. In this technique the needle will be inserted in-plane and advanced from lateral to medial in the transverse plane of the image. After piercing the fascia iliaca, inject 2 to 3 mL of saline to ensure the needle tip is beneath the fascia and the saline is spreading lateral to the femoral

artery and in the vicinity of the nerve before injecting the local anesthetics (Figs 14-10 to 14-15).

KEY POINTS

- High-resolution linear ultrasound (30- to 40-mm footprint) is preferred for the femoral nerve block.
- In some patients, the femoral nerve at the inguinal crease is already branched into superficial and deep divisions along with femoral artery division into superficial and profunda femoris branches. Therefore it is better to scan proximally to place the probe at the common femoral artery in order to ensure blocking the main trunk of the femoral nerve.

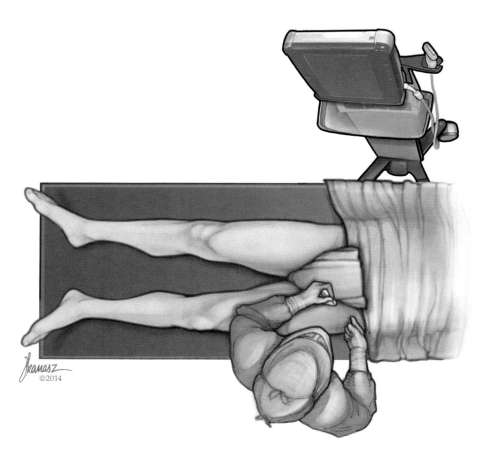

Figure 14-10. Position of the patient and ultrasound machine.

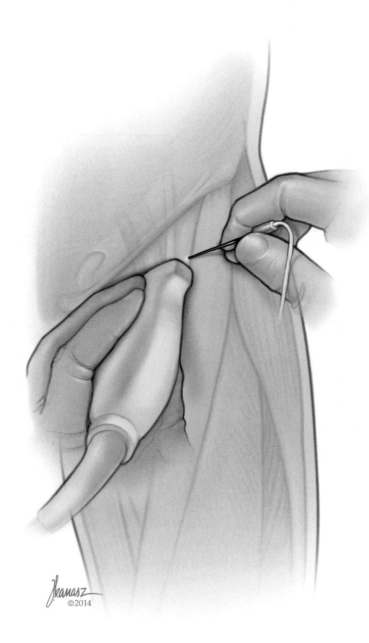

Figure 14-11. Note the needle in-plane and the needle direction from lateral to medial.

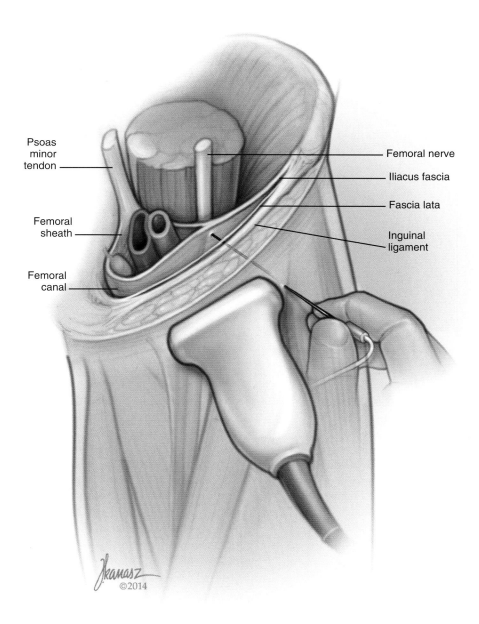

Psoas
minor
tendon

Femoral nerve

Iliacus fascia

Fascia lata

Femoral
sheath

Inguinal
ligament

Femoral
canal

Figure 14-12. The needle should pierce the iliacus fascia in order to have a successful block.

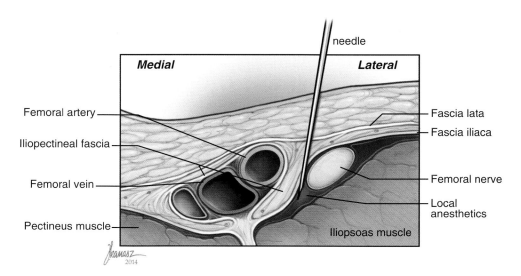

Medial

Lateral

needle

Femoral artery

Fascia lata

Fascia iliaca

Iliopectineal fascia

Femoral vein

Femoral nerve

Pectineus muscle

Local
anesthetics

Iliopsoas muscle

Figure 14-13. The needle and the local anesthetics are beneath the fascia iliaca.

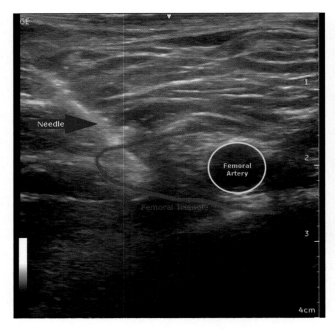

Figure 14-14. Ultrasound still of femoral block procedure.

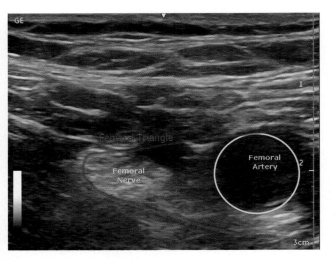

Figure 14-15. Ultrasound still of anatomy of femoral block.

- For catheter insertion, the Tuohy needle is used. The proper position of the tip of the needle beneath the fascia iliaca can be identified by injecting 2 to 3 mL of saline, which appears laterally to the artery and in the vicinity of the nerve. Then the catheter will be inserted 3 to 4 cm beyond the tip of the needle. For further confirmation of the location of the catheter tip, a small volume of air, which appears as a hyperechoic artifact, can be injected through the catheter.

PEARLS

- The femoral nerve can be confused in the short-axis view with inguinal lymph nodes, which also appear hyperechoic.

- If you are not able to identify the femoral nerve, injection in the hyperechoic triangle lateral to the femoral artery will suffice to produce successful block.
- After inserting the catheter through the Tuohy needle, keep the needle in situ and inject through the catheter 2 to 3 mL of saline or local anesthetic solution to identify the position of the catheter tip. This technique will help modify the catheter position by readjusting the needle and ensuring the catheter position in the vicinity of the nerve.
- The concentration of local anesthetic used in this block usually depends on the aim. For analgesic purposes, ropivacaine 0.1% to 0.2% is quite sufficient; however, ropivacaine 0.5% is ideal for anesthetic purposes.

Lateral Femoral Cutaneous Block

15

David L. Brown

Lateral Femoral Cutaneous Block 15

PERSPECTIVE

When this block is combined with other lower extremity blocks, it allows lower leg procedures to be carried out with fewer complaints of tourniquet pain. It also allows superficial procedures on the lateral thigh, including skin graft harvesting. In a pain practice, it allows the diagnosis of myalgia paresthetica, which is a neuralgia involving the lateral femoral cutaneous nerve.

Patient Selection.   Like femoral nerve block, this block is carried out with the patient in the supine position. Thus almost any patient is a candidate for a lateral femoral cutaneous block.

Pharmacologic Choice.   The same concerns about local anesthetic choice that were outlined for sciatic and femoral blocks (*Chapters 13 and 14* respectively) apply to the lateral femoral cutaneous block. If multiple lower extremity blocks are being used, the operator must consider the total dosage being administered. Because the lateral femoral cutaneous nerve does not have motor components, a lower concentration of 10 to 15 mL of local anesthetic is effective.

PLACEMENT

Anatomy.   As shown in Figure 15-1, the lateral femoral cutaneous nerve emerges along the lateral border of the psoas muscle immediately caudad to the ilioinguinal nerve. It courses deep to the iliac fascia and anterior to the iliacus muscle to emerge from the fascia immediately inferior and medial to the anterosuperior iliac spine, as shown in Figure 15-2. After passing beneath the inguinal ligament, it crosses or passes through the origin of the sartorius muscle and travels beneath the fascia lata, dividing into anterior and posterior branches at variable distances below the inguinal ligament. The anterior branch supplies the skin over the anterolateral thigh, whereas the posterior branch supplies the skin over the lateral thigh from the greater trochanter to the midthigh.

Position.   The patient is in a supine position with the anesthesiologist at the patient's side, similar to the position taken for the femoral nerve block.

Needle Puncture.   The anterosuperior iliac spine is marked in the supine patient, and a 22-gauge, 4-cm needle is inserted at a site 2 cm medial and 2 cm caudal to the mark (see Fig. 15-2). As shown in Figure 15-3, the needle is advanced until a "pop" is felt as the needle passes through the fascia lata. Local anesthetic is then injected in a fanlike manner above and below the fascia lata, from medial (position 1) to lateral (position 2), as illustrated in Figure 15-3.

POTENTIAL PROBLEMS

The superficial nature of this block allows one to avoid most problems associated with regional blocks.

PEARLS

An adequate volume of local anesthetic should be used for this block (i.e., 10 to 15 mL). Because this is a sensory nerve, low concentrations of local anesthetics are useful, such as 0.5% to 0.75% mepivacaine or lidocaine, 0.25% bupivacaine, or 0.2% ropivacaine. By keeping the concentration lower for this portion of a three- or four-nerve lower extremity block, adequate volumes and concentrations of local anesthetic can be maintained for the sciatic and femoral nerves. If this block is used to provide anesthesia for a skin graft harvest site on the lateral thigh, it is useful to perform the block, wait until sensory changes develop, and then outline the peripheral innervation of the lateral femoral cutaneous nerve in that specific patient before any skin is harvested.

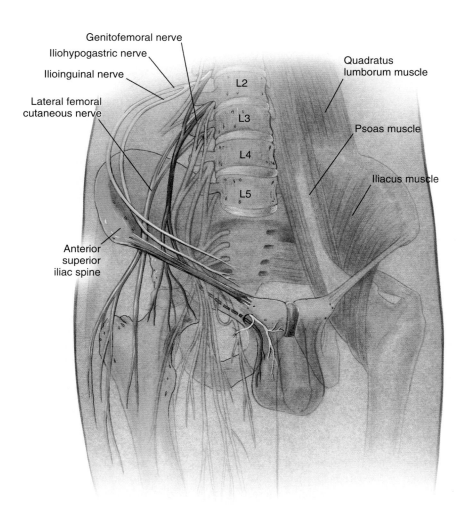

Figure 15-1. Lateral femoral cutaneous nerve: anatomy.

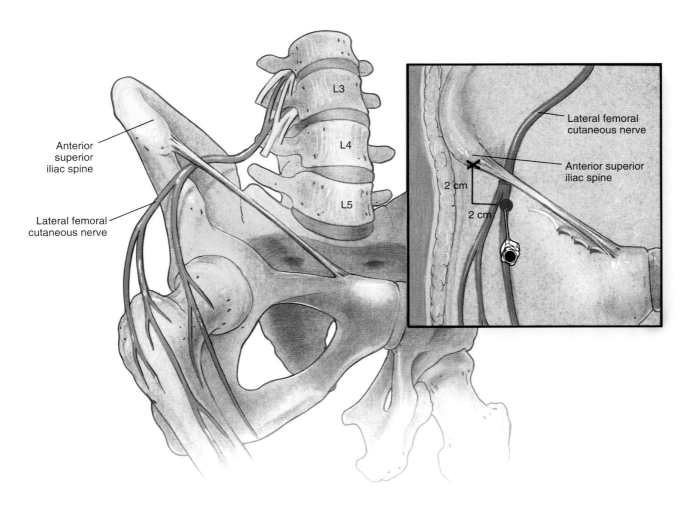

Figure 15-2. Lateral femoral cutaneous nerve block: technique.

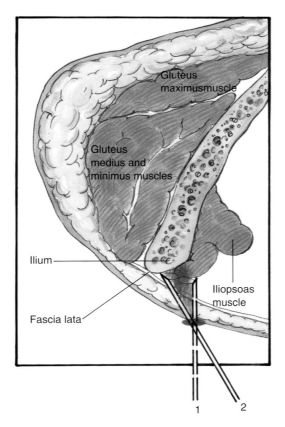

Figure 15-3. Lateral femoral cutaneous nerve block: cross-sectional technique for local anesthetic injection.

Obturator Block 16

Loran Mounir-Soliman and David L Brown

PERSPECTIVE

This block is most often combined with the sciatic, femoral, and lateral femoral cutaneous nerve blocks to allow surgical procedures on the lower extremities. If an operation on the knee using these peripheral blocks is planned, the obturator block is often essential. Another use for this block is in patients who have hip pain. It can be used diagnostically to help identify the cause of pain because obturator nerve block may provide considerable pain relief if the nerve's articular branch to the hip is involved in pain transmission. The block also may be useful in the evaluation of lower extremity spasticity or chronic pain syndromes.

Patient Selection. As with femoral and lateral femoral cutaneous nerve blocks, elicitation of paresthesias is not essential for obturator block. Any patient able to lie supine is a candidate.

Pharmacologic Choice. Motor blockade is most often not necessary for surgical patients receiving obturator nerve block; thus lower concentrations of local anesthetics are appropriate for obturator block: 0.75% to 1.0% lidocaine or mepivacaine, 0.25% bupivacaine, or 0.2% ropivacaine.

PLACEMENT

Anatomy. The obturator nerve emerges from the medial border of the psoas muscle at the pelvic brim and travels along the lateral aspect of the pelvis anterior to the obturator internus muscle and posterior to the iliac vessels and ureter. It enters the obturator canal cephalad and anterior to the obturator vessels, which are branches from the internal iliac vessels. In the obturator canal, the obturator nerve divides into anterior and posterior branches (Fig. 16-1). The anterior branch supplies the anterior adductor muscles and sends an articular branch to the hip joint and a cutaneous area on the medial aspect of the thigh. The posterior branch innervates the deep adductor muscles and sends an articular branch to the knee joint. In 10% of patients, an accessory obturator nerve may be found.

Position. The patient should be supine with the legs in a slightly abducted position. The genitalia should be protected from antiseptic solutions.

Needle Puncture. The pubic tubercle should be located and an "X" marked 1.5 cm caudad and 1.5 cm lateral to the tubercle (Fig. 16-2). The needle is inserted at this point, and at a depth of approximately 1.5 to 4 cm it contacts the horizontal ramus of the pubis. The needle is then withdrawn, redirected laterally in a horizontal plane, and inserted 2 to 3 cm deeper than the depth of the initial contact with bone. The needle tip now lies within the obturator canal (see Fig. 16-2). With the needle in this position, 10 to 15 mL of local anesthetic solution is injected while the needle is advanced and withdrawn slightly to ensure development of a "wall" of local anesthetic in the canal.

POTENTIAL PROBLEMS

The obturator canal is a vascular location; thus the potential exists for intravascular injection or hematoma formation, although these are more theoretical than clinical concerns.

PEARLS

This block, even in trained hands, has a variable success rate. Our experience suggests that one must rely on volume of anesthetic delivered rather than on absolute accuracy of needle position. Fortunately, use of an obturator block with the other lower extremity peripheral nerve blocks is not an absolute requirement for most surgical procedures. If this block is used diagnostically for patients with chronic pain, it is helpful to use a nerve stimulator to guide needle placement. This will minimize diagnostic confusion when pain relief is produced with a small volume of local anesthetic. Large-volume injections (approximately 15 mL) are performed with this block for many surgical procedures.

SONOANATOMY

The obturator nerve is formed from the anterior primary rami of the L2 to L4 roots as a branch of the lumbar plexus within the psoas muscle. The nerve exits the pelvis through the obturator foramen then typically divides into an anterior and posterior branch before entering the thigh. The anterior branch provides sensory supply to a variable area of the medial aspect of the thigh, as well as motor fibers to the adductor muscles. The posterior branch provides primarily motor fibers to the adductor muscles and occasional

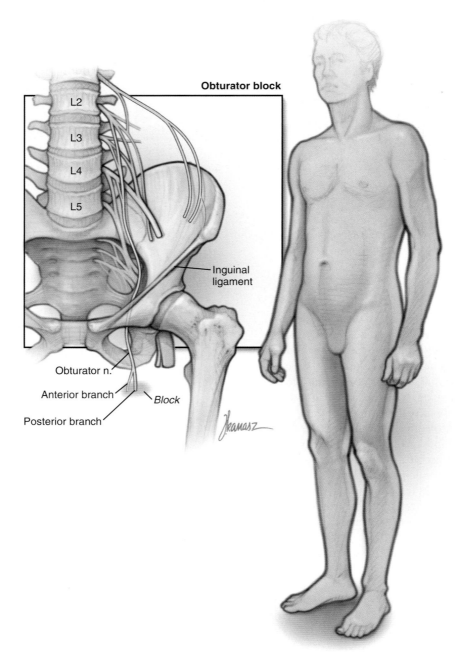

Obturator block

L2

L3

L4

L5

Inguinal ligament

Obturator n.

Anterior branch

Posterior branch

Block

Figure 16-1. Obturator nerve: functional anatomy.

articular sensation to the medial aspect of the knee joint. Notably, the articular branch of the hip joint provided by the obturator nerve usually originates from the main obturator nerve before division.

In the thigh, the two nerves run within the adductor compartment and medial to the femoral compartment. The anterior branch has a more superficial course between the fascia of the pectineus and adductor brevis muscles, whereas the posterior branch runs at a deeper level between the adductor brevis and adductor magnus muscles (Fig. 16-3).

INDICATIONS

- Avoid adductor muscle contractions during transurethral bladder surgery under spinal anesthesia

or when administration of muscle relaxants is undesirable.

- Provide complementary analgesia for major knee and thigh surgeries as a reliable alternative to 3-in-1 block, in conjunction with femoral and lateral femoral cutaneous nerve block. 3-in-1 block is a large volume local anesthetic injected near the femoral nerve.

TECHNIQUE

With the patient in the supine position, the thigh is slightly abducted and laterally rotated to better access the adductor compartment on the medial side of the thigh. The ultrasound probe is positioned in a transverse orientation to the

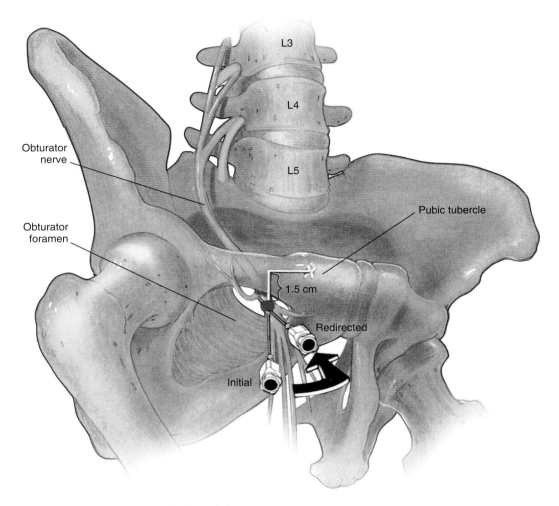

Figure 16-2. Obturator nerve block: technique.

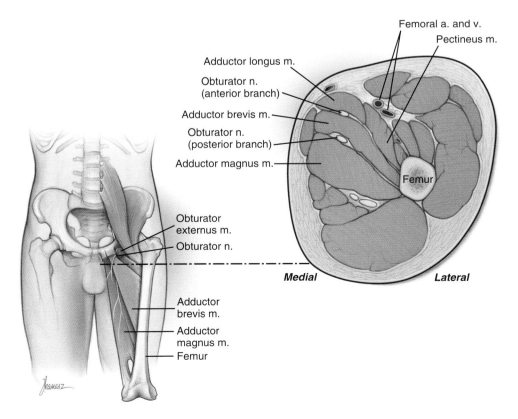

Figure 16-3. Obturator anatomy.

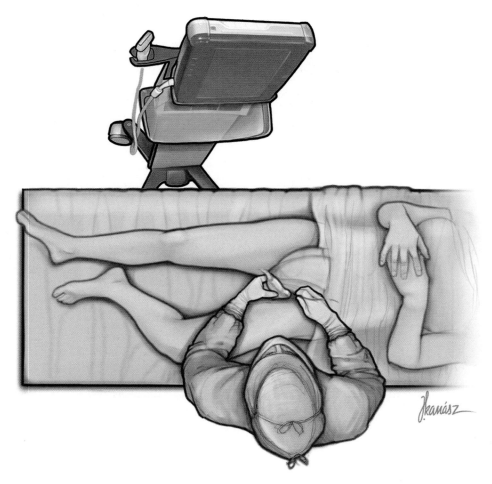

Figure 16-4. Obturator nerve block: position.

thigh (short-axis view to the adductor muscles) (Fig. 16-4). Usually, the pectineus muscle is medial to the femoral vessels slightly below the inguinal crease. Moving the probe farther medially to the pectineus muscle identifies the three adductor muscles aligned from superficial to deep: adductor longus, adductor brevis, and adductor magnus. The anterior and posterior branches of the obturator nerve are identified as hyperechoic and "white bands" superficial and deep to the adductor brevis muscle, respectively. Sometimes, the nerves are difficult to identify, especially in morbidly obese patients—the goal of the block is to install 10 to 15 mL of local anesthetic both superficially and deeply into the adductor brevis muscle. The posterior division of the obturator nerve can be blocked by installing the local anesthetic deeper to the adductor brevis in the fascial plane between the adductor brevis and adductor magnus muscles. The anterior branch is blocked superficially to the adductor brevis in the fascial plane between the pectineus or adductor longus and the adductor brevis muscle (known as the *interfascial injection technique*) (Fig. 16-5).

KEY POINTS

- The success of the block depends on the appropriate spread of local anesthetics in the appropriate fascial planes superficially and deeply to the adductor brevis muscle.

- Care should be taken to confirm the spread in the intermuscular fascial planes and not intramuscular.
- Change in adductor strength is the best assessment method for the block since the sensory distribution is variable.
- With a successful block, some residual adductor strength is secondary to the formal innervation to the pectineus, as well as some sciatic innervation to the adductor magnus.

PEARLS

- Both out-of-plane and in-plane approaches of the needle have been used successfully.
- When approaching the needle from the lateral side of the probe (in-plane technique), care must be taken to avoid vascular injury of the femoral or profunda femoris vessel or its branches.
- Separate injection of both branches in the thigh is mandatory because the obturator externus muscle separates both branches.
- Confirmation of the identified nerve-by-nerve stimulation inducing adduction is reassuring but not necessary for successful blocks.

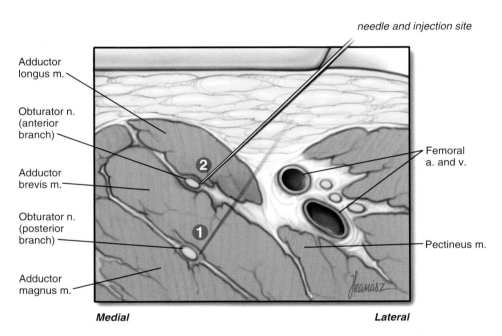

needle and injection site

Adductor longus m.

Obturator n. (anterior branch)

Adductor brevis m.

Obturator n. (posterior branch)

Adductor magnus m.

Femoral a. and v.

Pectineus m.

Medial   **Lateral**

Figure 16-5. Obturator ultrasound.

Popliteal and Saphenous Block 17

Maria Yared and David L. Brown

PERSPECTIVE

The nerves blocked in the popliteal fossa—the tibial and peroneal nerves—are extensions of the sciatic nerve. The principal use of this block is for foot and ankle surgery. The addition of a saphenous nerve block improves comfort because medial lower leg and ankle sensory blockade makes tourniquets and medial ankle surgery more comfortable.

Patient Selection.   To use the classic form of this block, the patient must be able to assume the prone position. Elicitation of paresthesia or a motor response is desirable but not essential; however, block effectiveness decreases without these endpoints.

Pharmacologic Choice.   The principal use of these blocks is to provide sensory analgesia; thus lower concentrations of a local anesthetic are practical in contrast to situations in which motor blockade is essential. Concentrations of 1% lidocaine, 1% mepivacaine, 0.25% to 0.5% bupivacaine, and 0.2% to 0.5% ropivacaine are effective.

TRADITIONAL BLOCK TECHNIQUE

PLACEMENT

Anatomy.   As illustrated in Figure 17-1, the cephalad popliteal fossa is defined by the semimembranosus and semitendinosus muscles medially and the biceps femoris muscle laterally. Its caudad extent is defined by the gastrocnemius muscles both medially and laterally. If this quadrilateral area is bisected, as shown in Figure 17-1, the area of interest to the anesthesiologist is the cephalolateral quadrant (hatched area). Here, both tibial and common peroneal nerve block is possible. The tibial nerve is the larger of these two nerves; it separates from the common peroneal nerve at the upper limit of the popliteal fossa and sometimes higher. The tibial nerve continues the straight course of the sciatic nerve and runs lengthwise through the popliteal fossa immediately under the popliteal fascia. Inferiorly, it passes between the heads of the gastrocnemius muscles. The common peroneal nerve follows the tendon of the biceps femoris muscle along the cephalolateral margin of the popliteal fossa, as illustrated in Figure 17-2. After the common peroneal nerve leaves the popliteal fossa, it travels around the head of the fibula and divides into the superficial peroneal and deep peroneal nerves.

Position.   The patient is placed in a prone position, and the anesthesiologist stands at the patient's side to allow palpation of the borders of the popliteal fossa.

Needle Puncture.   With the patient in the prone position, he or she is asked to flex the leg at the knee, which allows more accurate identification of the popliteal fossa. Once the popliteal fossa has been defined, it is divided into equal medial and lateral triangles, as shown in Figure 17-1. An "X" is placed 5 to 7 cm superior to the skin crease of the popliteal fossa and 1 cm lateral to the midline of the triangles, as shown in Figure 17-1. Through this site, a 22-gauge, 4- to 6-cm needle is advanced at an angle of 45 to 60 degrees to the skin while being directed anterosuperiorly (Fig. 17-3). Paresthesia or a motor response is sought; when obtained, 30 to 40 mL of local anesthetic is injected.

When a saphenous block is added for foot and ankle surgery, the patient's knee is bent at approximately a 45-degree angle and the medial aspect of the leg is exposed. Two primary techniques are used for saphenous block. A superficial ring of local anesthetic may be injected just distal to the medial surface of the tibial condyle. Often 5 to 10 mL of local anesthetic is needed. Conversely, a more proximal technique at the cross-sectional level of the superior border of the patella is possible (Fig. 17-4). In this case, a 22- to 25-gauge, 3- to 4-cm needle is inserted immediately deep to the sartorius muscle in the plane between the vastus medialis and the sartorius muscles, and 10 mL of local anesthetic is injected.

POTENTIAL PROBLEMS

Although vascular structures also occupy the popliteal fossa, intravascular injection should be infrequent if the usual precautions are taken. Hematoma formation is possible.

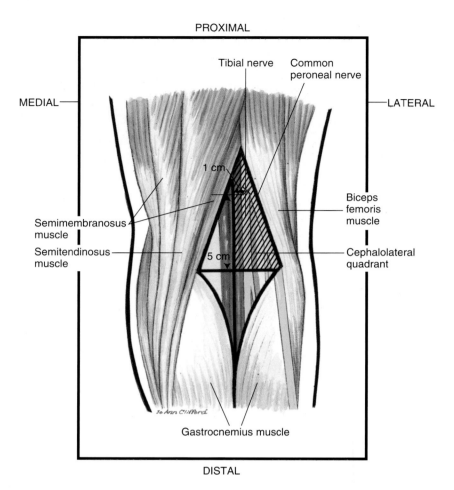

Figure 17-1. Popliteal fossa: surface anatomy and technique for popliteal block.

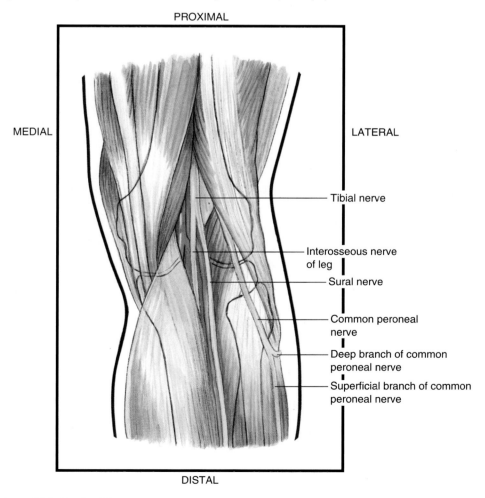

Figure 17-2. Popliteal fossa: neural anatomy.

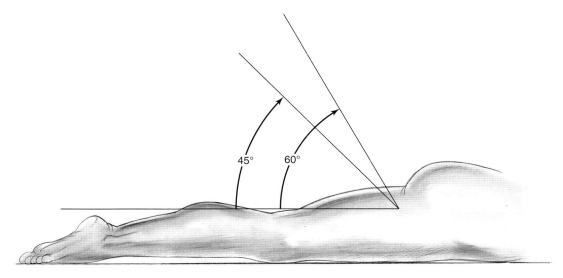

Figure 17-3. Popliteal fossa: needle angle technique for popliteal block.

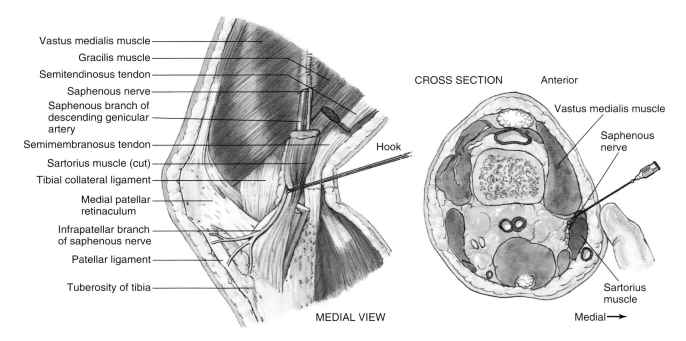

Vastus medialis muscle
Gracilis muscle
Semitendinosus tendon
Saphenous nerve
Saphenous branch of
descending genicular
artery
Semimembranosus tendon
Sartorius muscle (cut)
Tibial collateral ligament
Medial patellar
retinaculum
Infrapatellar branch
of saphenous nerve
Patellar ligament
Tuberosity of tibia

Hook

MEDIAL VIEW

CROSS SECTION   Anterior

Vastus medialis muscle

Saphenous
nerve

Sartorius
muscle

Medial →

Figure 17-4. Saphenous nerve block: anatomy and proximal technique.

ULTRASONOGRAPHY-GUIDED TECHNIQUE

SONOANATOMY

The sciatic nerve courses through the popliteal fossa where it is blocked. It is beneficial to use ultrasound for this block because the division of the sciatic nerve into posterior tibial and common peroneal nerves occurs at variable distances from the popliteal crease. The goal is to block the sciatic nerve before it divides and inject the local anesthetic within the epineurium. This allows for a more consistent blockade of both divisions and use of lower volumes of local anesthetic. The same anatomic land-marks that are used for the nerve stimulator–guided technique are also used for the ultrasound-guided block. However, with the ultrasound, the goal is to find the popliteal vessels first (Figs 17-5 and 17-6).

INDICATIONS

The sciatic nerve block at the popliteal fossa is done when the goal is to block the distal leg and foot (S2 to S4) for the following:

- Tibia or fibula repair
- Achilles tendon repair
- Calf tourniquet pain
- Ankle and toe surgeries

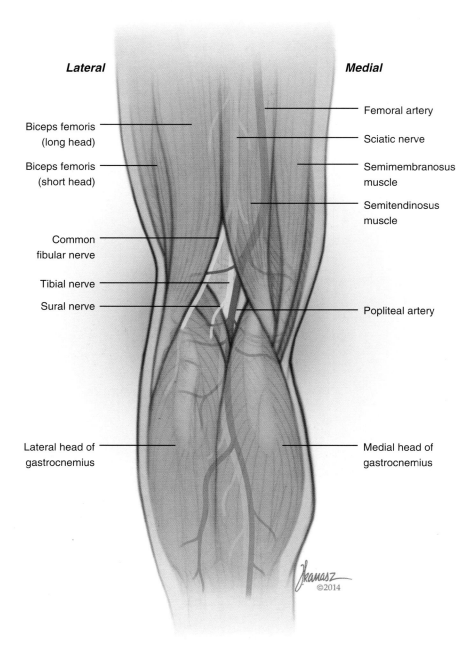

Figure 17-5. Anatomy of the popliteal fossa.

- Below-the-knee amputations
- Posterior knee pain

To have full surgical anesthesia of the area below the knee, one must also block the saphenous nerve, which is the terminal branch of the femoral nerve and innervates the skin of the medial portion of the lower leg.

TECHNIQUE

The popliteal block can be done with the patient in the prone, lateral decubitus, or supine position. We find the prone position to be easiest because it allows us to easily rest and stabilize the hand that is holding the ultrasound probe on the patient's leg once the desired image has been achieved. However, if the patient has a cast, external fixation device, or fracture making positioning difficult, then it may be preferable to place the patient lateral decubitus (operative site being superior and placing pillows between the knees) or supine (hip and knee are flexed with blankets serving as a footrest). Whichever approach you decide to use, the ultrasound image will be the same; it is the needle path that changes.

After identifying the popliteal fossa, place the linear ultrasound probe, which is 8 to 13 MHz, in the transverse position at the crease and ensure that the left side of the screen corresponds to the lateral side of the patient (where the biceps femoris muscle will lie). Then scan medially and laterally to find the popliteal artery, which tends to be about 4 cm deep. The popliteal vein, which is a compressible hypoechoic structure, can be lateral or deep to the artery. The posterior tibial nerve usually lies superficial and lateral

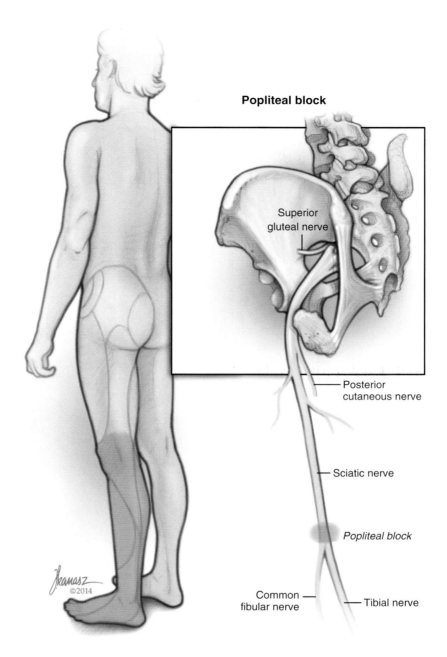

Figure 17-6. Anatomy of the popliteal block.

to the artery. The posterior tibial nerve will be a hyper-echoic oval with a honeycomb interior. Once the posterior tibial nerve is identified, slowly move the ultrasound probe cephalad. Adjust the probe as you scan to maintain a good view of the nerves. As you move cephalad, the popliteal artery tends to course deeper (more anteriorly) and may disappear from the ultrasound view. The common peroneal nerve, usually smaller in size than the tibial nerve, will emerge laterally and move medially to join the posterior tibial nerve until they are enveloped within a common epineural sheath. Their unity forms the sciatic nerve and usually occurs around 5 to 10 cm from the crease, but the distance varies.

We usually prefer the in-line approach when performing this block. For a single-shot nerve block, after the posterior tibial and common peroneal nerves join, we usually move the probe 1 to 2 cm more cephalad to ensure that the injected local anesthetic will surround both nerves. When

placing a continuous nerve catheter, we insert a 17-gauge Tuohy needle. Once the tip is located near the 6 o'clock position in relation to the nerve, we insert the catheter through the Tuohy needle and follow its trajectory by visualizing the catheter or tissue movement caused by the catheter in order to ensure that it does not migrate. Insert the catheter 5 cm beyond the tip of the Tuohy needle (Figs 17-7 through 17-12). Please refer to Chapter 18 for a review of the ultrasound-guided adductor canal block.

KEY POINTS

- Use a linear transducer probe (8 to 13 MHz), starting at a depth of 4 cm.
- For a single-shot nerve block, use a 21-gauge, 4-inch or 100-mm needle (stimulating or nonstimulating).

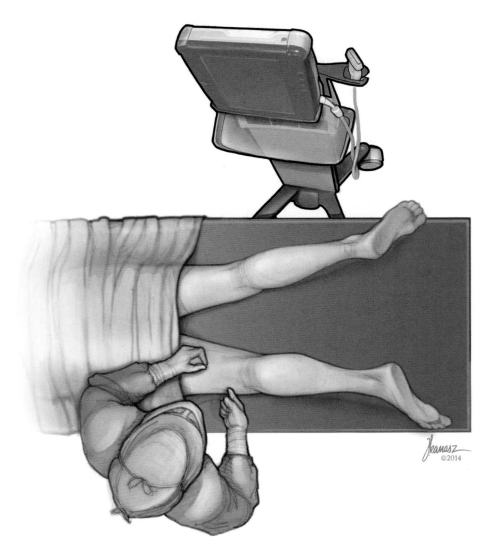

Figure 17-7. Patient position and ultrasound machine for the popliteal block in prone position.

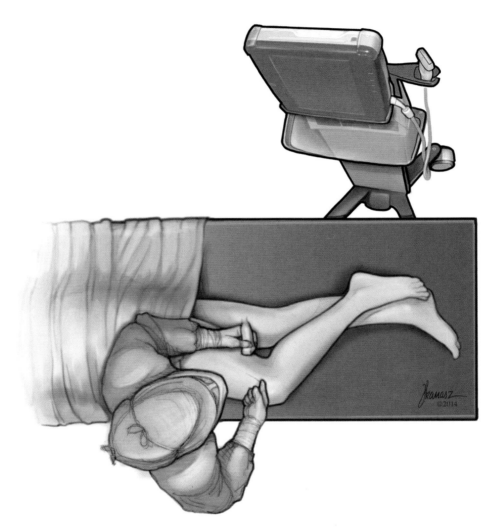

Figure 17-8. Patient position and ultrasound machine for the popliteal block in lateral position.

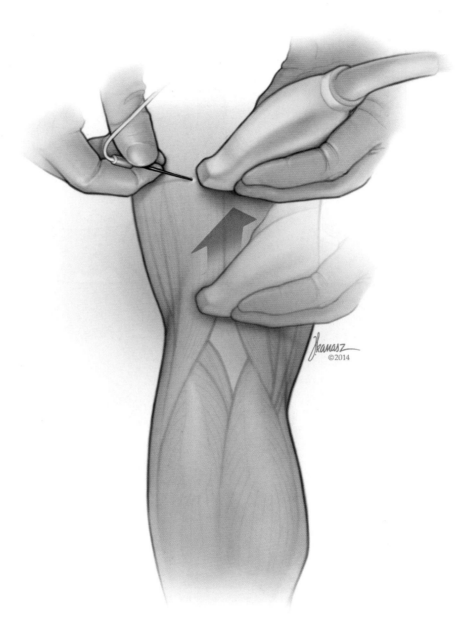

Figure 17-9. This illustration demonstrates the movement of the ultrasound probe as you move it cephalad from the popliteal crease. Within the popliteal fossa, the popliteal artery and the sciatic nerve's two main terminal branches (posterior tibial and common peroneal nerves) are visualized. One scans proximally/cephalad until the two branches unite together to form the sciatic nerve. Note that the ultrasound probe is in the transverse position; also note the in-plane technique, with the needle directed from lateral to medial, parallel to the ultrasound probe.

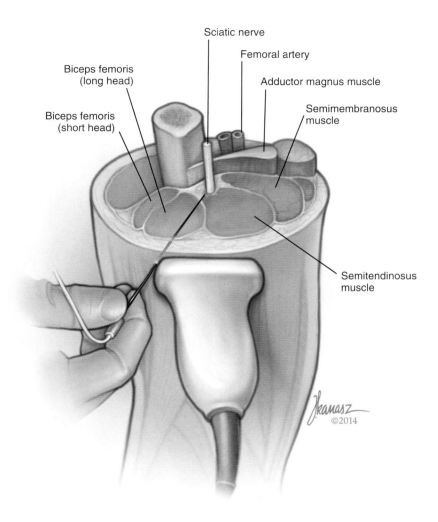

Figure 17-10. In-plane technique for the popliteal block with needle from lateral to medial.

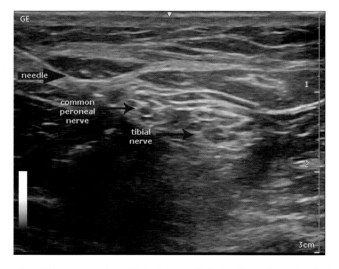

Figure 17-11. Ultrasound still of popliteal block procedure. Note the needle is in-plane, thus visualizing the entire needle shaft.

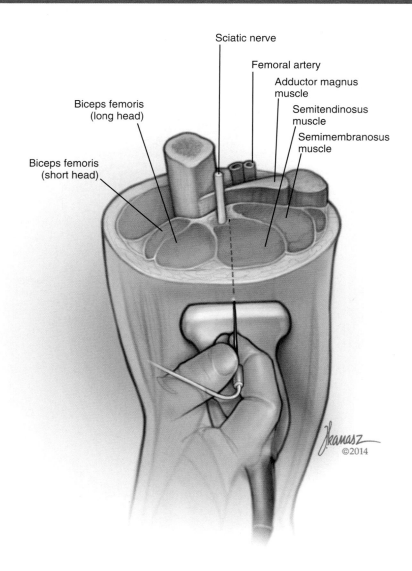

Figure 17-12. Out-of-plane technique for popliteal block.

- For local anesthetic solution in a single shot nerve block, bupivacaine or ropivacaine 0.5% 20 to 30 mL can be used.
- For a continuous nerve block, use a 17-gauge, 3.5-inch Tuohy needle with a 20-gauge catheter (stimulating or nonstimulating). You can inject ropivacaine 0.2% or bupivacaine 0.25% 20 mL and use a bag of solution containing ropivacaine 0.2% running at 8 mL per hour with a 12-mL bolus every 60 minutes.
- Confirm local anesthetic injection within the epineurium by tracking the local anesthetic spread proximally and distally from the site of injection around the nerves.
- If you are having trouble finding the artery, use color Doppler (artery pulsates and is hypoechoic).

PEARLS

- If you are having trouble getting a good image of the nerves, try tilting the ultrasound probe caudad to ensure that the ultrasound beams are hitting the nerves at a 90-degree angle.
- As you move the probe cephalad and the nerve tracks deeper, it may be more difficult to visualize the nerve and needle tip despite various attempts at probe manipulation. In this scenario, using the combined technique of ultrasound and nerve stimulation is helpful, or try hydrodissecting with dextrose.
- Muscle tendons may be mistaken for nerves. As you track the course of the tendon cephalad, it will disappear as it turns into muscle. Nerves will stay constant. Furthermore, asking the patient to dorsiflex the ankle will make the nerves rotate or move in relation to their surroundings.

Adductor Canal Block

Ehab Farag

SONOANATOMY

The saphenous nerve, a terminal branch of the posterior division of the femoral nerve, provides sensory innervation to the medial, anteromedial, and posteromedial aspects of the lower extremity from the distal thigh to the medial malleolus. It travels along the lateral aspect of the superficial femoral artery in the proximal artery within the adductor canal (Hunter's canal). It then crosses over the superficial femoral artery anteriorly just proximal of the lower end of the adductor magnus muscle and runs medially alongside the superficial femoral artery until emerging from the canal with the saphenous branch of the descending genicular artery. After leaving the adductor canal, the saphenous nerve divides into the infrapatellar branch, which provides a sensory branch to the peripatellar plexus of the knee, and the sartorial branch, which perforates the superficial fascia between the gracilis and sartorius muscles and emerges to lie in the subcutaneous tissue below the knee fold. It then descends along the medial tibial border with the saphenous vein giving cutaneous branches to the medial aspect of the leg, ankle, and the forefoot. The nerve to the vastus medialis is also a branch of the posterior division of the femoral nerve. It travels lateral to the superficial femoral artery within the adductor canal and sends multiple branches to the vastus medialis and supplies the anteromedial portion of the knee capsule.

The adductor canal is an aponeurotic tunnel in the middle third of the thigh. It courses between the anterior–medial compartment of the thigh and is covered by strong aponeurosis, the vastoadductor membrane. The canal contains the superficial femoral artery, vein, saphenous nerve, nerve to the vastus medialis, and the terminal nerve endings of the posterior branch of the obturator nerve.

The short-axis ultrasound image of the adductor canal at the midthigh usually shows the sartorius muscle and the saphenous nerve as a hyperechoic structure which lies lateral to the artery and anterior to the vein. The vastus medialis muscle lies laterally to the saphenous nerve, and the adductor longus and adductor magnus muscles are on its medial side (Figs 18-1 and 18-2).

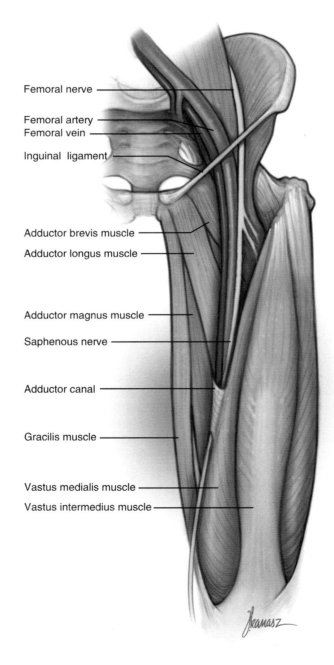

Figure 18-1. Anatomy of the adductor canal.

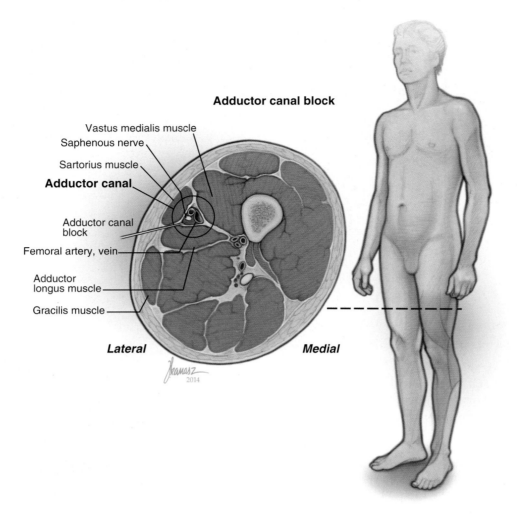

Figure 18-2. Cross-sectional anatomy of the adductor canal.

TECHNIQUE

At the midthigh level, approximately halfway between the superoanterior iliac spine and the patella, a high-frequency linear ultrasound transducer will be placed in the transverse cross-sectional view to obtain the short-axis view of the adductor canal and its contents. The femoral artery will be identified underneath the sartorius muscle with the vein just underneath the artery. The saphenous nerve usually appears at this position lateral to the artery as a hyperechoic structure. The block needle is usually inserted in plane from the lateral side of the transducer, through the sartorius muscle, with the tip of the needle placed lateral to the artery. After careful aspiration, 20 mL of local anesthetics will be injected lateral to the artery (Figs 18-3 through 18-6).

KEY POINTS

- A high-frequency transducer is preferred for this block.
- This approach is the most effective and easiest one for saphenous nerve block.

- This approach can be used in lieu of femoral nerve block after total knee arthroplasty to avoid quadriceps muscle weakness.
- This approach can be used as a block for the saphenous nerve after surgeries in the medial side of the foot and the ankle.

PEARLS

- This block is very useful as an alternative to the femoral nerve block after total knee arthroplasty to avoid quadriceps weakness. However, an injection of a high volume of local anesthetics in the adductor canal can spread as far as the anterior and posterior divisions of the femoral nerve to induce quadriceps weakness. Moreover, it has been demonstrated that there is no boundary between the apex of the femoral triangle and the adductor canal.
- The saphenous nerve block via the adductor canal approach can be successfully used to block the medial sides of the foot and the ankle after foot and

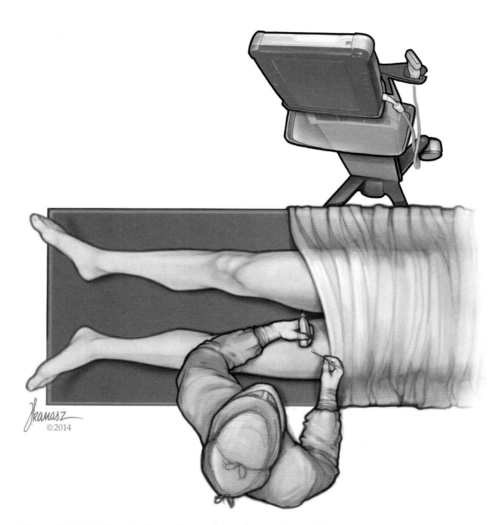

Figure 18-3. Position for the patient and the ultrasound machine.

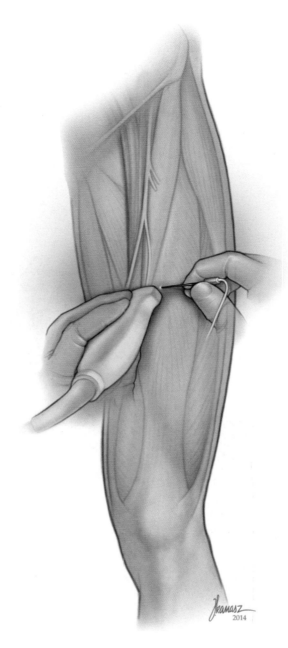

Figure 18-4. In-plane technique with needle direction from lateral to medial.

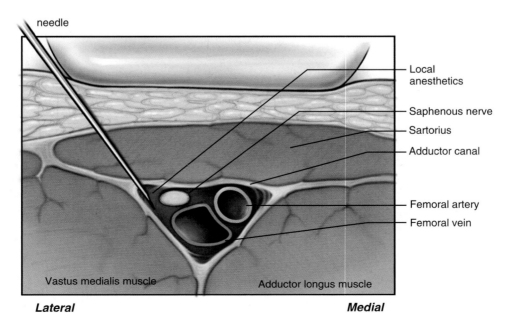

needle

Local anesthetics

Saphenous nerve

Sartorius

Adductor canal

Femoral artery

Femoral vein

Vastus medialis muscle

Adductor longus muscle

Lateral

Medial

Figure 18-5. Position of the needle with local anesthetic in the adductor canal. Note there should be separation of the artery from the fascia by the local anesthetic.

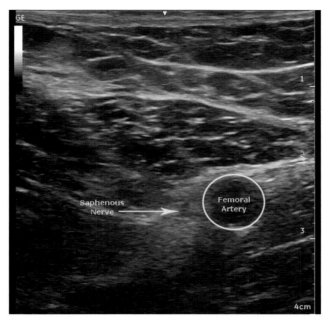

Figure 18-6. Ultrasound image of adductor canal.

ankle surgeries, either as a solo block or in addition to the popliteal nerve block.

- In morbidly obese patients, it can be difficult to identify the adductor canal and the femoral artery at the midthigh level. Therefore we usually identify the femoral artery at the inguinal crease and follow it distally into the adductor canal.

- The combination of vastoadductor membrane and vessel sheaths within the adductor canal can appear as hyperechoic structures resembling the saphenous nerve during ultrasound imaging. However, placing the needle tip through the vastoadductor membrane, within the adductor canal, may result in the successful localization of the saphenous nerve.

- For catheter insertion, with the Tuohy needle placed just lateral to the artery and the saphenous nerve, the catheter will be inserted 5 to 8 cm through the needle. To obtain the correct position of the catheter tip, the catheter will be slowly withdrawn during injection of 10 mL of normal saline under ultrasound guidance, until an expansion between the fascia and the vessels is visualized. Then the local anesthetics will be injected after careful aspiration through the catheter.

- Because the femoral artery lies above the vein in the adductor canal, I usually apply firm pressure with the ultrasound transducer to occlude the vein for better nerve visualization and to decrease the incidence of inadvertent vascular injection.

Ankle Block 19

David L. Brown

David L. Brown

PERSPECTIVE

This block is often used for surgical procedures carried out on the foot, especially for those not requiring high lower-leg tourniquet pressure.

Patient Selection. The ankle block is principally an infiltration block and does not require elicitation of paresthesia. Thus patient cooperation is not mandatory. Although the block is most efficient for the anesthesiologist if the patient can assume the prone as well as the supine position, this is not essential.

Pharmacologic Choice. Because motor blockade is not often needed for procedures carried out during ankle block, lower concentrations of local anesthetics may be used. Practical choices are 1% lidocaine, 1% mepivacaine, 0.25% to 0.5% bupivacaine, and 0.2% to 0.5% ropivacaine. Many physicians suggest that epinephrine not be used during ankle block, especially if injection is circumferential.

PLACEMENT

Anatomy. The peripheral nerves requiring block are derived from the sciatic nerve, with the exception of a terminal branch of the femoral nerve—the saphenous nerve. The saphenous nerve is the only branch of the femoral nerve below the knee; it courses superficially anterior to the medial malleolus, providing cutaneous innervation to an area of the medial ankle and foot. The remaining nerves requiring block at the ankle are terminal branches of the sciatic nerve—the common peroneal and tibial nerves. The tibial nerve divides into the posterior tibial and sural nerves, which provide cutaneous innervation as outlined in Figure 19-1. The common peroneal nerve divides into its terminal branches—the superficial and deep peroneal nerves—in the proximal portion of the lower leg. Their cutaneous innervation is also illustrated in Figure 19-1. Figure 19-2 identifies the locations of these nerves in a cross-sectional view at the level of ankle block.

Needle Puncture: General. It is often helpful (although not necessary) to have the patient in the prone position initially to facilitate block of the posterior tibial and sural nerves. Once these two nerves have been blocked, the patient assumes the supine position so that block of the saphenous and peroneal nerves can be carried out. The block can be performed with the patient in the supine position if the lower leg is placed on a padded support, and this position facilitates appropriate intravenous sedation.

Needle Puncture: Posterior Tibial Nerve. With the patient in the prone position, the ankle to be blocked is supported on a pillow. A 22-gauge, 4-cm needle is directed anteriorly at the cephalad border of the medial malleolus, just medial to the Achilles tendon, as shown in Figure 19-2. The needle is inserted near the posterior tibial artery, and if paresthesia is obtained, 3 to 5 mL of local anesthetic is injected. If paresthesia is not obtained, the needle is allowed to contact the medial malleolus, and 5 to 7 mL of local anesthetic is deposited near the posterior tibial artery.

Needle Puncture: Sural Nerve. The sural nerve is blocked with the patient positioned as for the posterior tibial nerve block. As illustrated in Figure 19-2, the sural nerve is blocked by inserting a 22-gauge, 4-cm needle anterolaterally immediately lateral to the Achilles tendon at the cephalad border of the lateral malleolus. If paresthesia is not obtained, the needle is allowed to contact the lateral malleolus, and 5 to 7 mL of local anesthetic is injected as the needle is withdrawn.

Needle Puncture: Deep Peroneal, Superficial Peroneal, and Saphenous Nerves. After the patient assumes the supine position, the anterior tibial artery pulsation is located at the superior level of the malleoli. A 22-gauge, 4-cm needle is advanced posteriorly and immediately lateral to this point (see Fig. 19-2). An alternative is to insert the needle between the tendons of the anterior tibial and the extensor hallucis longus muscles. Approximately 5 mL of local anesthetic is injected into this area. From this midline skin wheal, a 22-gauge, 8-cm needle is advanced subcutaneously laterally and medially to the malleoli, injecting 3 to 5 mL of local anesthetic in each direction. These lateral and medial approaches block the superficial peroneal and saphenous nerves, respectively.

POTENTIAL PROBLEMS

Although the ankle block can be painful if the patient is not adequately sedated, this should not be an issue because an alert patient is not essential for the block.

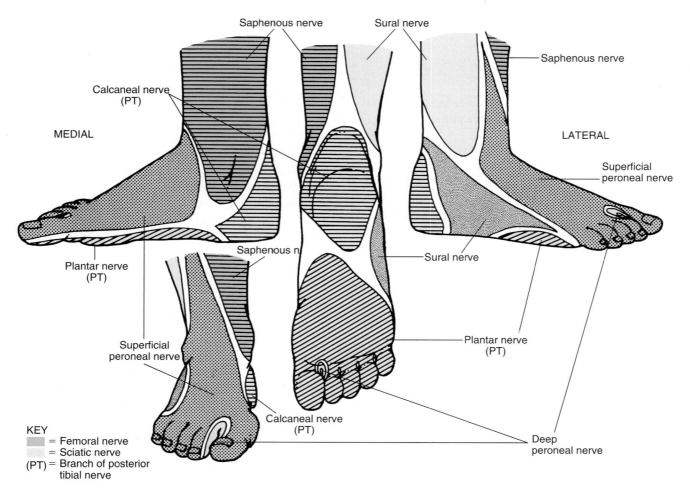

KEY
▦ = Femoral nerve
░ = Sciatic nerve
(PT) = Branch of posterior tibial nerve

Figure 19-1. Ankle block: peripheral innervation.

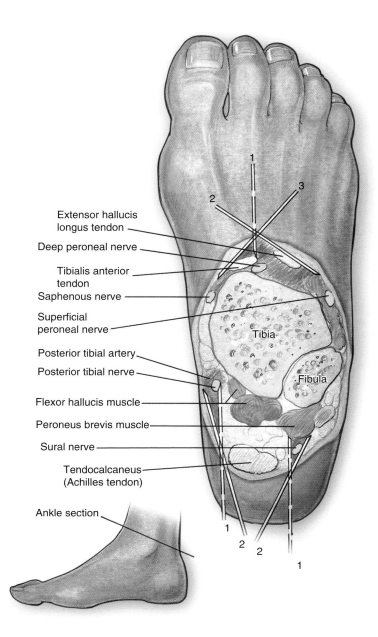

Extensor hallucis
longus tendon

Deep peroneal nerve

Tibialis anterior
tendon

Saphenous nerve

Superficial
peroneal nerve

Posterior tibial artery

Posterior tibial nerve

Flexor hallucis muscle

Peroneus brevis muscle

Sural nerve

Tendocalcaneus
(Achilles tendon)

Tibia

Fibula

Ankle section

Figure 19-2. Ankle block: cross-sectional anatomy and technique.

PEARLS

As mentioned, patients should be adequately sedated during this block because it is primarily a "volume" block. Although the medial and lateral malleoli approaches to an ankle block appear similar, there are differences. The sural nerve (lateral ankle) is found in a more superficial position relative to the malleolus than is the tibial nerve (medial ankle). The anesthesiologist should make sure to perform the sural portion of the block with this distinction in mind. The block should not be chosen if high tourniquet pressures are required to carry out the surgical procedure. Epinephrine-containing solutions should be avoided in circumferential injections of the ankle. Outpatient foot surgery patients often can walk with assistance after ankle block, which facilitates earlier discharge of these patients from the outpatient surgery center, while still experiencing effective postoperative analgesia.

SECTION IV
Head and Neck Blocks

Head and Neck Block Anatomy

20

David L. Brown

Use of regional anesthesia for head and neck surgery declined rapidly after general anesthesia and tracheal intubation became available and accepted. One reason for the decline is that small doses of local anesthetic can easily produce systemic toxicity. Nevertheless, in few other areas in the body can such small doses of local anesthetic provide such effective regional block. There are still circumstances in which head and neck block is useful. Many of these involve the diagnosis or treatment of pain syndromes. Also, many plastic surgical procedures on superficial structures can be managed easily with effective block of the nerves of the head and neck. One crucial aspect of head and neck block for anesthesiologists is expertise in airway anatomy and innervation. In some circumstances in an anesthetic practice, proper airway management, including airway blocks, can be lifesaving.

Sensory innervation of the face is provided by the trigeminal nerve. Three branches of the trigeminal—the ophthalmic, maxillary, and mandibular—provide innervation, as illustrated in Figure 20-1. The cutaneous innervation of the posterior head and neck is from the cervical nerves. The dorsal ramus of the second cervical nerve ends in the greater occipital nerve, which provides cutaneous innervation to the larger portion of the posterior scalp (see Fig. 20-1). The greater occipital nerve is a continuation of the medial branch of the dorsal ramus of the second cervical nerve and ascends from the cervical vertebrae to the muscles of the neck in company with the occipital artery. The greater occipital nerve becomes subcutaneous in its course with the occipital artery immediately lateral to the inion, slightly inferior to the superior nuchal line (Fig. 20-2). The ventral rami of cervical nerves II, III, and IV provide the majority of cutaneous innervation to the anterior and lateral portions of the neck, with cervical nerve II providing innervation to the scalp through both the lesser occipital and the posterior auricular nerves (see Fig. 20-1). The superficial cervical plexus is formed as cervical nerves II, III, and IV leave the vertebral transverse processes and follow a course in which they become subcutaneous at the midpoint of the posterior border of the sternocleidomastoid muscle (see Fig. 20-2). At this point, the superficial cervical plexus can be easily blocked by infiltration.

The trigeminal nerve is a mixed motor and sensory nerve, although the majority of it involves sensory innervation. The only motor fibers are the branches that supply the muscles of mastication through the mandibular nerve. The trigeminal nerve is organized in the cranium within the trigeminal ganglion (gasserian or semilunar ganglion). From this ganglion, the ophthalmic nerve exits from the cranium through the superior orbital fissure, the maxillary nerve through the foramen rotundum, and the mandibular nerve through the foramen ovale (Fig. 20-3). After leaving these foramina, the maxillary and mandibular nerves follow courses that place them in the immediate proximity of the lateral pterygoid plate. The pterygoid plate is an important landmark for effective maxillary or mandibular block (Fig. 20-4). The terminal branches of the trigeminal nerve end in the supraorbital, infraorbital, and mental nerves. These exit through bony foramina that occur on a line perpendicular through the pupil, as illustrated in Figure 20-5.

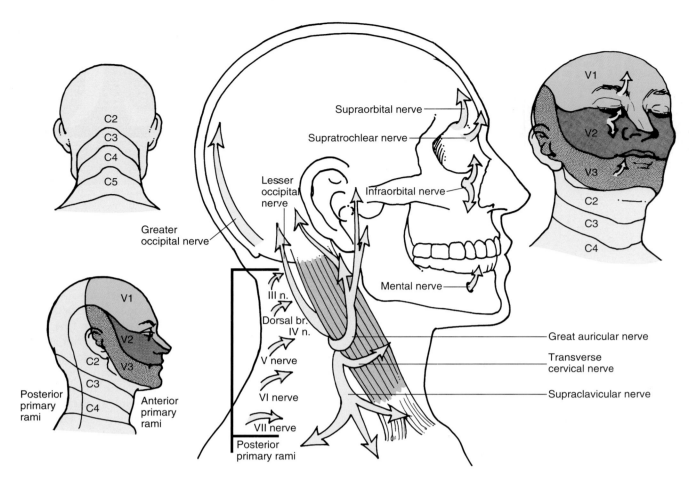

Figure 20-1. Head and neck anatomy: innervation.

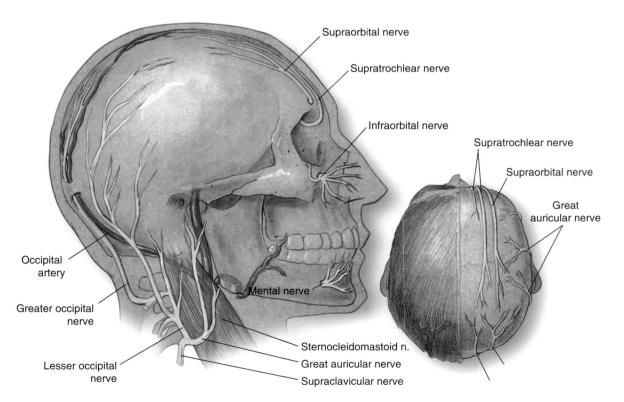

Figure 20-2. Head and neck anatomy: peripheral nerves.

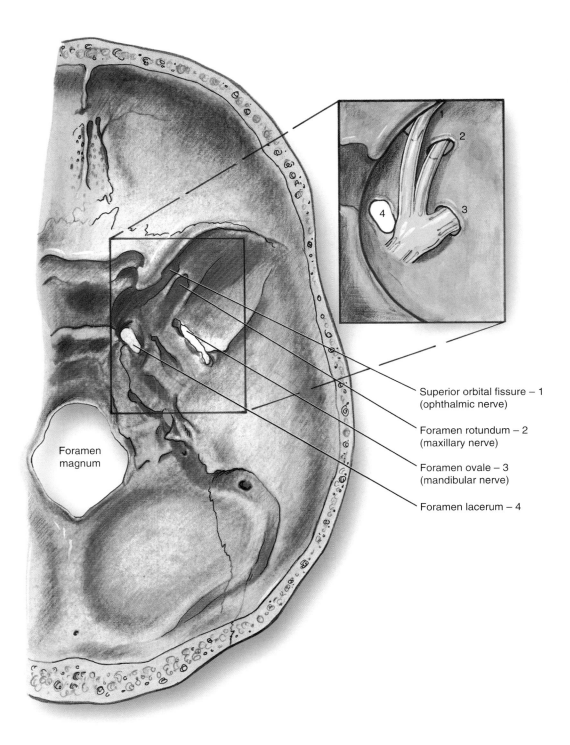

Figure 20-3. Intracranial anatomy: trigeminal nerve and branches.

Foramen
magnum

Superior orbital fissure – 1
(ophthalmic nerve)

Foramen rotundum – 2
(maxillary nerve)

Foramen ovale – 3
(mandibular nerve)

Foramen lacerum – 4

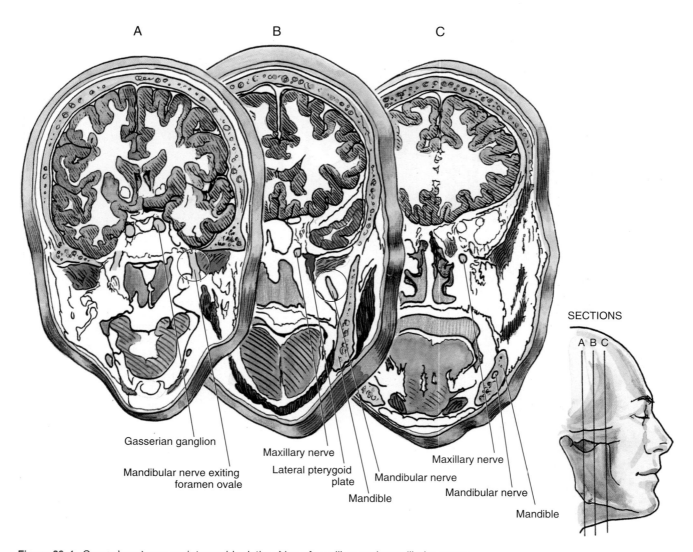

Figure 20-4. Coronal anatomy: peripterygoid relationships of maxillary and mandibular nerves.

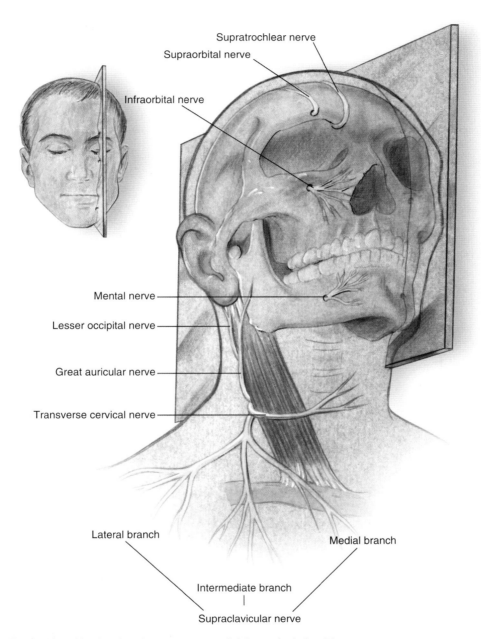

Figure 20-5. Head and neck anatomy: superficial neural relationships.

Occipital Block 21

David L. Brown

PERSPECTIVE

Occipital nerve block is most frequently used in the diagnosis and treatment of occipital neuralgia. It is also useful when combined with other head and neck blocks to provide scalp anesthesia when infiltration alone will not suffice.

Patient Selection. Most candidates for occipital nerve block will be experiencing symptoms consistent with occipital neuralgia. These patients are often at the end of a long and frustrating medical evaluation and thus may need a detailed explanation of what to expect during the block.

Pharmacologic Choice. This block requires only 3 to 5 mL of local anesthetic, so virtually any local anesthetic can be used.

PLACEMENT

Anatomy. The greater occipital nerve arises from the dorsal rami of the second cervical nerve and travels deep to the cervical musculature until it becomes subcutaneous slightly inferior to the superior nuchal line. It emerges on this line in association with the occipital artery, which is the most useful landmark for locating the greater occipital nerve (Fig. 21-1).

Position. The most effective patient position for the greater occipital block is the sitting position, with the chin flexed on the chest. A short, 25-gauge needle is inserted through the skin at the level of the superior nuchal line to develop a "wall" of local anesthetic surrounding the posterior occipital artery. The artery is commonly found approximately one-third of the distance between the external occipital protuberance and the mastoid process on the superior nuchal line. Injection of 3 to 5 mL of local anesthetic in this area will produce satisfactory anesthesia.

POTENTIAL PROBLEMS

The superficial nature of this block should make complications infrequent. However, it is important to ask the patient whether he or she has undergone any posterior cranial surgery because total spinal anesthesia has occurred after occipital nerve block in patients who have had such surgery.

PEARLS

To make this block effective for pain diagnosis and therapy, the anesthesiologist must make the expectations for the block clear to the patient before performing it. Often patients reach the anesthesiologist only after a long and arduous trial of alternative pain therapies; thus it is as important for the anesthesiologist to handle the psychosocial implications of the procedure as it is to discuss the technical features.

When a diagnostic block is planned, it is important to keep the dose of local anesthetic small to minimize confusion with relief of myofascial pain. Similarly, relief of ipsilateral retroorbital or temporal pain after an occipital block does not rule out the possibility of occipital neuralgia as the cause of the pain syndrome because pain relief is produced outside the typical sensory distribution of the occipital nerve. In some of these cases, due to brainstem and spinal cord interneuronal connections between the trigeminal nucleus and the second cervical spinal nerve, retroorbital pain is frequently relieved with a greater occipital nerve block.

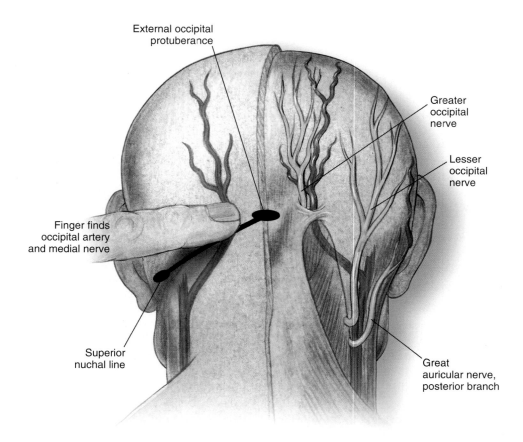

Figure 21-1. Occipital nerve block: anatomy and technique.

Trigeminal (Gasserian) Ganglion Block

David L. Brown

PERSPECTIVE

Although the trigeminal ganglion block can be used for surgical procedures involving the face, its principal use is as a diagnostic block before trigeminal neurolysis in patients with facial neuralgia. Even after the anesthesiologist successfully identifies the trigeminal nerve as the cause of facial pain, neurolysis is most often carried out today using thermocoagulation techniques rather than neurolytic solutions.

Patient Selection. Current practice patterns virtually guarantee that patients undergoing this block will be experiencing facial neuralgia. Patients with severe underlying cardiopulmonary disease who require more than minor facial surgery may be candidates for local anesthetic trigeminal ganglion blocks.

Pharmacologic Choice. Trigeminal ganglion block can be carried out with 1 to 3 mL of local anesthetic; thus almost any of the local anesthetics is an option.

PLACEMENT

Anatomy. The trigeminal ganglion is located intracranially and measures approximately 1 × 2 cm. In its intracranial location, it lies lateral to the internal carotid artery and cavernous sinus and slightly posterior and superior to the foramen ovale, through which the mandibular nerve leaves the cranium (Fig. 22-1). From the trigeminal ganglion, the fifth cranial nerve divides into its three principal divisions: the ophthalmic, maxillary, and mandibular nerves. These nerves provide sensation to the region of the eye and forehead, upper jaw (midface), and lower jaw, respectively (see Fig. 22-1). The mandibular division carries motor fibers to the muscles of mastication, but otherwise these nerves are wholly sensory. The trigeminal ganglion is partially contained within a reflection of dura mater—Meckel's cave. Figures 22-2 and 22-3 show that the foramen ovale is approximately in the horizontal plane of the zygoma, and in the frontal plane it is roughly at the level of the mandibular notch. The foramen ovale is slightly less than 1 cm in diameter and is situated immediately dorsolateral to the pterygoid process.

Position. Patients are placed in a supine position and asked to fix their gaze straight ahead, as if they were looking off into the distance. The anesthesiologist should be positioned at the patient's side, slightly below the level of the shoulder, so that by looking toward the patient's face, the perspective shown in Figure 22-4 is observed.

Needle Puncture. A skin wheal is raised immediately medial to the masseter muscle, which can be located by asking the patient to clench his or her teeth. (It will most often be located approximately 3 cm lateral to the corner of the mouth.) Through this site, as illustrated in Figure 22-5, a 22-gauge, 10-cm needle is inserted as shown at *position 1*, aided by fluoroscopic guidance. The plane of insertion should be in line with the pupil, as illustrated in Figure 22-4. This will allow the needle tip to contact the infratemporal surface of the greater wing of the sphenoid bone, immediately anterior to the foramen ovale. This occurs at a depth of 4.5 to 6 cm. Once the needle is firmly positioned against this infratemporal region, it is withdrawn and redirected in a stepwise manner until it enters the foramen ovale at a depth of approximately 5 to 7 cm, or 1 to 1.5 cm past the needle length required to contact the bone initially (*position 2*).

As the foramen is entered, a mandibular paresthesia is often elicited. By advancing the needle slightly, one may also elicit paresthesia in the distribution of the ophthalmic or maxillary nerves. These additional paresthesias should be sought in order to verify a periganglionic position of the needle tip. If the only paresthesia obtained is in the mandibular distribution, the needle tip may not have entered the foramen ovale, but may be inferior to it while it abuts the mandibular nerve.

Before injection of local anesthetic, careful aspiration of the needle should be performed to check for cerebrospinal fluid (CSF) because the ganglion's posterior two-thirds is enveloped in a reflection of dura—Meckel's cave. If trigeminal block is being undertaken diagnostically before neurolysis, 1 mL of local anesthetic should now be injected. Nerve block should develop within 5 to 10 minutes; if the block is incomplete, an additional 1 to 2 mL of local anesthetic can be injected or the needle can be repositioned in an effort to obtain a more complete block.

POTENTIAL PROBLEMS

Subarachnoid injection of local anesthetic is possible with this block due to the close anatomic relationship between the trigeminal ganglion and the dural reflection—Meckel's cave. Likewise, the needle will pass through highly vascular regions on its way to the foramen ovale, and hematoma

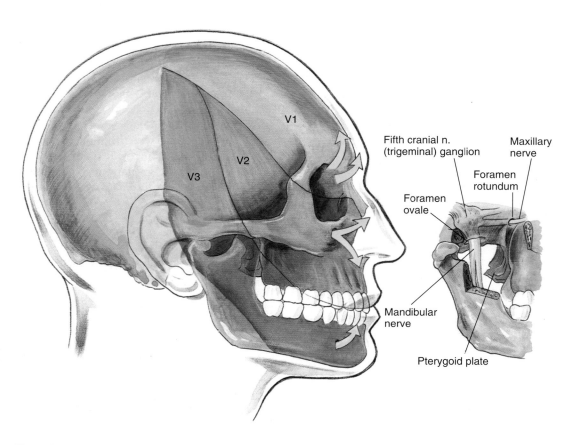

Figure 22-1. Fifth cranial nerve (trigeminal) ganglion anatomy: innervation and peripterygoid relationships.

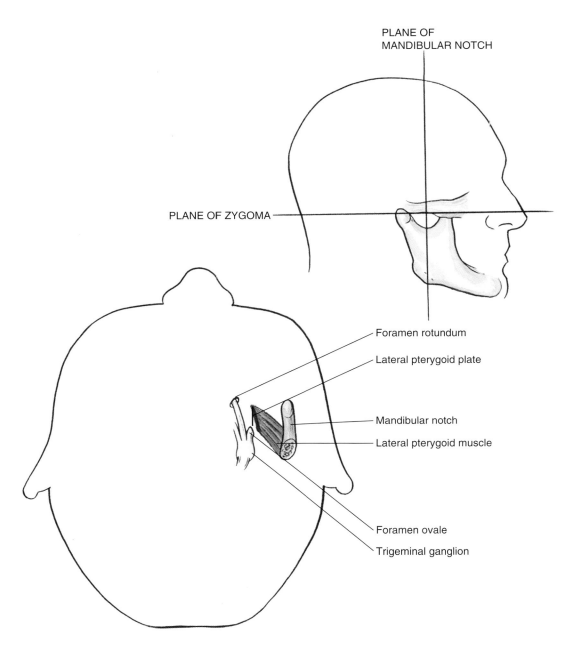

PLANE OF
MANDIBULAR NOTCH

PLANE OF ZYGOMA

Foramen rotundum

Lateral pterygoid plate

Mandibular notch

Lateral pterygoid muscle

Foramen ovale

Trigeminal ganglion

Figure 22-2. Cross-sectional anatomy: fifth cranial nerve (trigeminal) ganglion and foramen ovale.

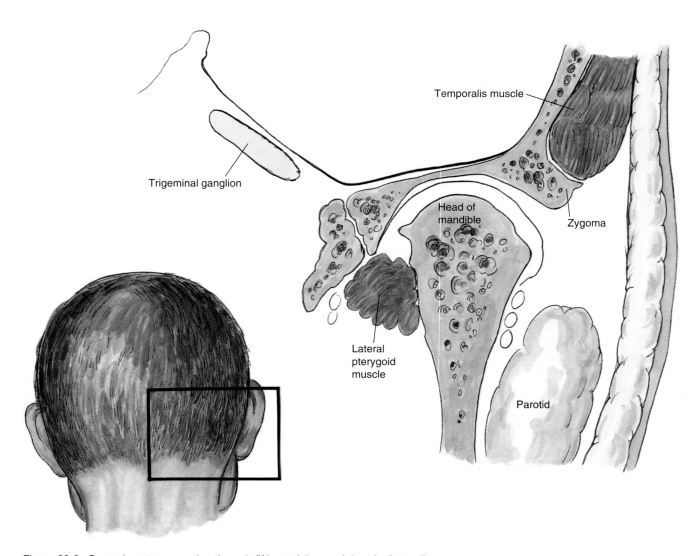

Figure 22-3. Coronal anatomy: section through fifth cranial nerve (trigeminal) ganglion.

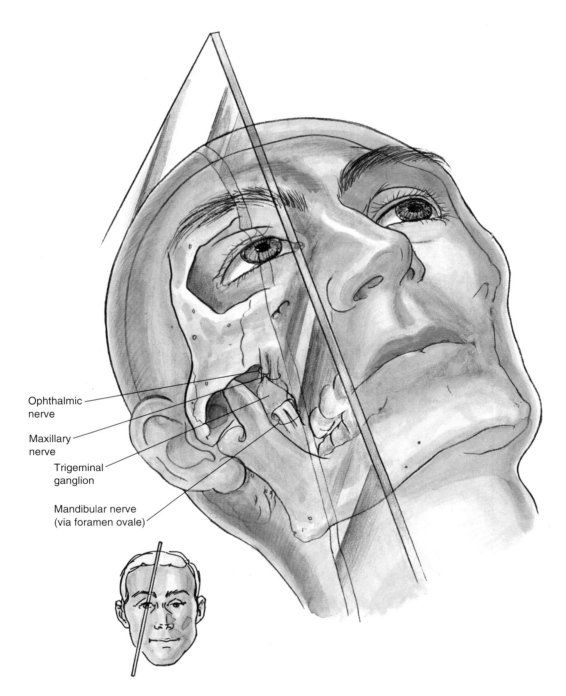

Ophthalmic
nerve

Maxillary
nerve

Trigeminal
ganglion

Mandibular nerve
(via foramen ovale)

Figure 22-4. Trigeminal ganglion block: anatomy and needle insertion plane.

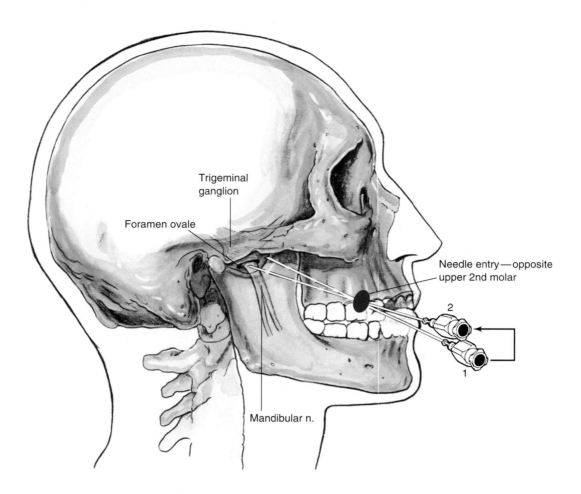

Figure 22-5. Trigeminal ganglion block: anatomy and technique.

formation is a possibility. The block can also be painful for the patient and may require effective sedation before final needle placement.

PEARLS

As with all regional block techniques, it is important not to develop a sense of "time pressure" when performing this block. This is especially pertinent to trigeminal ganglion block because doses of 1% lidocaine as small as 0.25 mL have produced unconsciousness when unintentionally injected into the CSF during the block. Because this block can be uncomfortable, sufficient time is needed to allow the patient to become comfortable with the approach and appropriate sedation to occur. In addition, skill with fluoroscopic guidance of the technique should be developed.

Maxillary Block 23

David L. Brown

PERSPECTIVE

Local anesthetic block of the maxillary nerve in its peripterygoid location is most commonly used to evaluate facial neuralgia. However, it can be used to facilitate surgical procedures in the nerve's cutaneous distribution (Fig. 23-1). Injection of neurolytic solution from the lateral approach to the maxillary nerve in its peripterygoid location should be undertaken with extreme caution due to its location near the orbit.

Patient Selection. This block is principally used diagnostically in the workup of facial neuralgia. For patients with significant cardiopulmonary disease who require a surgical procedure in the distribution of the maxillary nerve, it can be used for surgical anesthesia.

Pharmacologic Choice. The maxillary nerve can be blocked with a low volume of local anesthetic (<5 mL); thus virtually any local anesthetic can be chosen.

PLACEMENT

Anatomy. The maxillary nerve is entirely sensory and passes through the foramen rotundum to exit from the cranium. The nerve passes through the pterygopalatine fossa, medial to the lateral pterygoid plate, on its way to the infraorbital fissure. As illustrated in Figure 23-2, it is accessible to the anesthesiologist through a lateral approach as it passes into the pterygopalatine fossa.

Position. The patient is placed in the supine position with the head and neck rotated away from the side to be blocked. While the anesthesiologist palpates the mandibular notch, the patient is asked to open and close his or her mouth gently to make the notch even more obvious.

Needle Puncture. A 22-gauge, 8-cm needle is inserted through the mandibular notch in a slightly cephalomedial direction, as illustrated in Figure 23-3. This allows the needle to impinge on the lateral pterygoid plate at a depth of approximately 5 cm (*position 1*). The needle is then withdrawn and redirected in a stepwise manner toward *position 2* (the pterygopalatine fossa). The needle should not be advanced more than 1 cm past the depth of initial contact with the pterygoid plate. As the needle is "walked off" the pterygoid plate, a sense of walking into the pterygopalatine fossa should be appreciated. Once the needle is adequately positioned, 5 mL of local anesthetic is injected.

POTENTIAL PROBLEMS

Due to the close proximity of the maxillary nerve to the infraorbital fissure, some spill of local anesthetic into the orbit is possible; thus patients should be warned that eye movement or vision might be affected. The lateral approach to the maxillary nerve also involves insertion of the needle through a vascular region, and hematoma formation is possible. Again, due to the close association of the pterygopalatine fossa with the orbit, patients frequently develop a "black eye" after this block.

PEARLS

To become comfortable and clinically successful with this block, the anesthesiologist should find the time to examine the relationship of the foramen rotundum, pterygoid plate, and pterygopalatine fossa. An understanding of the peripterygoid anatomy will promote the anesthesiologist's confidence and the clinical efficacy of this block.

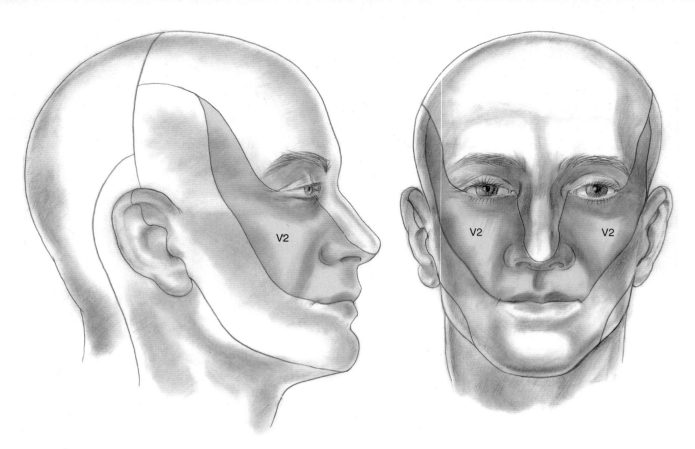

Figure 23-1. Maxillary nerve (V2): cutaneous innervation.

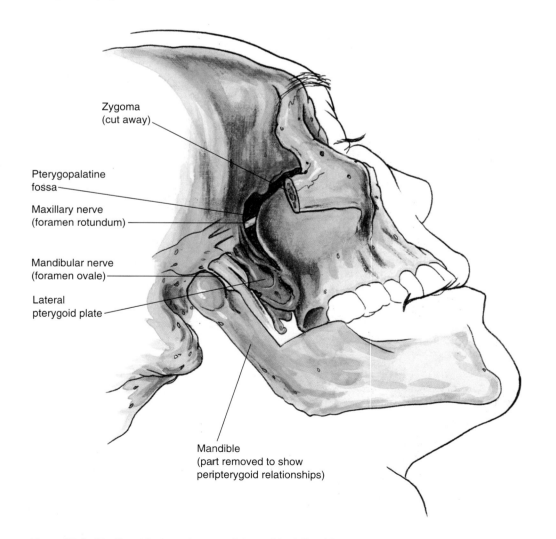

Zygoma
(cut away)

Pterygopalatine
fossa

Maxillary nerve
(foramen rotundum)

Mandibular nerve
(foramen ovale)

Lateral
pterygoid plate

Mandible
(part removed to show
peripterygoid relationships)

Figure 23-2. Maxillary block anatomy: peripterygoid relationships.

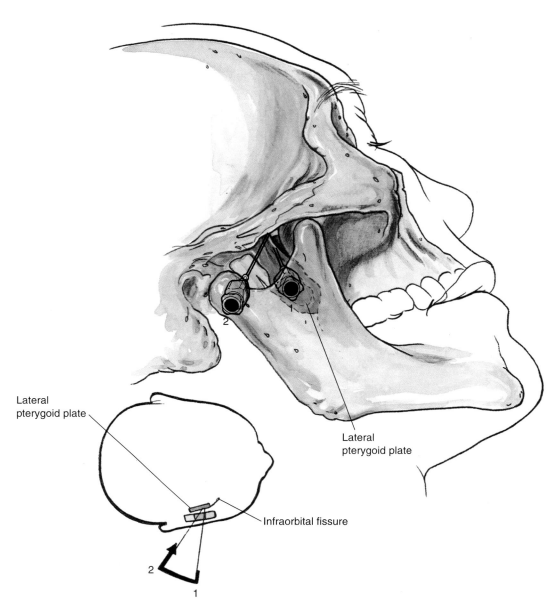

Lateral
pterygoid plate

Lateral
pterygoid plate

Infraorbital fissure

Figure 23-3. Maxillary block anatomy: needle insertion technique.

Mandibular Block 24

David L. Brown

PERSPECTIVE

This block is most often used for diagnosis of facial neuralgias; however, it can be used for surgical procedures on the skin overlying the lower jaw, except at the jaw's angle. Dental procedures on the lower jaw can also be carried out, although dentists more commonly use the intraoral approach to the mandibular nerve to perform this block.

Patient Selection. Patients appropriate for this block are those with facial neuralgias and those with significant cardiopulmonary disease who require a surgical procedure in the region innervated by the mandibular nerve.

Pharmacologic Choice. Because small volumes (5 mL) of local anesthetic will produce regional block of the mandibular nerve, virtually any local anesthetic agent is an acceptable choice.

PLACEMENT

Anatomy. The mandibular nerve is a mixed motor-sensory nerve, although it is primarily sensory. It exits from the cranium through the foramen ovale and parallels the posterior margin of the lateral pterygoid plate as it descends inferiorly and laterally toward the mandible (Figs. 24-1 and 24-2). The anterior division of the mandibular nerve is principally motor and supplies the muscles of mastication, whereas the posterior division is principally sensory and supplies the skin and mucous membranes overlying the lower jaw and skin anterior and superior to the ear (Fig. 24-3).

Sensory branches of the mandibular nerve are the buccal, auriculotemporal, lingual, and inferior alveolar nerves. The *buccal nerve* is exclusively sensory and supplies the mucous membranes of the cheek. The *auriculotemporal nerve* passes posterior to the neck of the mandible to supply the skin anterior to the ear and extends into the scalp's temporal region. The *lingual nerve* is joined by the chorda tympani branch of the facial nerve, and together they supply taste and general sensation to the anterior two-thirds of the tongue and sensation to the floor of the mouth, including the lingual aspect of the lower gingivae. The *inferior alveolar nerve* supplies the lower teeth and terminates as the mental nerve, which supplies sensation to the lower labial mucous membranes and skin of the chin.

Position. The patient is placed in the supine position, with the head and neck turned away from the side to be blocked. As in the approach used for maxillary block, the patient is asked to open and close his or her mouth gently while the anesthesiologist palpates the mandibular notch to identify it more clearly.

Needle Puncture. The needle is inserted in the midpoint of the mandibular notch and directed to reach the lateral pterygoid plate by taking a slightly cephalomedial angle through the notch, as shown in Figure 24-4. The 24-gauge, 8-cm needle will impinge on the lateral pterygoid plate at a depth of approximately 5 cm (*needle position 1*). The needle is then withdrawn and redirected in small steps to "walk off" the posterior border of the lateral pterygoid plate in a horizontal plane (*needle position 2*), as shown in Figure 24-4. The needle should not be advanced more than 0.5 cm past the depth of the pterygoid plate because the superior constrictor muscle of the pharynx is easily pierced; thus the needle will enter the pharynx if it is inserted more deeply. Once the needle tip is appropriately positioned, 5 mL of local anesthetic is administered.

POTENTIAL PROBLEMS

As with maxillary nerve block, the lateral approach to the mandibular nerve requires needle insertion through a vascular region. Thus hematoma formation is possible. If a hematoma does occur, most often watchful waiting is all that is required. Although it is more difficult to enter the cerebrospinal fluid (CSF) through the foramen ovale from the lateral approach, one must be constantly aware that if a needle is inserted through the foramen ovale into Meckel's cave, small doses of local anesthetic in the CSF can produce unconsciousness.

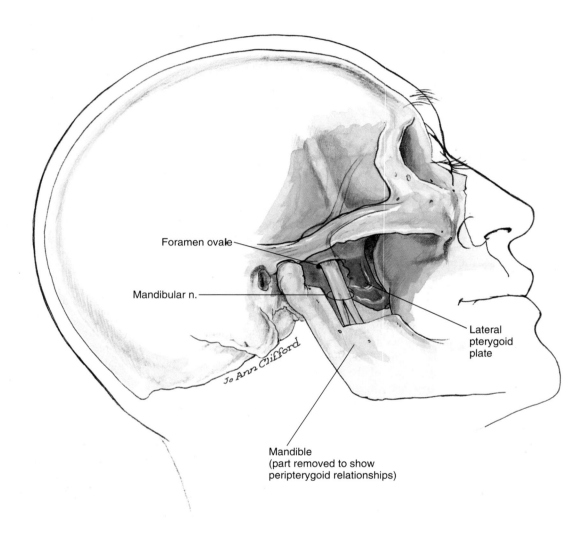

Foramen ovale

Mandibular n.

Lateral pterygoid plate

Mandible
(part removed to show peripterygoid relationships)

Figure 24-1. Mandibular block anatomy: peripterygoid relationships.

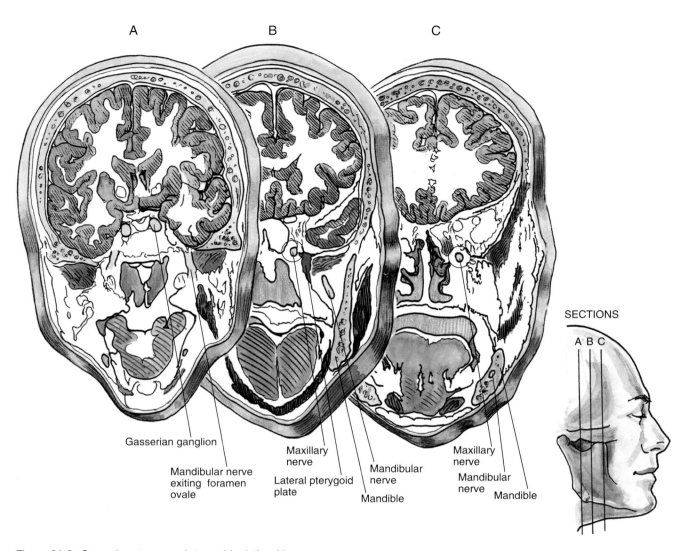

A   B   C

SECTIONS

A B C

Gasserian ganglion

Mandibular nerve
exiting foramen
ovale

Maxillary
nerve

Lateral pterygoid
plate

Mandibular
nerve

Mandible

Maxillary
nerve

Mandibular
nerve

Mandible

Figure 24-2. Coronal anatomy: peripterygoid relationships.

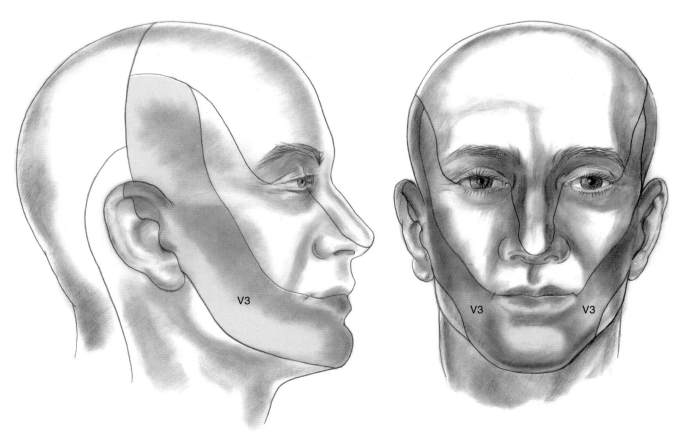

V3

V3   V3

Figure 24-3. Mandibular nerve (V3): cutaneous innervation.

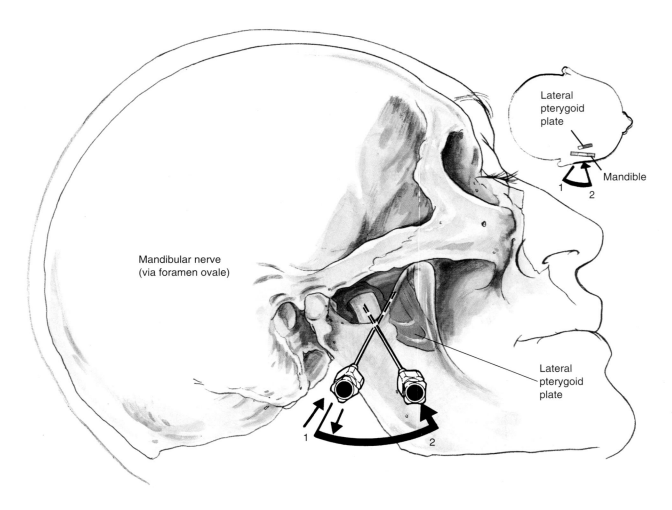

Figure 24-4. Mandibular block anatomy: needle insertion technique.

PEARLS

As with maxillary nerve block, anesthesiologists should develop a thorough understanding of the peripterygoid anatomy before carrying out this block. Needle movements with the mandibular block involve fewer planes than with the maxillary block because the needle is moved primarily in the horizontal plane once it has made contact with the pterygoid plate. Therefore in some ways, this block is less complex than the maxillary block. Also, because the mandibular nerve is more distant from the orbital structures, there is less risk in using neurolytic solutions with this block.

Distal Trigeminal Block 25

David L. Brown

PERSPECTIVE

This block can be used for the diagnosis of facial neuralgia; however, more frequently it is used for superficial surgical procedures that require more than simple infiltration for anesthesia.

Patient Selection. Almost all patients are candidates for distal trigeminal blocks because the bony foramina—supraorbital, infraorbital, and mental—are easily palpable.

Pharmacologic Choice. Due to the small volumes of local anesthetic necessary for this block, almost any local anesthetic agent may be chosen.

PLACEMENT

Anatomy. The distal branches of the three divisions of the trigeminal nerve—ophthalmic (supraorbital), maxillary (infraorbital), and mandibular (mental)—exit from the skull through their respective foramina on a line that runs almost vertically through the pupil (Fig. 25-1).

Position. The patient is placed in the supine position with the anesthesiologist at the patient's side, approximately at the level of the shoulder.

Needle Puncture. For this block, as illustrated in Figure 25-2, once the respective foramina are identified by palpation, a short, 25-gauge needle is inserted in a cephalomedial direction near each foramen, and approximately 2 to 3 mL of local anesthetic is injected at each site. If paresthesia is obtained, the local anesthetic can be deposited at that point.

POTENTIAL PROBLEMS

This block is superficial and thus carries with it few complications. One should be cautious about entering the foramina to inject the local anesthetic because intraneural injection is probably more frequent with that approach.

PEARLS

The anesthesiologist should ensure that the patient is properly sedated and should clearly identify the foramina to be blocked so that accurate needle placement is achieved.

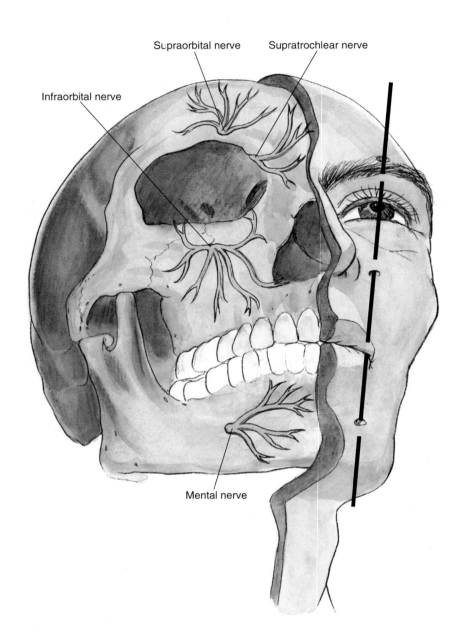

Infraorbital nerve

Supraorbital nerve

Supratrochlear nerve

Mental nerve

Figure 25-1. Distal trigeminal nerve: anatomy.

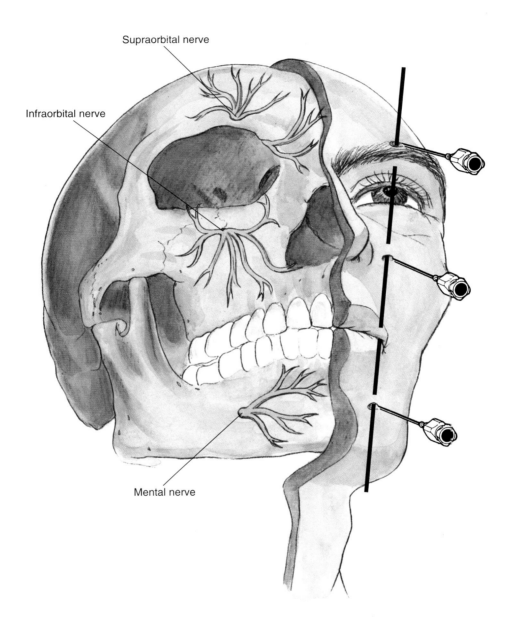

Figure 25-2. Distal trigeminal nerve block: technique.

Retrobulbar (Peribulbar) Block 26

David L. Brown

PERSPECTIVE

This block is performed more often by ophthalmologists than by anesthesiologists. The combination of retrobulbar anesthesia and block of the orbicularis oculi muscle allows most intraocular surgery to be performed. This regional block is most useful for corneal, anterior chamber, and lens procedures.

Patient Selection. Patients who require retrobulbar (peribulbar) anesthesia are principally older patients who are undergoing ophthalmic operations.

Pharmacologic Choice. If retrobulbar block is used, 2 to 4 mL of local anesthetic is all that is required to produce adequate retrobulbar anesthesia. Conversely, if the peribulbar approach is chosen (i.e., the needle tip is not purposely inserted through the cone of extraocular muscles), slightly larger volumes—4 to 6 mL—may be necessary. Almost any of the local anesthetic agents are applicable, with many ophthalmic anesthetists using combinations of bupivacaine and lidocaine.

PLACEMENT

Anatomy. Sensation to the eye is provided by the ophthalmic nerve through the long and short posterior ciliary nerves. Autonomic innervation is provided by the same nerves, and sympathetic fibers traveling with the arteries and parasympathetic fibers carried by the inferior branch of the oculomotor nerve provide additional autonomic innervation. Because the innervation of the orbicularis oculi muscle is through the facial nerve, blockade of these fibers is required to ensure a quiet eye during ophthalmic operations. The ciliary ganglion, measuring approximately 2 to 3 mm in length, lies deep in the orbit just lateral to the optic nerve and medial to the lateral rectus muscle. From this ganglion, the long and short ciliary nerves extend forward in the orbit. Immediately posterior to the ciliary ganglion, the ophthalmic artery can be found at the lateral side of the optic nerve as it crosses superior to it and passes forward medially (Fig. 26-1).

Position. Patients are placed in the supine position and are instructed to maintain their primary gaze directly ahead, not "up and in" as in earlier recommendations. With the globe in primary gaze, the optic nerve position minimizes potential intraneural injection. The anesthesiologist is positioned for the injection as illustrated in Figure 26-2.

Needle Puncture. While the patient's gaze is directed cephalad and opposite to the site of injection, a 27-gauge, 31-mm, sharp-beveled needle is inserted at the inferolateral border of the bony orbit and directed toward the apex of the orbit, as illustrated in Figure 26-3. The needle should be oriented so that the bevel opening faces toward the globe. A "pop" may be appreciated as the needle tip traverses the bulbar fascia and enters the orbital muscle cone. Before 2 to 4 mL of local anesthetic is injected, careful needle aspiration should be carried out. After retrobulbar block, 5 to 10 minutes should be allowed to pass before the operation is started. This helps avoid operating on patients who develop retrobulbar hematomas. During these 5 to 10 minutes, the anesthesiologist can apply gentle pressure to the globe, principally to facilitate lowering the intraocular pressure. If a peribulbar technique is chosen, needle insertion begins like that used for retrobulbar (inferotemporal) injection; however, the operator inserts the needle parallel and lateral to the lateral rectus muscle and bulbar fascia rather than making an effort to puncture it. Many practitioners also now suggest making a second injection of 3 to 5 mL for a peribulbar block either in the superomedial orbit or at the extreme medial side of the palpebral fissure. To complete the local block for ocular surgery, the orbicularis oculi muscle must be blocked to produce an immobile eye. This is carried out by blocking the facial nerve fibers that innervate the muscle.

There are many ways of performing blocks of these facial nerve fibers, and the method illustrated in Figure 26-4 is the example of Van Lint. In this block, a 25-gauge, 4-cm needle is inserted at *needle position 1* until the lower inferolateral orbital rim is reached. When the needle tip contacts the bony surface, 1 mL of local anesthetic is injected. Through this skin wheal, the needle is repositioned along the lateral and inferior margins of the orbit (*needle positions 2 and 3*), and 2 to 3 mL of local anesthetic is injected along each needle path.

POTENTIAL PROBLEMS

The most common complication with retrobulbar block is hematoma formation. This can be minimized by using

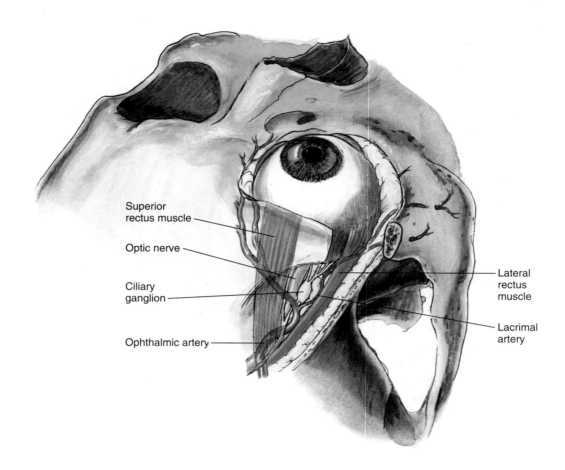

Superior
rectus muscle

Optic nerve

Ciliary
ganglion

Ophthalmic artery

Lateral
rectus
muscle

Lacrimal
artery

Figure 26-1. Orbital anatomy.

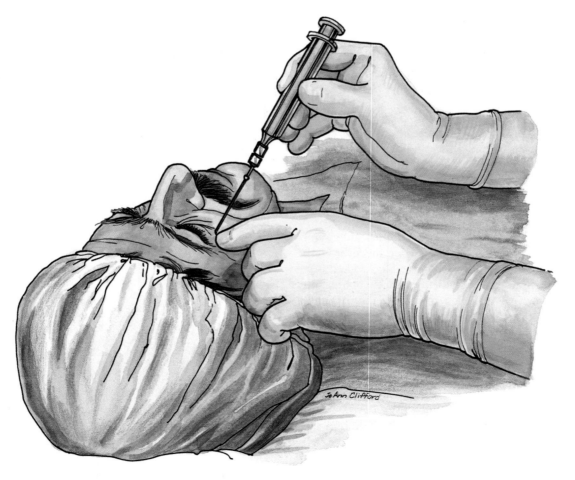

Figure 26-2. Retrobulbar (peribulbar) block: position.

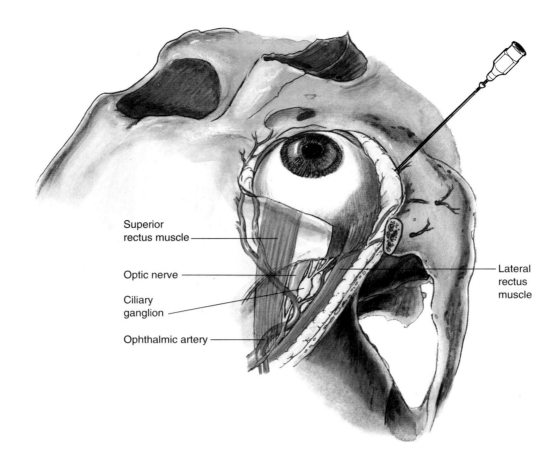

Superior
rectus muscle

Optic nerve

Ciliary
ganglion

Ophthalmic artery

Lateral
rectus
muscle

Figure 26-3. Retrobulbar (peribulbar) block: needle puncture.

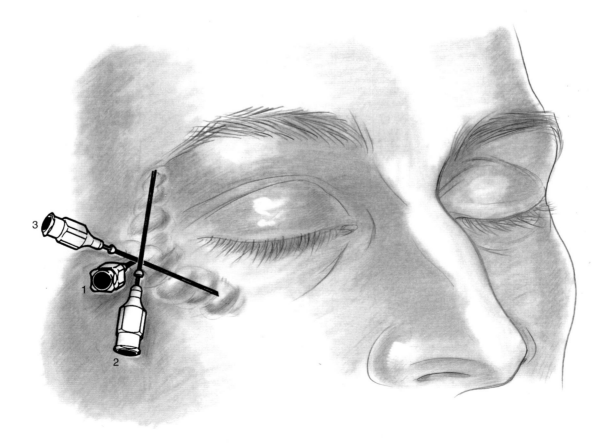

Figure 26-4. Regional block of orbicularis oculi muscle: Van Lint method.

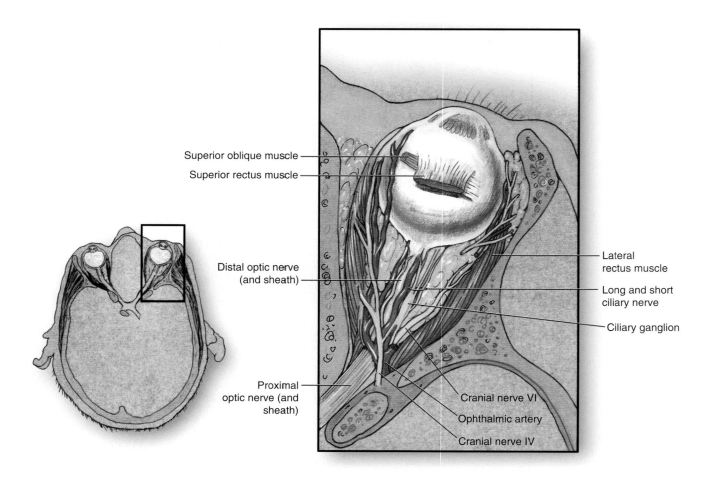

Superior oblique muscle
Superior rectus muscle
Distal optic nerve (and sheath)
Proximal optic nerve (and sheath)
Lateral rectus muscle
Long and short ciliary nerve
Ciliary ganglion
Cranial nerve VI
Ophthalmic artery
Cranial nerve IV

Figure 26-5. Orbital functional anatomy.

a needle shorter than 31 mm. Hematoma formation is more likely if a longer needle is used and the needle tip rests in the vicinity of the ophthalmic artery as it crosses the optic nerve. Hematoma can also be minimized by using a peribulbar approach. Other complications that can accompany retrobulbar block include local anesthetic toxicity, development of the oculocardiac reflex, and cases of sudden apnea and obtundation after retrobulbar injection. The latter two results are probably related to injection within the optic nerve sheath, resulting in unexpected spinal anesthesia, or intravascular injection affecting the respiratory centers in the midbrain, as illustrated in Figure 26-5.

PEARLS

If anesthesiologists carry out retrobulbar anesthesia, they must work with ophthalmologists who are supportive and willing to share this part of their practice. Theoretically, many of the complications of retrobulbar anesthesia can be avoided if peribulbar block is carried out. This can be produced by placing the needle along the muscular cone of extraocular muscles rather than within the muscular cone. Although slightly larger volumes of local anesthetic are required with this technique, most of the major complications can be avoided.

Cervical Plexus Block 27

David L. Brown

PERSPECTIVE

Cervical plexus blocks are used to carry out both superficial and deep operations in the region of the neck and supra-clavicular fossa. The choice of deep or superficial block depends on the surgical procedure.

Patient Selection. This block can be performed easily in a supine patient; thus almost any patient is a candidate. Bilateral deep cervical plexus block should be avoided because the phrenic nerve may be partially blocked with this technique. Examples of procedures that are suitable for this technique are carotid endarterectomy, lymph node biopsy, and plastic surgical procedures.

Pharmacologic Choice. Most procedures carried out with cervical plexus block do not demand significant motor relaxation. Thus lower concentrations of local anesthetics, such as 0.75% to 1% lidocaine or mepivacaine, 0.25% bupivacaine, or 0.2% ropivacaine, are appropriate with these techniques.

PLACEMENT

Anatomy. Cervical plexus block can be divided into superficial and deep techniques. The cutaneous innerva-tion of the cervical nerves is schematically illustrated in Figure 27-1. The cervical nerves have both dorsal and ventral rami, and those illustrated in Figure 27-2 represent the ventral rami of C1 to C4. In addition, there are both sensory and motor branches from the dorsal rami of C1 to C4 that are not shown. Before regrouping to form the cer-vical plexus, the cervical nerves exit from the cervical ver-tebrae through a gutter in the transverse process in an anterocaudolateral direction, immediately posterior to the vertebral artery.

To simplify understanding the cervical plexus, it can be divided into (1) the cutaneous branches of the plexus, (2) the ansa cervicalis complex, (3) the phrenic nerve, (4) con-tributions to the accessory nerve, and (5) direct muscular branches (see Fig. 27-2). The *cutaneous branches of the plexus* are the lesser occipital, greater auricular, transverse cervical, and supraclavicular nerves (see Fig. 27-1). The first three arise from the second and third cervical nerves, and the supraclavicular nerves arise from the third and fourth cervical nerves. The *ansa cervicalis complex* provides innervation to the infrahyoid and geniohyoid muscles. The

phrenic nerve is the sole motor nerve to the diaphragm and also provides sensation to its central portion. The nerve arises from a large root from the fourth cervical nerve, reinforced by smaller contributions from the third and fifth nerves. Its course takes it to the lateral border of the ante-rior scalene muscle before it descends vertically over the ventral surface of this muscle and enters the chest along its medial border. The *accessory nerve* (cranial nerve XI) receives contributions from the cervical plexus at several points and provides innervation to the sternocleidomas-toid muscle as well as the trapezius muscles. The *direct muscular branches* of the plexus supply prevertebral muscles in the neck. The superficial plexus becomes subcutaneous at the midpoint of the posterior border of the sternocleido-mastoid muscle (Fig. 27-3, and see Fig. 27-5).

Position. The patient is placed in the supine position, with the head and neck turned opposite the side to be blocked. The anesthesiologist should stand at the patient's side, approximately at the level of the shoulder.

Needle Puncture: Deep Cervical Plexus Block. The patient should be positioned with the neck slightly extended and the head turned away from the side to be blocked. A line should be drawn on the skin between the tip of the mastoid process and Chassaignac's tubercle (i.e., the most easily palpable transverse process of the cervical vertebra, C6). A second line should be drawn parallel and 1 cm posterior to the first line, as illustrated in blue in Figure 27-4. The C4 transverse process should be located by first finding the C2 transverse process 1 to 2 cm caudal to the mastoid process and then identifying C3 and subsequently C4. Each of these transverse processes is palpable approximately 1.5 cm caudal to the immediately more cephalad process. Ultraso-nographic guidance can also assist in locating the C4 trans-verse process. Once the C4 transverse process is identified, a 22-gauge, 5-cm needle is inserted immediately over the C4 transverse process so that it will contact that process at a depth of approximately 1.5 to 3 cm. If paresthesia is obtained, 10 to 12 mL of local anesthetic is injected at this site. It is helpful to obtain paresthesia with this technique before injection because one is relying on the continuity of the paravertebral space in the neck to facilitate local anes-thetic spread. If paresthesia is not elicited on the first pass, the needle should be withdrawn and "walked" in a stepwise fashion in an anteroposterior manner. Again, ultrasono-graphic guidance will allow you to observe the spread of local anesthetic in the paravertebral space.

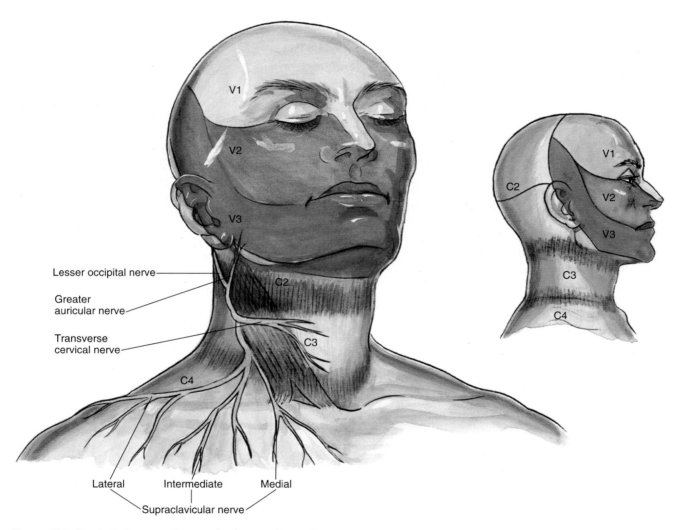

Lesser occipital nerve

Greater
auricular nerve

Transverse
cervical nerve

V1

V2

V3

C2

C3

C4

Lateral   Intermediate   Medial

Supraclavicular nerve

Figure 27-1. Cervical plexus: anatomy and cutaneous innervation.

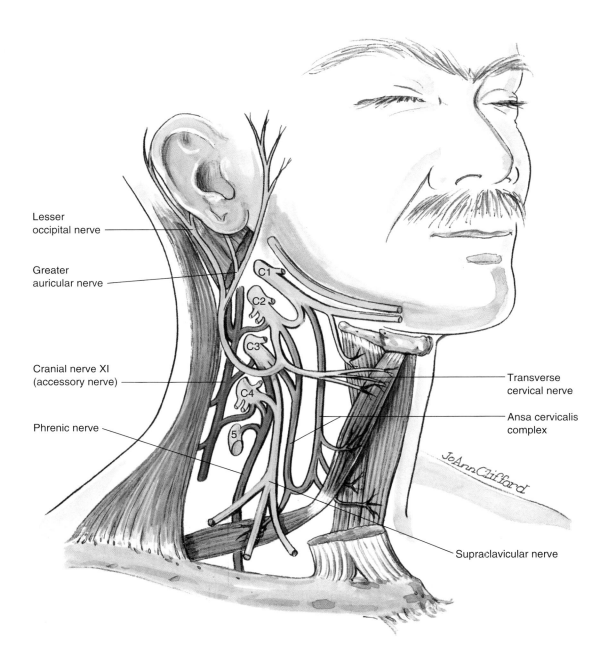

Lesser
occipital nerve

Greater
auricular nerve

Cranial nerve XI
(accessory nerve)

Phrenic nerve

C1

C2

C3

C4

5

Transverse
cervical nerve

Ansa cervicalis
complex

Supraclavicular nerve

JoAnnClifford

Figure 27-2. Cervical plexus: functional anatomy of the ventral rami of C1 to C4.

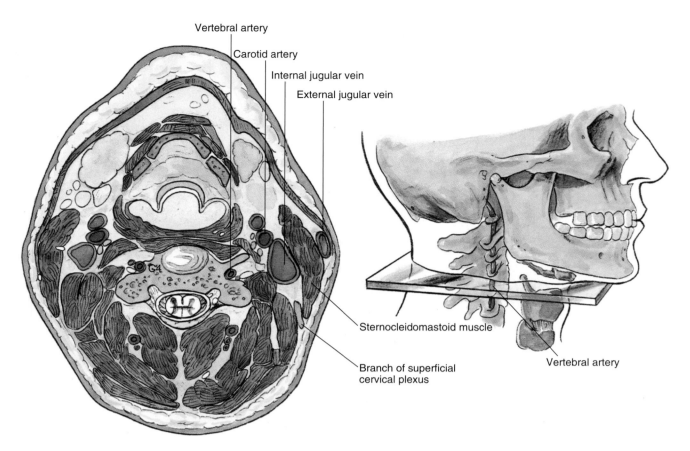

Figure 27-3. Cervical plexus: cross-sectional anatomy at the midpoint of the sternocleidomastoid muscle.

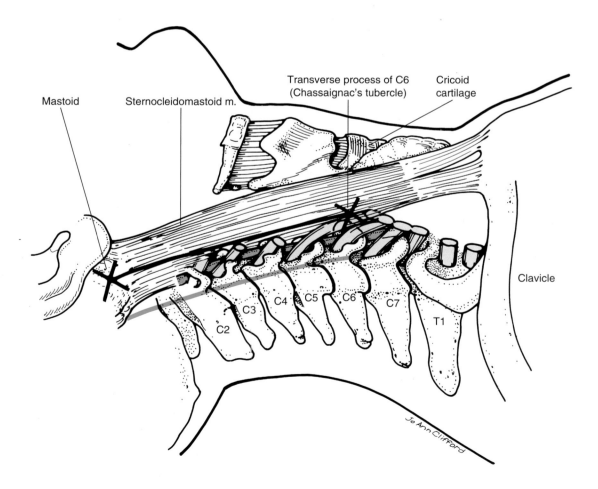

Figure 27-4. Deep cervical plexus block: technicue.

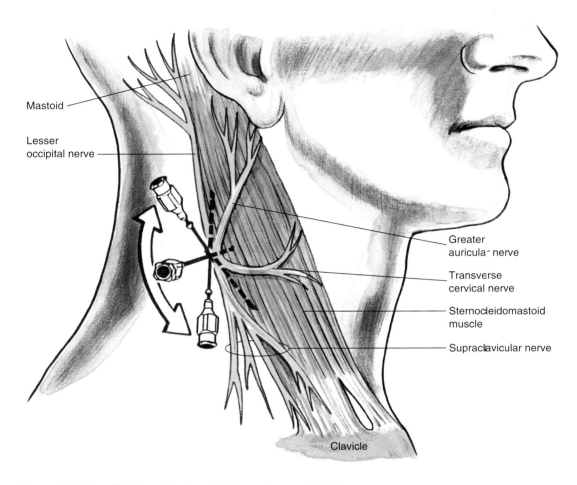

Figure 27-5. Superficial cervical plexus block: anatomy and technique.

Needle Placement: Superficial Cervical Plexus Block. The superficial cervical plexus block, as illustrated in Figure 27-5, relies on local anesthetic "volume" to be effective. At the midpoint on the posterior border of the sternocleidomastoid muscle, the superficial cervical plexus is arranged such that infiltration deep to the posterior border of the sternocleidomastoid muscle will produce a block. To perform the block, a 22-gauge, 4-cm needle is inserted subcutaneously posterior and immediately deep to the sternocleidomastoid muscle, and 5 mL of local anesthetic is injected. The needle is then redirected both superiorly and inferiorly along the posterior border of the sternocleidomastoid, and 5 mL of solution is injected along each of these sites. In this fashion, a field block of the superficial plexus is created.

POTENTIAL PROBLEMS

Deep cervical plexus block is often accompanied by at least partial phrenic nerve block, so bilateral blocks should be used with caution. The block also places the needles near the vertebral artery and other neuraxial structures. When carrying out the superficial block, one should simply avoid the external jugular vein, which often overlies the block site. Likewise, intravascular injection through the internal jugular vein can occur if the needle is inserted too deeply during performance of the field block.

PEARLS

If patients are properly positioned for this block, the superficial block should rarely result in problems. If the deep block is carried out and proper palpation is used to limit the amount of tissue between the anesthesiologist's fingertips and the transverse process, very short needles can help minimize the occurrence of errant deep injections. If a deep cervical plexus block is to be carried out for carotid endarterectomy, the anesthesiologist should consult with his or her surgical colleagues to learn their expectations so that anesthesia is adequate. Superficial cervical plexus block can be used effectively in addition to interscalene block during shoulder surgery to ensure the presence of cutaneous anesthesia when the surgical procedure is started soon after the block.

Stellate Block 28

David L. Brown

PERSPECTIVE

The primary use of stellate block is in the diagnosis and treatment of complex regional pain syndromes of the upper extremity. It may also be used in clinical situations when increased perfusion to the upper extremity is desired, although this can also be accomplished with the brachial plexus blocks.

Patient Selection. Patients for this block are primarily those with complex regional pain syndromes of the upper extremity or those with impaired perfusion to the upper extremity after trauma.

Pharmacologic Choice. Even during diagnostic use of stellate ganglion block, it is often desirable to produce a long-lasting block. Therefore a solution of 0.25% bupivacaine or 0.2% ropivacaine with 1:200,000 epinephrine is often my first choice.

PLACEMENT

Anatomy. The cervical sympathetic trunk is a cephalad continuation of the thoracic sympathetic trunk. It is composed of three ganglia: the superior cervical ganglion, generally opposite the first cervical vertebra; the middle cervical ganglion, usually opposite the sixth cervical vertebra; and the stellate (cervicothoracic) ganglion, generally opposite the seventh cervical and first thoracic vertebrae near the head of the first rib. The stellate ganglion is a fusion of the inferior cervical ganglion and the first thoracic ganglion—hence the name *cervicothoracic ganglion* (Fig. 28-1). The cervical part of the sympathetic chain and ganglion lies on the anterior surface of, and is separated from, the transverse processes of the cervical vertebrae by the thin prevertebral musculature (primarily the longus colli muscle), as illustrated in Figure 28-2. Because the anterior approach to the stellate ganglion is often made at the level of the sixth cervical vertebral (Chassaignac's) tubercle, it can be seen that the term *stellate block* is really a misnomer. To produce stellate (cervicothoracic) ganglion block, the anesthesiologist must rely on spread of the local anesthetic solution along the prevertebral muscles, or place the needle at the level of the seventh cervical vertebra with the use of ultrasonography or fluoroscopy.

Position. The patient should be in the supine position, with the neck in slight extension (Fig. 28-3). This is often facilitated by removing the patient's pillow before positioning. The anesthesiologist should stand beside the patient's neck and identify the sixth cervical vertebral tubercle with palpation. This can be accomplished by locating the cricoid cartilage and moving the fingers laterally until they contact this easily palpable vertebral tubercle.

Needle Puncture. Once the sixth cervical vertebral tubercle is identified as shown in Figure 28-3, the anesthesiologist should place the index and third fingers between the carotid artery laterally and the trachea medially at the level of C6. A short, 22- or 25-gauge needle is inserted until it contacts the transverse process of C6. The needle is then withdrawn approximately 1 to 2 mm, and 5 to 10 mL of local anesthetic is injected (Fig. 28-4).

POTENTIAL PROBLEMS

As illustrated in Figure 28-2, the vertebral artery runs close to the transverse process of C6, and intravascular injection must be avoided. The recurrent laryngeal and phrenic nerves may also be blocked if the needle position is not ideal. Patients should be cautioned that they may experience a lump in the throat or a sense of dyspnea. Reassurance is usually all that is necessary.

PEARLS

The most useful maneuver to facilitate this block is to use the index and third fingers of the palpating hand to compress the tissues overlying the sixth cervical vertebral tubercle. The patient will experience some deep pressure discomfort from this maneuver, but clear identification of the tubercle will make this block efficient, and most patients are willing to accept the deep discomfort if the block is

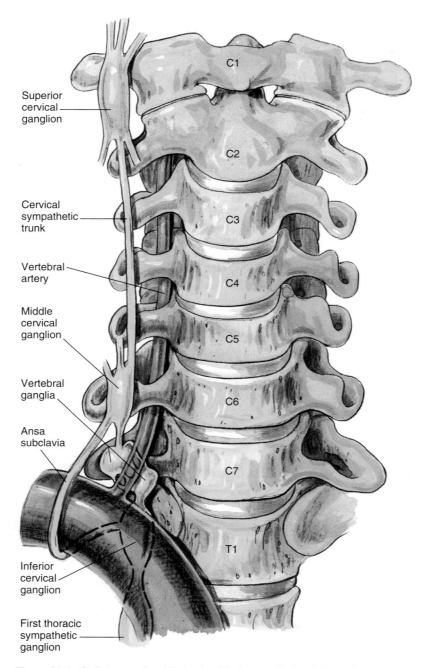

Superior cervical ganglion

Cervical sympathetic trunk

Vertebral artery

Middle cervical ganglion

Vertebral ganglia

Ansa subclavia

Inferior cervical ganglion

First thoracic sympathetic ganglion

C1
C2
C3
C4
C5
C6
C7
T1

Figure 28-1. Stellate ganglion block: simplified sympathetic chain anatomy.

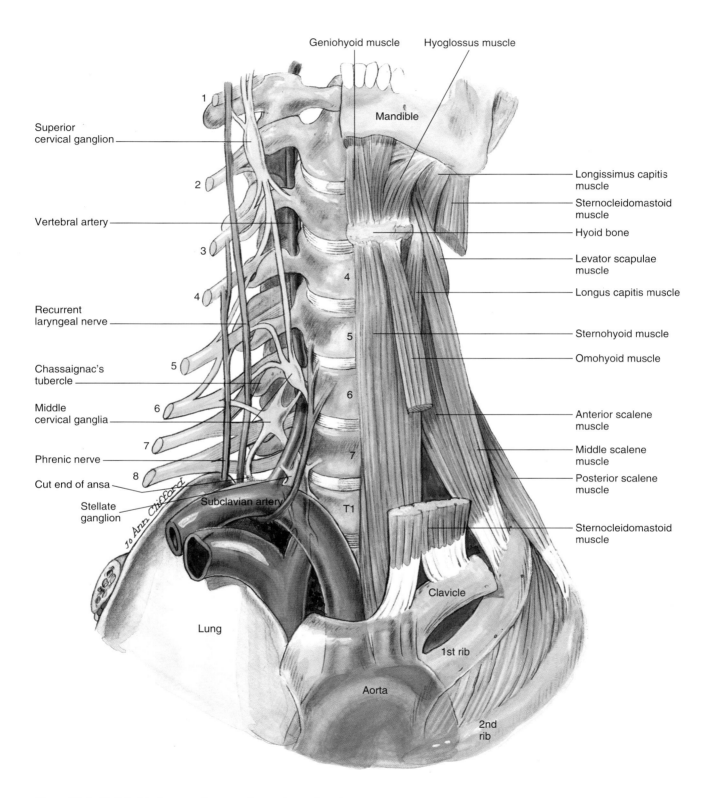

Figure 28-2. Stellate block: muscular, vascular, and neural anatomy.

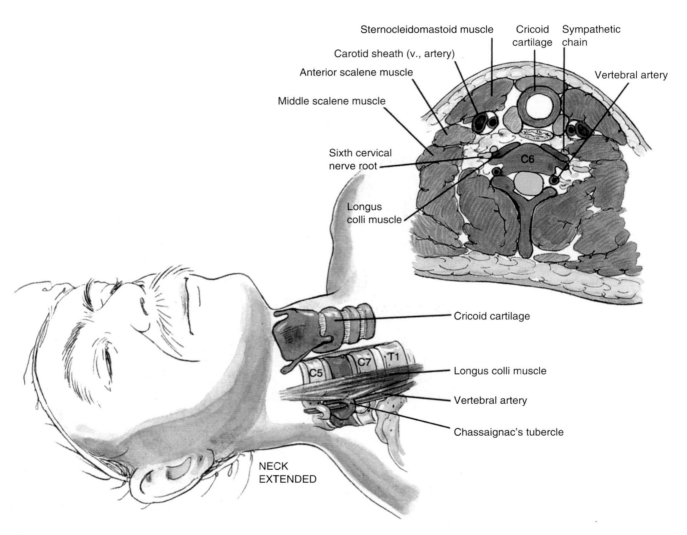

Figure 28-3. Stellate block: surface and cross-sectional anatomy.

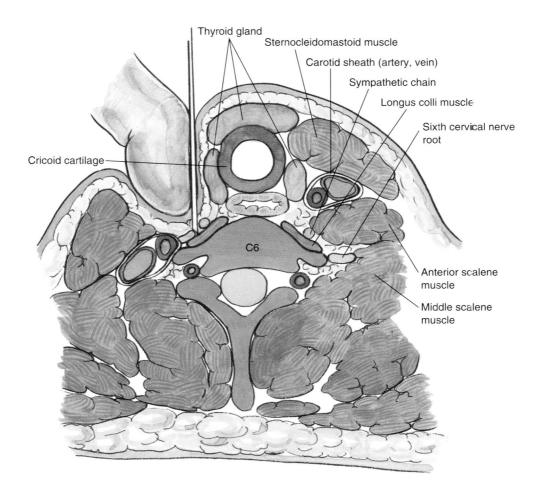

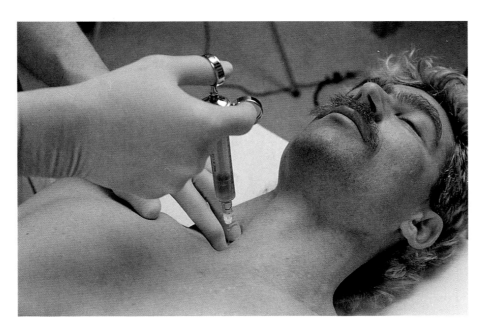

Figure 28-4. Stellate block: anatomy and technique.

carried out efficiently. In a small number of patients (<5%), a motor block of the ipsilateral upper extremity may develop after a stellate block performed without imaging guidance. Most likely this is because a prominent posterior tubercle at the posterior aspect of the transverse process is mistaken on palpation for the typically more prominent anterior portion of the sixth cervical vertebra. It is important to inform patients undergoing a stellate block about this possibility to minimize disappointment if it does develop.

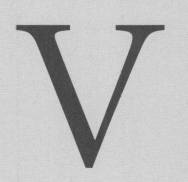

SECTION
Airway Blocks

Airway Block Anatomy

29

David L. Brown

If there is one set of regional blocks that an anesthesiologist should master, it is airway blocks. Even those anesthesiologists who prefer to use general anesthesia for the majority of their cases will be faced with the need to provide airway blocks before anesthetic induction in patients who may have airway compromise, trauma to the upper airway, or unstable cervical vertebrae. As illustrated in Figure 29-1, innervation of the airway can be separated into three principal neural pathways: trigeminal, glossopharyngeal, and vagus. If nasal intubation is planned, some method of anesthetizing the maxillary branches from the trigeminal nerve will need to be carried out. Because manipulations involve the pharynx and posterior third of the tongue, glossopharyngeal block will be required. Structures more distal in the airway to the epiglottis will require block of vagal branches.

Specific glossopharyngeal nerves that are of interest to anesthesiologists who undertake airway anesthesia are the pharyngeal nerves, which are primarily sensory to the pharyngeal mucosa; the tonsillar nerves, which provide sensation to the mucosa overlying the palatine tonsil and contiguous parts of the soft palate; and sensory branches to the posterior third of the tongue. The glossopharyngeal nerve exits the skull through the jugular foramen in close contact with the spinal accessory nerve. As the glossopharyngeal nerve exits the jugular foramen, it is also in close contact with the vagus nerve, which likewise travels within the carotid sheath in the upper portion of the neck.

The vagus nerve supplies innervation to the mucosa of the airway from the level of the epiglottis to the distal airways through both the superior and the recurrent laryngeal nerves, as illustrated in Figures 29-2 and 29-3. Although the vagus is primarily a parasympathetic nerve, it also contains some fibers from the cervical sympathetic chain, as well as motor fibers to laryngeal muscles. The superior laryngeal nerve provides sensation to the surfaces of the epiglottis and to the airway mucosa to the level of the vocal cords. It provides innervation to the mucosa after entering the thyrohyoid membrane just inferior to the hyoid bone between the greater and the lesser cornua of the hyoid. This mucosal innervation is carried out through the internal laryngeal nerve, a branch of the superior laryngeal nerve. The superior laryngeal nerve also continues as the external laryngeal nerve along the exterior of the larynx; it provides motor innervation to the cricothyroid muscle.

The recurrent laryngeal nerve is a branch of the vagus nerve that ascends along the posterolateral margin of the trachea after looping under the right subclavian artery as it leaves the vagus nerve on the right, or around the left side of the arch of the aorta, lateral to the ligamentum arteriosum, on the left. The recurrent nerves ascend and innervate the larynx and the trachea caudal to the vocal cords. This anatomy is illustrated in Figures 29-2, 29-3, and 29-4. Figure 29-5 shows a sagittal magnetic resonance image with an interpretive illustration of airway innervation keyed to the colors used in Figure 29-1.

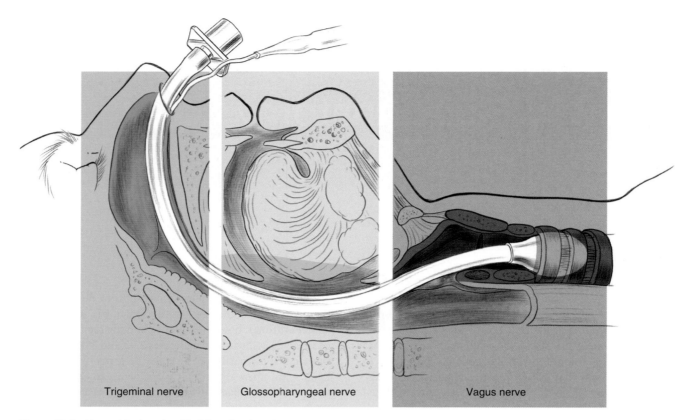

Trigeminal nerve   Glossopharyngeal nerve   Vagus nerve

Figure 29-1. Airway blocks: simplified functional anatomy.

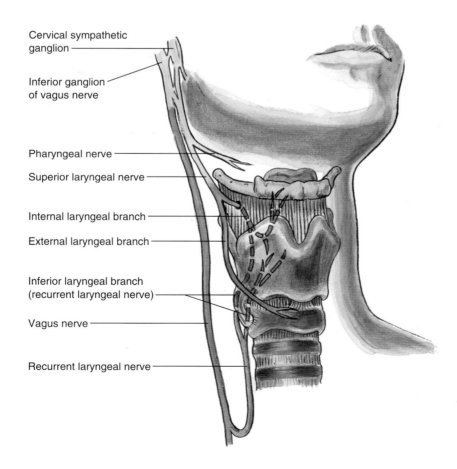

Cervical sympathetic ganglion

Inferior ganglion of vagus nerve

Pharyngeal nerve

Superior laryngeal nerve

Internal laryngeal branch

External laryngeal branch

Inferior laryngeal branch (recurrent laryngeal nerve)

Vagus nerve

Recurrent laryngeal nerve

Figure 29-2. Airway blocks: anatomy of laryngeal innervation.

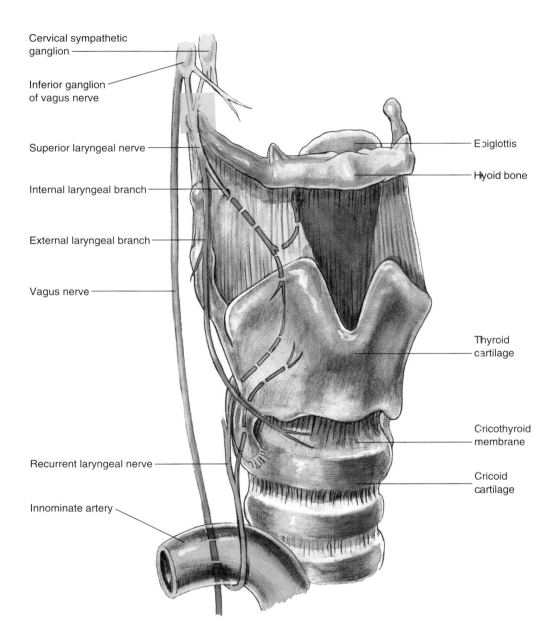

Figure 29-3. Airway blocks: anatomy of laryngeal, vagal, and sympathetic connections.

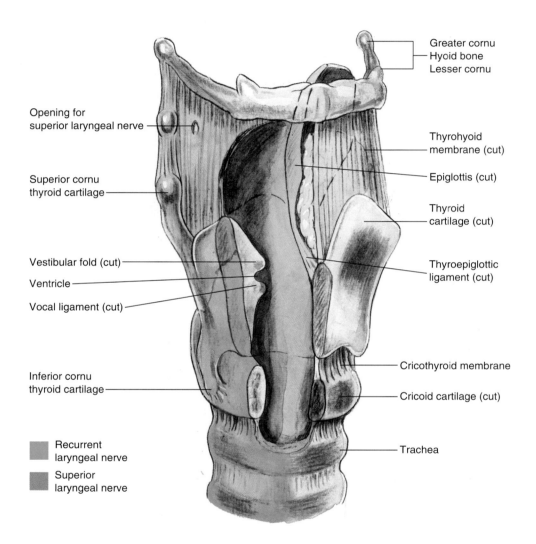

Greater cornu
Hyoid bone
Lesser cornu

Opening for
superior laryngeal nerve

Thyrohyoid
membrane (cut)

Epiglottis (cut)

Superior cornu
thyroid cartilage

Thyroid
cartilage (cut)

Vestibular fold (cut)

Ventricle

Vocal ligament (cut)

Thyroepiglottic
ligament (cut)

Cricothyroid membrane

Inferior cornu
thyroid cartilage

Cricoid cartilage (cut)

Recurrent
laryngeal nerve

Superior
laryngeal nerve

Trachea

Figure 29-4. Airway blocks: anatomy of laryngeal structures and simplified innervation.

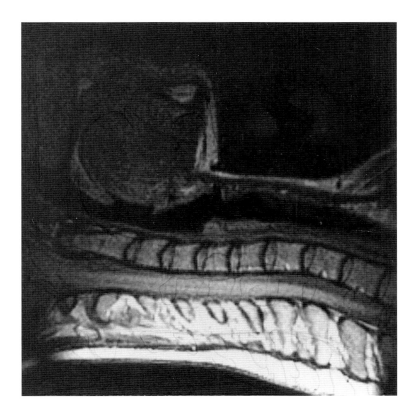

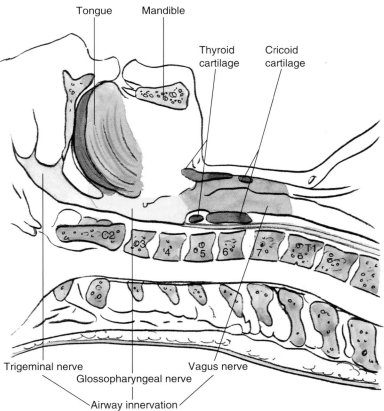

Figure 29-5. Airway blocks: sagittal anatomy on magnetic resonance imaging and an interpretive line drawing.

Glossopharyngeal Block

30

David L. Brown

PERSPECTIVE

Glossopharyngeal block is useful for anesthesia of the mucosa of the pharynx and soft palate, as well as for eliminating the gag reflex that results when pressure is applied to the posterior third of the tongue.

Patient Selection.   Glossopharyngeal block can be used in most patients who need atraumatic, sedated, spontaneously ventilating, "awake" tracheal intubation.

Pharmacologic Choice.   The local anesthetic chosen for glossopharyngeal block does not need to provide motor blockade. Lidocaine (0.5%) is an appropriate choice of local anesthetic.

PLACEMENT

Anatomy.   The glossopharyngeal nerve exits from the jugular foramen at the base of the skull, as illustrated in Figure 30-1, in close association with other structures of the carotid sheath, vagus nerve, and styloid process. The glossopharyngeal nerve descends in the neck, passes between the internal carotid and the external carotid arteries, and then divides into pharyngeal branches and motor branches to the stylopharyngeus muscle, as well as branches innervating the area of the palatine tonsil and the posterior third of the tongue. These distal branches of the glossopharyngeal nerve are located submucosally immediately posterior to the palatine tonsil, deep to the posterior tonsillar pillar.

Position.   Glossopharyngeal block can be carried out intraorally or in a peristyloid manner. If the block is to be carried out intraorally, the patient must be able to open the mouth, and sufficient topical anesthesia of the tongue must be provided to allow needle placement at the base of the posterior tonsillar pillar. If the block is to be carried out in a peristyloid manner, the patient does not need to be able to open the mouth.

Needle Puncture: Intraoral Glossopharyngeal Block.   After topical anesthesia of the tongue, the patient's mouth is opened widely and the posterior tonsillar pillar (palatopha-ryngeal fold) is identified by using a no. 3 Macintosh laryngoscope blade. An angled 22-gauge, 9-cm needle (see comment in Pearls section) is inserted in the caudad portion of the posterior tonsillar pillar. The needle tip is inserted submucosally and then, after careful aspiration for blood, 5 mL of local anesthetic is injected. The block is repeated on the contralateral side (Fig. 30-2).

Needle Puncture: Peristyloid Approach.   The patient lies supine with the head in a neutral position. Marks are placed on the mastoid process and the angle of the mandible, as illustrated in Figure 30-3. A line is drawn between these two marks, and at the midpoint of that line the needle is inserted to contact the styloid process. To facilitate styloid identification, a finger palpates the styloid process with deep pressure and, although this can be uncomfortable for the patient, the short 22-gauge needle is then inserted until it impinges on the styloid process. This needle is then withdrawn and redirected off the styloid process posteriorly. As soon as bony contact is lost and aspiration for blood is negative, 5 to 7 mL of local anesthetic is injected. The block can then be repeated on the contralateral side.

POTENTIAL PROBLEMS

Both the intraoral and the peristyloid blocks have few complications if careful aspiration for blood is carried out. In the peristyloid approach, the glossopharyngeal nerve is closely related to both the internal jugular vein and the internal carotid artery. In the intraoral approach, the terminal branches of the glossopharyngeal nerves are closely related to the internal carotid arteries, which lie immediately lateral to the needle tips if they are correctly positioned.

PEARLS

A frequent problem with the intraoral glossopharyngeal block is finding a needle to use for the block. This problem can be easily overcome by using a 22-gauge disposable

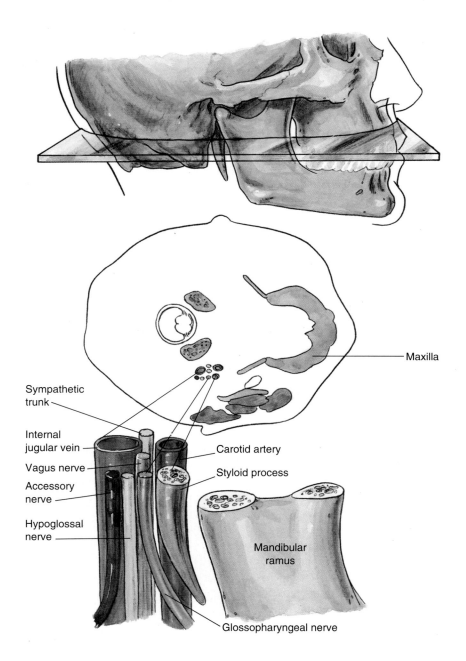

Figure 30-1. Glossopharyngeal block: cross-sectional view of peristyloid anatomy with detail.

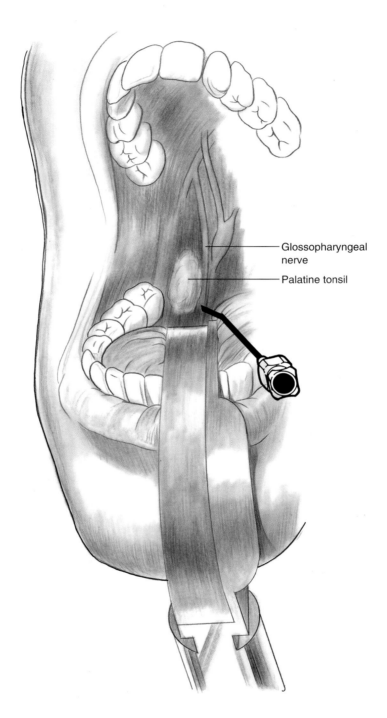

Figure 30-2. Glossopharyngeal block: intraoral anatomy and technique.

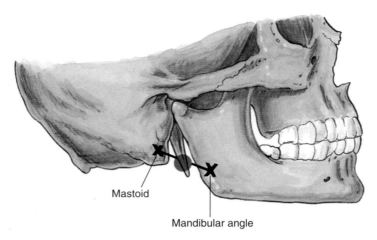

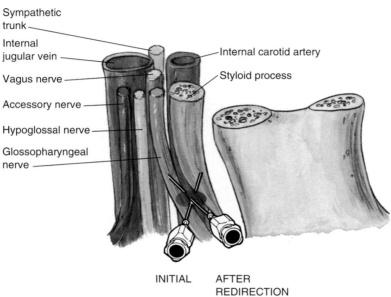

Figure 30-3. Glossopharyngeal block: peristyloid technique.

spinal needle. In an aseptic manner, the stylet should be removed from the disposable spinal needle and discarded. Subsequently, using the sterile container in which the 22-gauge spinal needle was packaged, the distal 1 cm of the needle is bent to allow more control during submucosal insertion.

This block is underused when airway anesthesia is needed for sedated, spontaneously ventilating, "awake" patients requiring tracheal intubation. I believe that the block is effective in further reducing the gag reflex that results from pressure on the posterior third of the tongue, even after adequate topical mucosal anesthesia has been obtained.

Superior Laryngeal Block 31

David L. Brown

PERSPECTIVE

The superior laryngeal nerve block is one of the methods of providing airway anesthesia. Block of the superior laryngeal nerve provides anesthesia of the larynx from the epiglottis to the level of the vocal cords.

Patient Selection.   This block may be appropriate for any patient requiring tracheal intubation before anesthetic induction.

Pharmacologic Choice.   Lidocaine (0.5%) is an appropriate local anesthetic for this block.

PLACEMENT

Anatomy.   The superior laryngeal nerve is a branch of the vagus nerve. After it leaves the main vagal trunk, it courses through the neck and passes medially, caudal to the greater cornu of the hyoid bone, at which point it divides into an internal branch and an external branch. The internal branch is the nerve of interest in superior laryngeal nerve block, and it is blocked where it enters the thyrohyoid membrane just inferior to the caudal aspect of the hyoid bone (Fig. 31-1).

Position.   The patient is placed supine with the neck extended. The anesthesiologist should displace the hyoid bone toward the side to be blocked by grasping it between the index finger and the thumb (Fig. 31-2). A 25-gauge, short needle is then inserted to make contact with the greater cornu of the hyoid. The needle is "walked off" the caudal edge of the hyoid and advanced 2 to 3 mm so that the needle tip rests between the thyrohyoid membrane laterally and the laryngeal mucosa medially. Two to 3 mL of the drug is then injected; an additional 1 mL is injected while the needle is withdrawn.

POTENTIAL PROBLEMS

It is possible to place the needle into the interior of the larynx with this approach, although that should not result in long-term problems. If the block is carried out as described, intravascular injection should be infrequent despite the presence of the superior laryngeal artery and vein, which pierce the thyrohyoid membrane with the internal laryngeal nerve.

PEARLS

One helpful maneuver when performing this block is to firmly displace the hyoid bone toward the side to be blocked, even if it causes the patient some minor discomfort. The discomfort usually can be minimized by using appropriate amounts of sedation. If a three-ring syringe is used, the sedation, coupled with an efficient block, provides an acceptable experience for both patient and anesthesiologist.

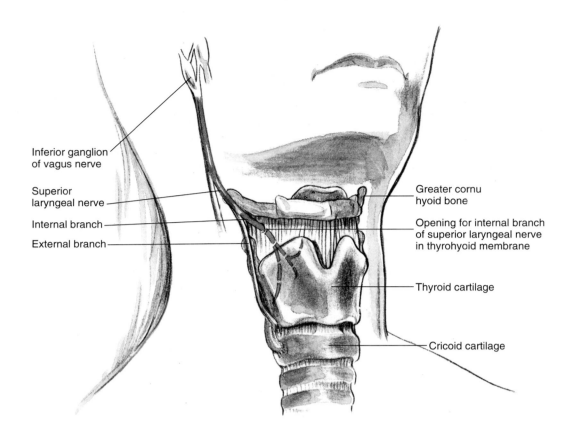

Figure 31-1. Superior laryngeal nerve block: anatomy.

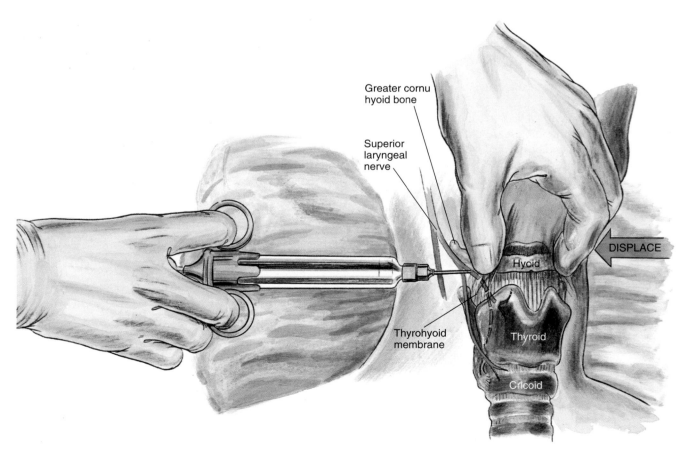

Figure 31-2. Superior laryngeal nerve block: technique.

Translaryngeal Block 32

David L. Brown

PERSPECTIVE

This block, like all airway blocks, can be useful in sedated, spontaneously ventilating, "awake" patients requiring tracheal intubation.

Patient Selection. Any patient is a candidate in whom it is desirable to avoid the Valsalva-like straining that may follow awake tracheal intubation (in which the patient is sedated and spontaneously ventilating).

Pharmacologic Choice. The local anesthetic most often chosen for this block is 3 to 4 mL of 4% lidocaine. When multiple airway blocks are administered, the anesthesiologist should be aware of the total dose of local anesthetic used.

PLACEMENT

Anatomy. Translaryngeal block is most useful in providing topical anesthesia to the laryngotracheal mucosa innervated by branches of the vagus nerve. Both surfaces of the epiglottis and laryngeal structures to the level of the vocal cords receive innervation through the internal branch of the superior laryngeal nerve, a branch of the vagus. The distal airway mucosa also receives innervation through the vagus nerve but through the recurrent laryngeal nerve. Translaryngeal injection of local anesthetic is helpful in providing topical anesthesia for both of these vagal branches because injection below the cords through the cricothyroid membrane results in the solution being spread onto the tracheal structures and coughed onto the more superior laryngeal structures (Fig. 32-1).

Position. The patient should be in a supine position, with the pillow removed and the neck slightly extended. As illustrated in Figure 32-2, the anesthesiologist should be in position to place the index and third fingers in the space between the thyroid and the cricoid cartilages (cricothyroid membrane).

Needle Puncture. The cricothyroid membrane should be localized, the midline identified, and the needle, 22-gauge or smaller, inserted into the midline until air can be freely aspirated. When air can be freely aspirated, 3 mL of local anesthetic is rapidly injected. The needle should be removed immediately because it is almost inevitable that the patient will cough at this point. Conversely, a needle-over-the-catheter assembly (intravenous catheter) can be used for the block. Once air has been aspirated, the inner needle is removed and the injection is performed through the catheter.

POTENTIAL PROBLEMS

This block can result in coughing, which should be considered in patients in whom coughing is clearly undesirable. The midline should be used for needle insertion because the area is nearly devoid of major vascular structures. The needle does not need to be misplaced far off the midline to encounter significant arterial and venous vessels.

PEARLS

This block is most effective after the patient has been appropriately sedated. There has long been a belief that this block should be used cautiously, if at all, in patients at high risk for gastric aspiration. My belief is that the block is more frequently misused by not being applied in appropriate situations than by being applied when the patient is at risk for gastric aspiration.

Another hint is to perform the local anesthetic injection after asking the patient to forcefully exhale. This forces the patient to initially inspire before coughing, making distal airway anesthesia predictable.

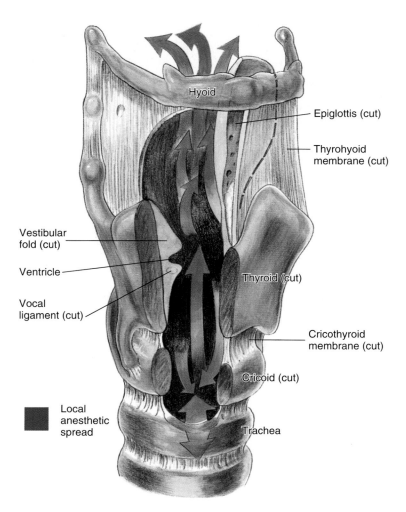

Figure 32-1. Translaryngeal block: anatomy and local anesthetic spread.

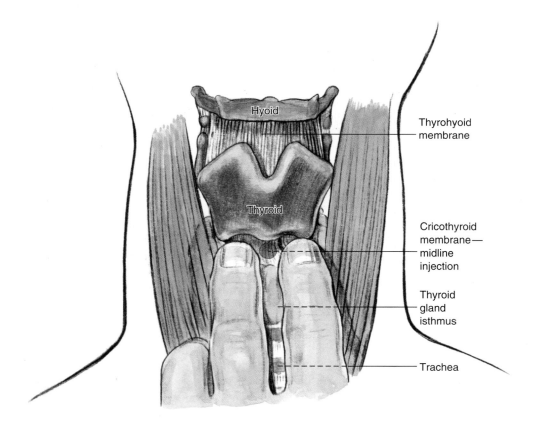

Figure 32-2. Translaryngeal block: anatomy and technique.

SECTION
Truncal Blocks

VI

Truncal Block Anatomy 33

David L. Brown

A number of regional anesthetic techniques rely on block of the thoracic or lumbar somatic (paravertebral) nerves. As illustrated in Figure 33-1, thoracic and lumbar somatic innervation extends from the chest and axilla to the toes. Although few major surgical procedures can be carried out under somatic block alone, appropriate use of somatic block with long-acting local anesthetics provides unique and useful analgesia. Also, when even longer-acting local anesthetics become available, possibly some form of thoracic or lumbar somatic nerve block, such as intercostal or paravertebral nerve block, will be able to provide even more useful postoperative analgesia. This is approaching clinical relevance with thoracic paravertebral use during care of patients undergoing breast surgery.

One of the advantages that somatic (paravertebral) block has over neuraxial blocks is the ability to avoid widespread interruption of the sympathetic nervous system. As shown in Figure 33-2, the major somatic nerves are the ventral rami of the thoracic and lumbar nerves. In addition, as shown in the inset in Figure 33-2, the nerves contribute preganglionic sympathetic fibers to the sympathetic chain through the white rami communicantes and receive postganglionic neurons from the sympathetic chain through gray rami communicantes. These rami from the sympathetic system connect to the spinal nerves near their exit from the intervertebral foramina. The dorsal rami of these spinal nerves provide innervation to dorsal midline structures. The medial branch of the dorsal primary ramus supplies the dorsal vertebral structures, including the supraspinous and intraspinous ligaments, the periosteum, and the fibrous capsule of the facet joint.

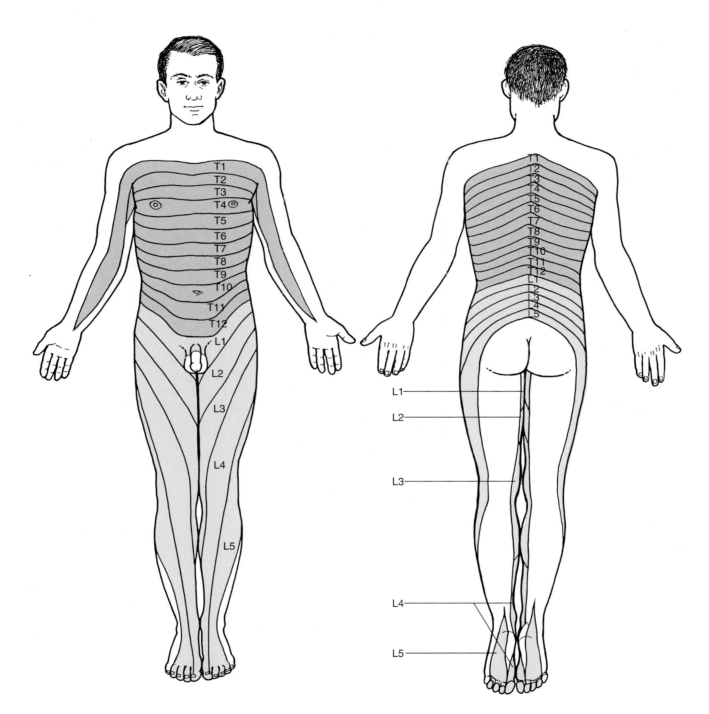

Figure 33-1. Truncal anatomy: dermatomes.

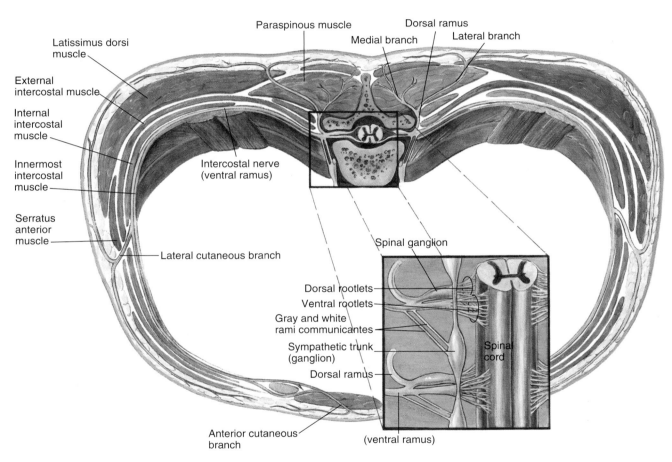

Figure 33-2. Truncal anatomy: cross-sectional view.

Breast Block 34

David L. Brown

There is increasing emphasis on carrying out "lesser" surgical procedures for breast cancer. These lesser procedures often consist of lumpectomy or simple mastectomy and avoid extensive chest wall procedures that in the past also involved shoulder structures. For this reason, breast blocks may become more appropriate for women undergoing operations for breast cancer.

Patient Selection.   Any individual requiring a breast surgical procedure is a candidate for breast block, although appropriate sedation for the block and procedure must be kept in mind.

Pharmacologic Choice.   This block is designed to provide sensory block rather than motor block. For this reason, lower concentrations of local anesthetic are possible. For example, 0.75% to 1% lidocaine or mepivacaine is appropriate, as is 0.25% bupivacaine or 0.2% ropivacaine if longer duration of postoperative analgesia is the goal.

PLACEMENT

Anatomy.   The nerves that must be blocked to carry out the breast block are the second through seventh intercostal (ventral rami for paravertebral) nerves and some terminal branches from the superficial cervical plexus (Fig. 34-1).

Position.   This block can be carried out with the patient in the supine position if block of the intercostal nerves is undertaken in the midaxillary line. Conversely, the same somatic nerves can be blocked from a posterior approach if the patient is placed in the prone position.

Needle Puncture.   This block can be carried out with the patient in the supine position by performing intercostal nerve block from T2 to T7 in the patient's midaxillary line, as shown in Figure 34-2A. Fewer intercostal nerves may be blocked if a limited breast procedure is planned, allowing a more tailored approach. In any event, the patient's arm should be abducted at the shoulder and placed on an arm board or "tucked under" the head, as shown in Figure 34-2A. The intercostal nerve block can be carried out by using a 22-gauge, short-beveled, 3-cm needle and placing 4 to 5 mL of local anesthetic solution inferior to each rib after "walking" the needle tip off each rib's inferior border. If insufficient analgesia is produced, subcutaneous infiltra-tion may have to be added because the lateral cutaneous branches of the intercostal nerve may have been missed. This is possible because the lateral cutaneous nerve may branch more posteriorly in some patients. In addition to the intercostal nerve block, subcutaneous infiltration of local anesthetic must be performed in an "upside-down L" pattern, as shown in Figure 34-2C. This infraclavicular infiltration must be added to interrupt those branches of the superficial cervical plexus that provide sensation to portions of the upper chest wall. Subcutaneous infiltration is also required in the midline to block those intercostal nerve fibers that cross the midline from the contralateral side. Subcutaneous infiltration is facilitated by using a 10- to 12-cm needle.

If a posterior approach to the intercostal nerves (or paravertebral block) is used, the patient must be placed in the prone position and intercostal nerve block carried out by "walking" the needle off, and immediately inferior to, the ribs from T2 through T7 (see Fig. 34-2B). This technique is described in Chapter 35, Intercostal Block. If a paravertebral block is planned, the technique is described in Chapter 39, Paravertebral Block. In any event, if the posterior approach is chosen, the subcutaneous infiltration, as previously outlined, must also be added.

POTENTIAL PROBLEMS

Pneumothorax can occur with this technique (or with paravertebral block), although it should be infrequent.

PEARLS

Due to the understandable anxiety that often accompanies breast surgery, patients should understand before undergoing this anesthetic approach that heavy sedation or light general anesthesia (total intravenous anesthesia, or TIVA) is most often appropriate in combination with the breast block. Patients who desire to maintain a sense of control during reconstructive or augmentation breast surgery are ideal candidates for a technique in which the loss of control accompanying general anesthesia is avoided. Finally, an emerging trend, thoracic paravertebral blocks (see Chapter 39, Paravertebral Block) are often used effectively in place of the intercostal portion of this nerve block.

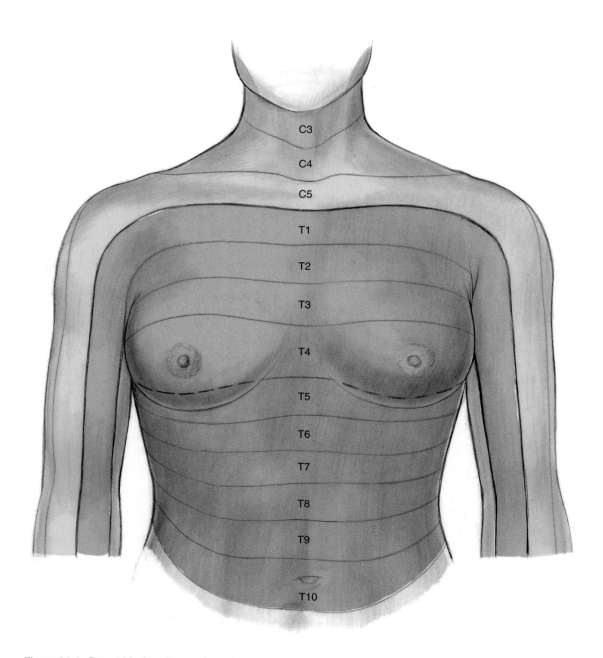

Figure 34-1. Breast block anatomy: dermatomes.

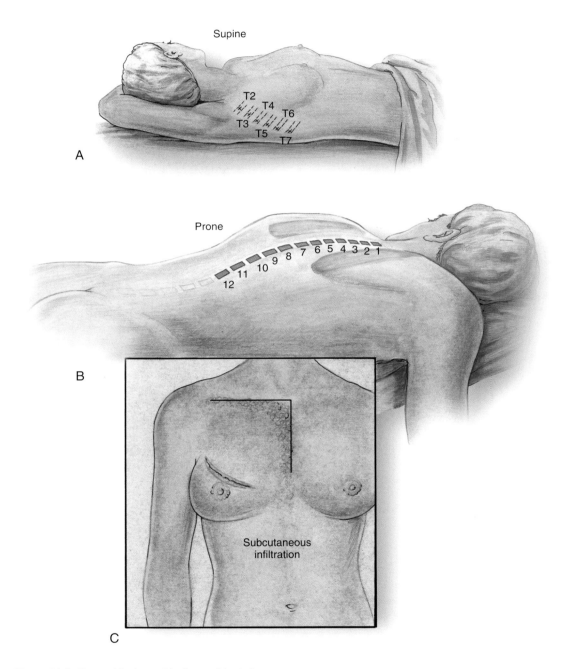

Figure 34-2. Breast block: positioning and technique.

Intercostal Block 35

David L. Brown

PERSPECTIVE

Intercostal nerve blocks provide unexcelled analgesia of the body wall. Thus it is appropriate to use the technique for analgesia after upper abdominal and thoracic surgery or for rib fracture analgesia. It is possible to perform minor surgical procedures on the chest or abdominal wall using only intercostal blocks, but most often some supplementation is appropriate. This block can also be used when chest tubes (thoracostomy tubes) are placed or when feeding gastrostomy tubes are inserted.

Patient Selection. All patients are candidates for this block, although as patients become more obese, the blocks are technically more difficult to carry out.

Pharmacologic Choice. As with any decision about the choice of local anesthetic, it must be decided whether motor blockade will be required for a successful block. If intercostal nerve block is combined with light general anesthesia for intraabdominal surgery and the intercostal block is prescribed to provide abdominal muscle relaxation, a higher concentration of local anesthetic will be needed. In this setting, 0.5% bupivacaine or ropivacaine, 1.5% lidocaine, or 1.5% mepivacaine is an appropriate choice. Conversely, if sensory analgesia is all that is necessary from the block, then 0.25% bupivacaine, 0.2% ropivacaine, 1% lidocaine, or 1% mepivacaine is appropriate.

PLACEMENT

Anatomy. The intercostal nerves are the ventral rami of T1 through T11. The twelfth thoracic nerve travels a subcostal course and is technically not an intercostal nerve. The subcostal nerve can provide branches to the ilioinguinal and iliohypogastric nerves. Some fibers from the first thoracic nerve also unite with fibers from C8 to form the lowest trunk of the brachial plexus. The other notable variation in intercostal nerve anatomy is the contribution of some fibers from T2 and T3 to the formation of the intercostobrachial nerve. The terminal distribution of this nerve is to the skin of the medial aspect of the upper arm.

Examination of an individual intercostal nerve shows that there are five principal branches (Fig. 35-1). The intercostal nerve contributes preganglionic sympathetic fibers to the sympathetic chain through the white rami communicantes *(branch 1)* and receives postganglionic neurons from the sympathetic chain ganglion through the gray rami communicantes *(branch 2).* These rami are joined to the spinal nerves near their exit from the intervertebral foramina. Also, shortly after exiting from the intervertebral foramina, the dorsal rami carrying posterior cutaneous and motor fibers *(branch 3)* supply skin and muscles in the paravertebral region. The lateral cutaneous branch of the intercostal nerve arises just anterior to the midaxillary line before sending subcutaneous fibers posteriorly and anteriorly *(branch 4).* The termination of the intercostal nerve is known as the anterior cutaneous branch *(branch 5).* Medial to the angle of the rib, the intercostal nerve lies between the pleura and the internal intercostal fascia. In the paravertebral region, there is loose areolar and fatty tissue between the nerve and the pleura. At the rib's posterior angle, the area most commonly used during intercostal nerve block, the nerve lies between the internal intercostal muscles and the intercostalis intimus muscle. Throughout the intercostal nerve's course, it traverses the intercostal spaces inferior to the intercostal artery and vein of the same space.

Position. To block the intercostal nerve in its preferred location (i.e., just lateral to the paraspinous muscles at the angle of the ribs), the patient ideally is placed in the prone position. A pillow should be placed under the patient's midabdomen to reduce lumbar lordosis and to accentuate the intercostal spaces posteriorly. The arms should be allowed to hang down from the edge of the block table (or gurney) to permit the scapula to rotate as far laterally as possible.

Needle Puncture. It is advisable to use a marking pen to outline the pertinent anatomy for most regional blocks, and in no block is this more important than in the intercostal nerve block. The midline should be marked from T1 to L5; then two paramedian lines should be drawn at the posterior angle of the ribs. These lines should angle medially in the upper thoracic region so that they parallel the medial edge of the scapula. By successfully palpating and marking the inferior edge of each rib along these two paramedian lines, a diagram like that shown in Figure 35-2 is created. Before needle puncture, appropriate intravenous sedation should be administered to produce amnesia and analgesia during the multiple injections needed for the block. Barbiturates, benzodiazepines, ketamine, or short-acting opioids can be combined. Skin wheals are raised with a 30-gauge needle at each of the previously marked sites of injection, and then intercostal block is carried out bilaterally. As illustrated in Figure 35-3, a 22-gauge,

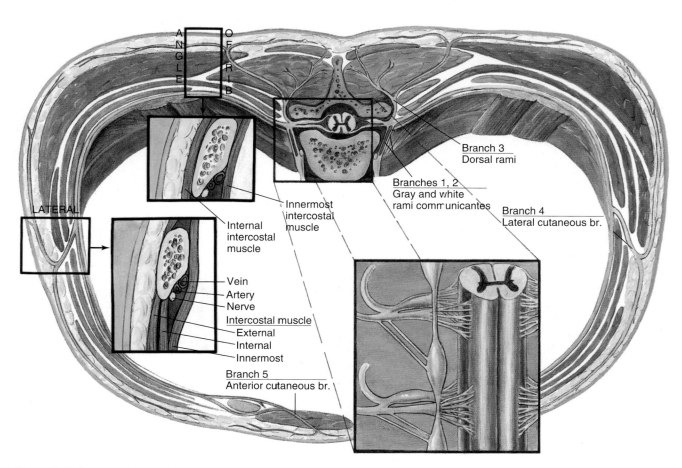

Branch 3
Dorsal rami

Branches 1, 2
Gray and white
rami communicantes

Branch 4
Lateral cutaneous br.

Innermost
intercostal
muscle

Internal
intercostal
muscle

Vein
Artery
Nerve
Intercostal muscle
External
Internal
Innermost

Branch 5
Anterior cutaneous br.

ANGLE OF RIB

LATERAL

Figure 35-1. Intercostal nerve block: cross-sectional anatomy.

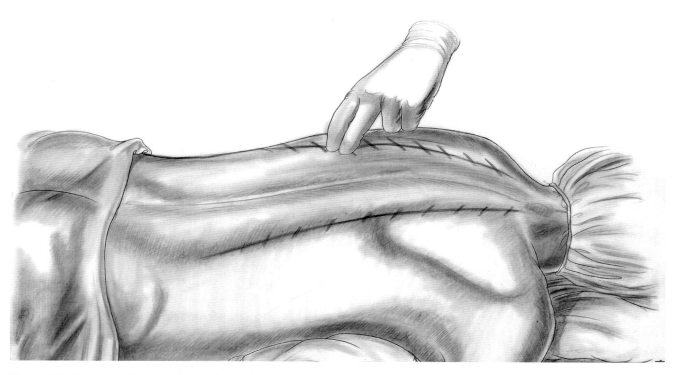

Figure 35-2. Intercostal block: position and technique.

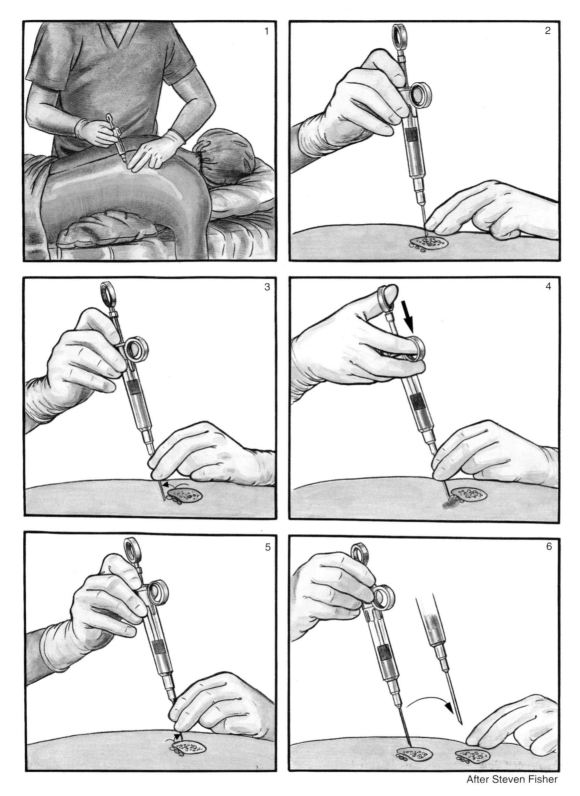

Figure 35-3. Intercostal block: stepwise technique (1 to 6).

After Steven Fisher

short-beveled, 3- to 4-cm needle is attached to a 10-mL control syringe. It is important that the anesthesiologist adhere to the hand and finger positions illustrated in Figure 35-3 and incorporate them into his or her systematic technique.

Beginning at the most caudal rib to be blocked, the index and third fingers of the left hand are used to retract the skin up and over the rib. The needle should be introduced through the skin between the tips of the retracting fingers and advanced until it contacts rib. It is important not to allow the needle to enter a depth greater than the depth that the palpating fingers define as rib. Once the needle contacts the rib, the right hand firmly maintains this contact while the left hand is shifted to hold the needle's hub and shaft between the thumb, the index finger, and the middle finger. The left hand's hypothenar eminence should be firmly placed against the patient's back. This hand placement allows maximal control of the needle

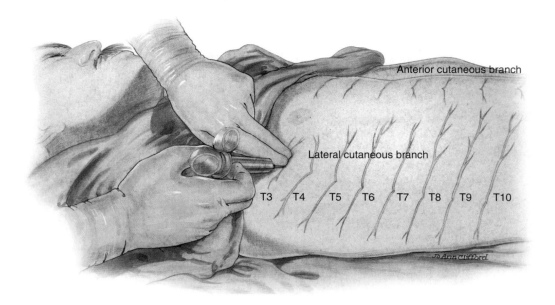

Figure 35-4. Intercostal block: lateral technique.

depth as the left hand "walks" the needle off the inferior margin of the rib and into the intercostal groove (i.e., a distance of 2 to 4 mm past the edge of the rib). With the needle in position, 3 to 5 mL of local anesthetic solution is injected. The process is then repeated for each of the nerves to be blocked. In certain patients with cachexia or a severe barrel chest deformity, the intercostal injection can be most effectively carried out with an even shorter 23- or 25-gauge needle.

Intercostal block at the posterior angle of the rib is not the only method applicable to clinical regional anesthesia. As outlined in Chapter 34, Breast Block, intercostal block also can be effectively carried out at the midaxillary line while the patient is in a supine position (Fig. 35-4). This position is clinically more convenient in many situations and probably underused. Some anesthesiologists are concerned that the lateral approach to the intercostal nerve may miss the lateral cutaneous branch of the intercostal nerve. This does not seem to be the case clinically, and computed tomographic studies show that injected solutions spread readily along the subcostal groove for a distance of many centimeters. Therefore even when lateral intercostal block is carried out, the lateral branch should most often be bathed with local anesthetic solution.

POTENTIAL PROBLEMS

The principal concern with intercostal nerve block is pneumothorax. Although the incidence of this complication is extremely low, many physicians avoid this block because of the imagined high frequency and seriousness of complications. Data suggest that the incidence of pneumothorax is less than 0.5%, and even when it occurs, careful clinical observation is usually all that is necessary. The incidence of symptomatic pneumothorax after intercostal block is even lower—approximately 1 in 1000. If treatment is deemed necessary, often needle aspiration can produce reexpansion of the lung. Chest tube drainage should be performed only if the lung fails to reexpand after observation or percutaneous aspiration.

Because of the vascularity of the intercostal space, blood levels of local anesthetic are higher for multiple-level intercostal block than for any other standard regional anesthetic technique. Because these peak blood levels may be delayed for 15 to 20 minutes, patients should be closely monitored after the completion of a block for at least that interval.

PEARLS

Effective intercostal nerve block requires adequate sedation so that patients are able to lie comfortably on the table during the block. Combinations of sedatives seem to be the most effective, and patients find a combination of benzodiazepine with a short-acting narcotic or ketamine acceptable. The anesthesiologist should develop a recipe for sedation; likewise, the anesthesiologist should develop a consistent method of maintaining hand and needle control for the block.

Interpleural Anesthesia

36

David L. Brown

PERSPECTIVE

Interpleural anesthesia is a technique developed in an attempt to simplify body wall and visceral anesthesia after upper abdominal or thoracic surgery. Although considerable research has been carried out on the technique, accurate stratification of the risks and benefits of interpleural anesthesia remains elusive, and it is primarily a technique of historical interest.

Patient Selection.   Patients undergoing upper abdominal or flank surgery or those recovering from fractured ribs have been most frequently selected for interpleural anesthesia. The appropriate selection of these patients remains ill defined.

Pharmacologic Choice.   Most commonly, 20 to 30 mL of local anesthetic solution is injected through the interpleural needle or catheter. The most common local anesthetic concentrations used have been 0.25% to 0.5% bupivacaine or 0.2% to 0.5% ropivacaine.

PLACEMENT

Anatomy.   The pleural space extends from the apex of the lung to the inferior reflection of the pleura at approximately L1. The pleural space also relates to the posterior and anterior mediastinal structures, as illustrated in Figure 36-1.

Position.   The patient is most often turned to an oblique position with the side to be blocked uppermost, as illustrated in Figure 36-2. The anesthesiologist stands facing the patient's back.

Needle Puncture.   Once the patient is positioned properly and supported by a pillow, a skin wheal is raised immediately superior to the eighth rib in the seventh intercostal space, approximately 10 cm lateral to the midline. If a continuous technique is selected, a needle allowing passage of a catheter (often epidural) is selected. If a single-injection technique is chosen, a short, beveled needle of sufficient length to reach the pleural space can be used. (The proponents of this block most often advocate intermittent injections by catheter; thus a single-injection technique is unusual.) Before inserting the needle, a syringe containing approximately 2 mL of saline solution is inserted immediately superior to the eighth rib, using a loss-of-resistance

technique much like that used during epidural anesthesia. When the needle tip is in the pleural space, it is very easy to inject local anesthetic solution.

Conversely, some clinicians are proponents of a modified hanging-drop technique to identify entry into the pleural space. These anesthesiologists suggest a new term, *falling column,* to describe this technique. If the syringe plunger shown in Figure 36-2 is removed and the column of solution in the syringe barrel is observed, entry of the needle tip into the pleural space is identified by a falling column of saline solution. The needle is then secured, and the procedure continues as it does with the loss-of-resistance method.

Once the needle is in position, either the local anesthetic is injected, if it is to be a single-injection technique, or a catheter is threaded through the needle. If a catheter is used, it should be threaded approximately 10 cm into the pleural space, taking care to minimize the volume of air entrained through the needle. The catheter is then taped in a position that will not interfere with the surgical procedure, and local anesthetic is injected. Typically, 20 to 30 mL of local anesthetic is injected, after which the patient is rolled into the supine position to allow distribution of the anesthetic.

POTENTIAL PROBLEMS

Although pneumothorax might seem to be associated with any technique that violates the pleural space, this complication is apparently infrequent with interpleural anesthesia. A second problem with interpleural anesthesia is the unpredictable nature of the analgesia accompanying what seems to be an otherwise acceptable technique. This may be a result of anesthesiologists' varying levels of experience with the technique, or perhaps it is the result of overzealous promotion of the technique.

PEARLS

The mechanism behind interpleural anesthesia remains uncertain. As illustrated in Figure 36-1, one mechanism proposed is that the local anesthetic diffuses from the pleural space through the intercostal membrane to reach the intercostal nerves along the chest wall. A second

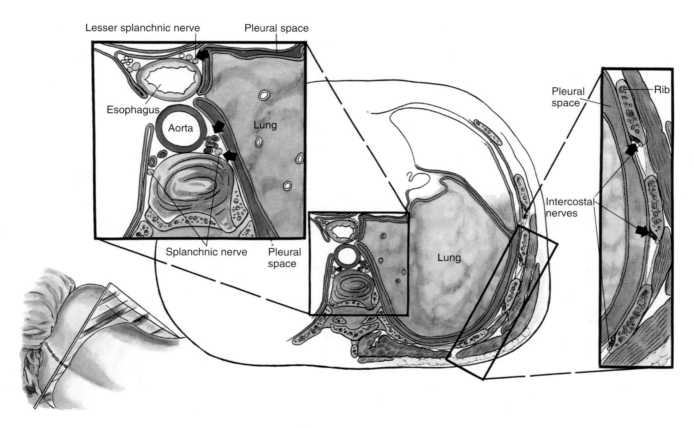

Figure 36-1. Interpleural block: anatomy.

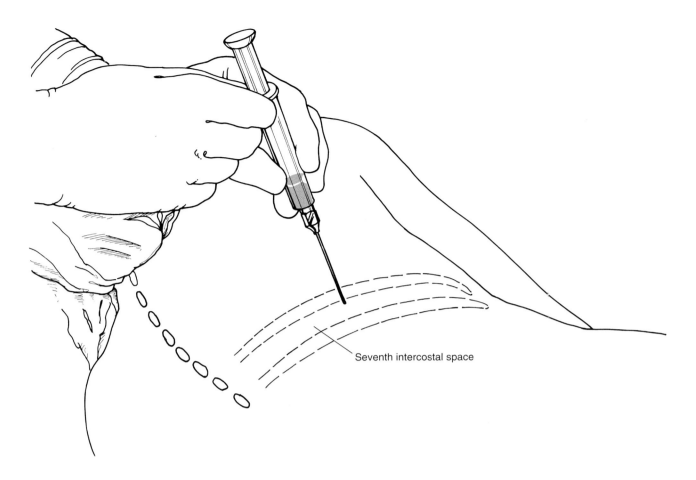

Seventh intercostal space

Figure 36-2. Interpleural block: position and technique.

mechanism is that the local anesthetic is distributed through the pleura and into the region of the posterior mediastinum, at which point the local anesthetic provides visceral analgesia by contacting the greater, lesser, and least splanchnic nerves. When more data are available, we will probably find that interpleural anesthesia results from a combination of these two mechanisms, plus the absorption of enough local anesthetic from the pleural space to produce blood levels that promote systemic analgesia.

Lumbar Somatic Block

David L. Brown

PERSPECTIVE

Lumbar somatic block is often used to complement multiple intercostal nerve blocks, thus allowing anesthesia for lower abdominal and even upper leg surgery. For example, lumbar somatic block of T12, L1, and L2 will cover most of the requirements for inguinal herniorrhaphy. Likewise, individual blocks of lumbar nerves (including block of T12 off the L1 spine) may allow differentiation of lower abdominal and postherniorrhaphy pain syndromes. Because this nerve block is carried out in a paravertebral location, it can be considered a form of paravertebral nerve block. The paravertebral block described in Chapter 39, Paravertebral Block, is a large-volume, single-injection method.

Patient Selection. Lumbar somatic block is often used in a pain clinic setting. In addition, some surgical patients, such as those undergoing herniorrhaphy, benefit from appropriate use of the block. Also, although the frequency of flank incision for renal surgical procedures has decreased since the advent of lithotripsy, patients undergoing flank incisions are well managed with a combination of lower intercostal and lumbar somatic block and light general anesthesia.

Pharmacologic Selection. The local anesthetic choice for lumbar somatic block is limited only by the extent of additional blockade and concerns over systemic toxicity. If pinpoint diagnostic accuracy is essential for chronic pain syndromes, local anesthetic volumes as small as 1 to 2 mL are appropriate; if surgical anesthesia is desired, volumes of 5 to 7 mL per lumbar root are appropriate.

PLACEMENT

Anatomy. It is useful to conceptualize paravertebral lumbar somatic block as an intercostal block in miniature. Using this concept, the short vertebral transverse process (a "rudimentary rib") becomes the principal focus and landmark for needle position. Lumbar somatic nerves leave the vertebral foramina slightly caudad and ventral to the transverse process of their respective vertebral level (Fig. 37-1).

As Figure 37-2 illustrates, from the intervertebral foramina, the lumbar somatic nerves angle caudad and anteriorly and hence pass anterior to the lateral extent of the trans-verse process of the next-lower vertebral body (see Fig. 37-1). For example, as the L1 somatic root leaves its intervertebral foramen, its route places it immediately anterior at the lateral border of the L2 transverse process. Similarly, the T12 somatic root (a subcostal nerve) is found immediately anterior at the lateral extent of the L1 transverse process.

Returning to the intercostal nerve analogy, each lumbar nerve gives off an immediate posterior branch to the paravertebral muscles and skin of the back. Again, as with intercostal nerve anatomy, the lumbar somatic nerve also receives white rami communicantes from the upper two or three lumbar nerves and gives rise to gray rami communicantes to all lumbar somatic nerves. After these connections to the sympathetic nervous system, the main somatic nerve passes directly into the psoas major muscle or comes to lie in a plane between the psoas and the quadratus lumborum muscles. Here the nerves intertwine to form the lumbar plexus. Figure 37-3 highlights this cross-sectional anatomy. Figure 37-4 illustrates the cutaneous distribution of the lumbar somatic nerves.

Position. The conceptual similarity of this block to an intercostal nerve block carries through to the actual performance of the technique. The most advantageous position is to have the patient prone with a pillow under the lower abdomen to reduce lumbar lordosis. Skin markings are made as illustrated in Figure 37-5 (i.e., the lumbar spinous process of each vertebra corresponding to the roots to be blocked is identified and marked). Then, from the cephalad edge of each of these lumbar posterior spines, lines are drawn horizontally, and marks are placed on the lines 2.5 to 3 cm from the midline (paravertebral in location). The anatomic rationale behind these markings is that the cephalad edge of each lumbar posterior spine is approximately on the same horizontal plane as its own vertebral transverse process. Skin wheals are made at the site 2.5 to 3 cm from the midline on the lines overlying the lower edge of the transverse process. Through the skin wheals an 8-cm, 22-gauge needle is inserted in a vertical plane without a syringe attached (Fig. 37-6). As the needle is advanced, it will contact the transverse process at a depth of 3 to 5 cm in the average adult (*needle position 1*). Failure to contact the transverse process at that depth implies that the needle has passed between the two transverse processes.

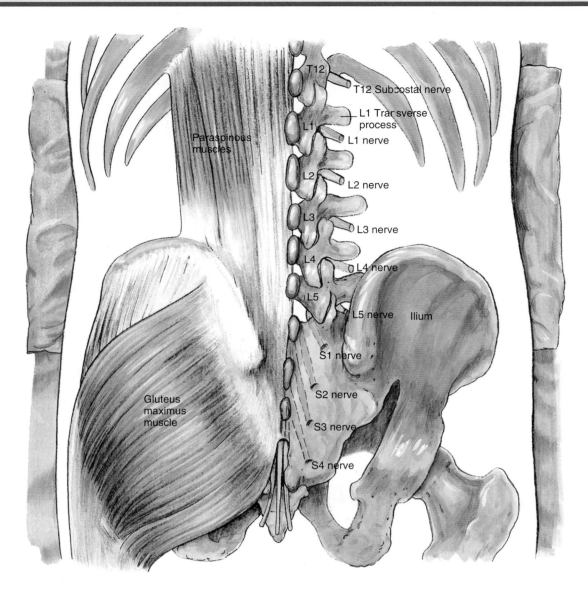

Figure 37-1. Lumbar somatic block: anatomy.

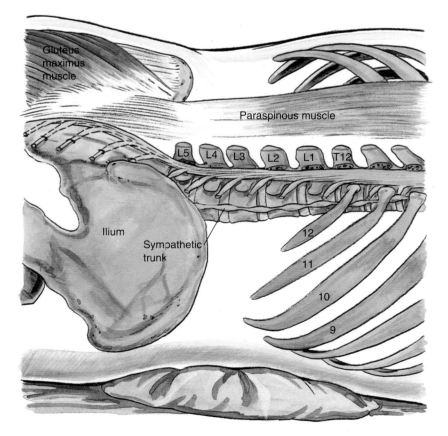

Figure 37-2. Lumbar somatic block: anatomy.

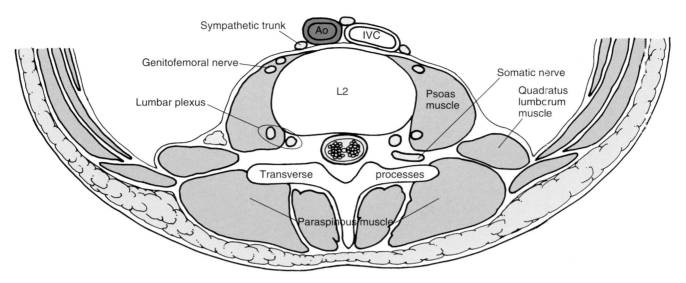

Figure 37-3. Lumbar somatic block: cross-sectional anatomy. Ao, aorta; IVC, inferior vena cava.

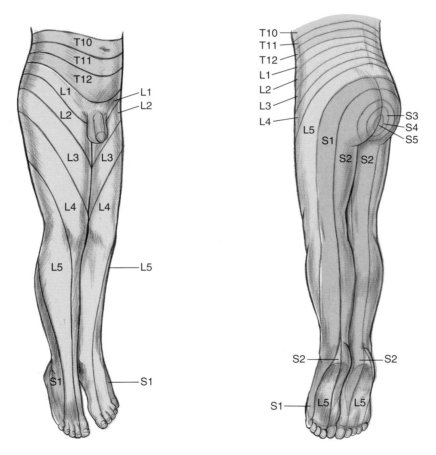

Figure 37-4. Lumbar somatic block: dermatomal anatomy.

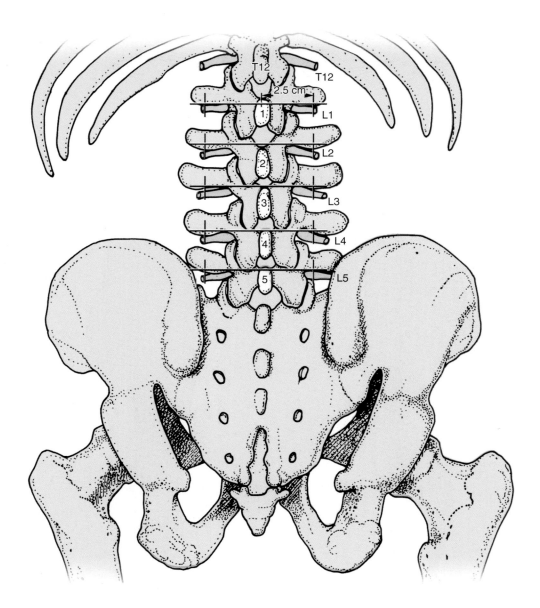

Figure 37-5. Lumbar somatic block: placement of skin markings.

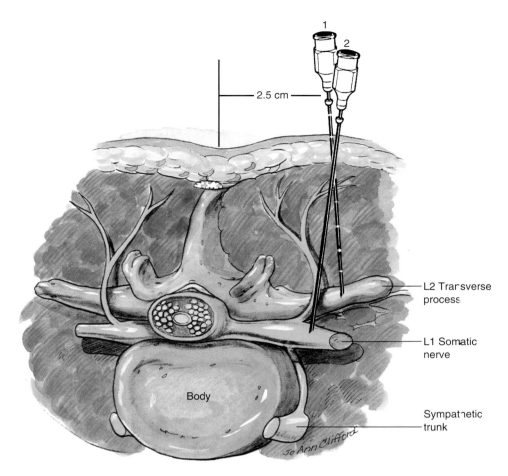

Figure 37-6. Lumbar somatic block: technique.

To contact bone, a repeat insertion is made through the same skin wheal, but with a slight cephalad angulation of the needle. Once the transverse process has been identified, the needle tip is withdrawn to a subcutaneous location before being reinserted to pass just caudad to the previously identified transverse process. This allows block of the lumbar root corresponding to the same lumbar vertebra. The needle is reinserted just cephalad to the corresponding transverse process in order to block the lumbar root one segment more cephalad. As the needle slides off and past the transverse process, it should be advanced approximately the thickness of the transverse process, or approximately 1 to 2 cm, after contact with bone is lost (*needle position 2*). This will place the tip in the plane immediately anterior to the transverse process. When the final needle position has been established, approximately 5 mL of local anesthetic solution is injected. The process should be repeated at each site at which local anesthetic block is desired.

POTENTIAL PROBLEMS

Because the lumbar roots are close to other neuraxial structures, epidural and subarachnoid anesthesia can be inadvertently produced with lumbar somatic block. It is most likely that in these cases the needle was angled medially during insertion rather than being maintained in a parasagittal plane. Likewise, because of the proximity of the sympathetic ganglion to the lumbar roots, if the needles are inserted too deeply, the volume of local anesthetic solution injected is often enough to cause lumbar sympathetic blockade. That may result in a decrease in blood pressure similar to that seen during low spinal anesthesia.

PEARLS

Blockade of the twelfth thoracic nerve is effectively carried out by blocking the root immediately superior to the L1 transverse process. This method is often preferable to attempts to block it like an intercostal nerve at the angle of the ribs. If these blocks are used for herniorrhaphy procedures, use of a long-acting local anesthetic of sufficient concentration to produce motor blockade may limit patients from walking normally for a number of hours, because some weakness of the hip flexors may be produced with blockade of the L1 and L2 roots. If this technique is chosen for pain clinic diagnostic evaluation, fluoroscopy is advised to minimize confusion over the vertebral level injected.

Inguinal Block 38

David L. Brown

Inguinal block is primarily a technique of peripheral block for inguinal herniorrhaphy.

Patient Selection. Increasing numbers of patients are undergoing inguinal herniorrhaphy as outpatients; thus this block may be incorporated in most practices.

Pharmacologic Choice. As with many of the peripheral regional blocks, motor blockade is not essential for success with inguinal block. Therefore lower concentrations of intermediate- to long-acting local anesthetics can be chosen. For example, 1% lidocaine or mepivacaine is appropriate, as is 0.25% bupivacaine or 0.2% ropivacaine. Often the surgeon must supplement inguinal block intraoperatively by injecting near the spermatic cord, so the volume of local anesthetic used during the initial block should not preclude additional intraoperative injection.

PLACEMENT

Anatomy. Innervation of the inguinal region arises from the distal extensions of the more cephalad lumbar plexus nerves: the iliohypogastric and ilioinguinal nerves, which have their origin from the first lumbar nerve, and the genitofemoral nerve, which has its origin from the first and second lumbar nerves (Fig. 38-1). These peripheral extensions of the lumbar plexus and the twelfth thoracic nerve follow a circular course that is influenced by the bowllike shape of the ilium. As these nerves course anteriorly, as illustrated in Figure 38-2, they pass near an important landmark for the block: the anterior superior iliac spine. Near the anterior superior iliac spine, the twelfth thoracic and iliohypogastric nerves lie between the internal and the external oblique muscles. The ilioinguinal nerve lies between the transversus abdominis muscle and the internal oblique muscle initially and then penetrates the internal oblique muscle some distance medial to the anterosuperior iliac spine. All these nerves continue anteriorly in a medial orientation and become superficial as they terminate in the skin and muscles of the inguinal region (Fig. 38-3). As also shown in Figure 38-3, the genitofemoral nerve follows a different course, and it is this nerve that must often be supplemented intraoperatively to make this regional block effective for inguinal herniorrhaphy.

Position. This block can be carried out with the patient in the supine position and the anesthesiologist at the patient's side in a position to use the anterosuperior iliac spine as a landmark.

Needle Puncture. The anterosuperior iliac spine should be marked while the patient is supine. Another mark should be made approximately 3 cm medial and inferior to the anterosuperior iliac spine (see Fig. 38-3). A skin wheal is created, and an 8-cm, 22-gauge needle is inserted in a cephalolateral direction (*needle position 1*) to contact the inner surface of the ilium, as illustrated in Figure 38-4. Ten mL of local anesthetic solution is injected as the needle is slowly withdrawn through the layers of the abdominal wall. The needle should then be reinserted at a steeper angle to ensure penetration of all three abdominal muscle layers (*needle position 2*). Again, the injection is repeated as the needle is withdrawn. In patients who are heavily muscled or obese, a third injection may be necessary at an even steeper angle. From the previously placed skin wheal, the injection is extended toward the umbilicus, creating a subcutaneous field block. This process is repeated from umbilicus to pubis (Fig. 38-5). Because the surgeon may need to inject additional local anesthetic into the cord, the anesthesiologist should allow for it to be added intraoperatively without concern over local anesthetic systemic toxicity.

POTENTIAL PROBLEMS

This block is primarily a superficial block and is associated with few major complications. Some proponents of this technique advocate making a preoperative injection in the region of the inguinal canal and spermatic cord. However, this additional injection may cause hematoma formation in the region of the cord. Although this does not harm the patient, it may make it difficult for the surgeon to perform an adequate surgical dissection.

PEARLS

The key to using this block successfully is to combine adequate sedation with a systematic method of injecting local anesthetic near the iliac crest. The system should be established to ensure that the anesthetic has been deposited at all body wall levels.

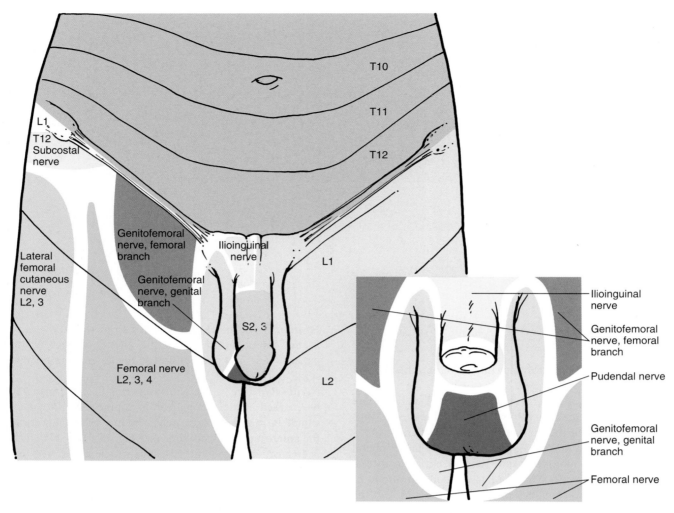

Figure 38-1. Inguinal block: dermatomal anatomy.

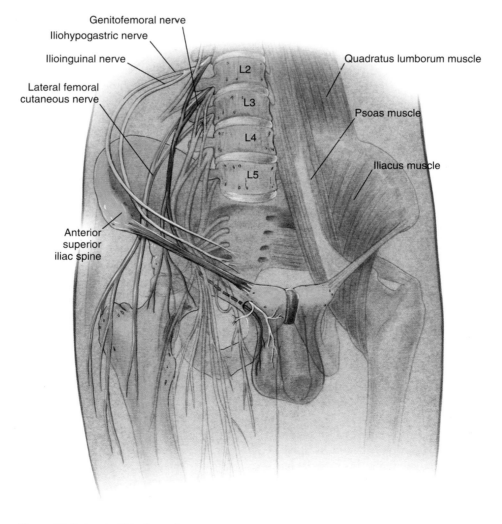

Figure 38-2. Inguinal block: anatomy.

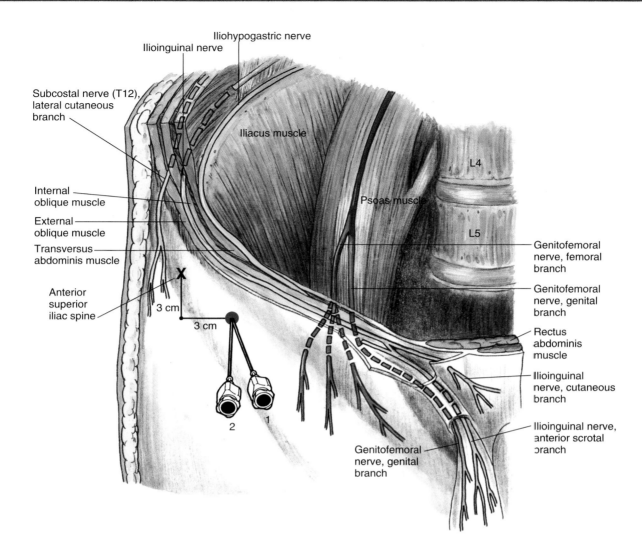

Figure 38-3. Inguinal block: anatomy and technique.

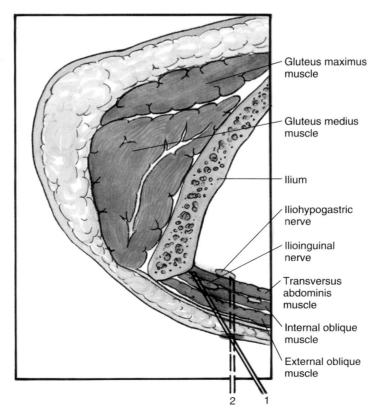

Figure 38-4. Inguinal block: cross-sectional anatomy and technique.

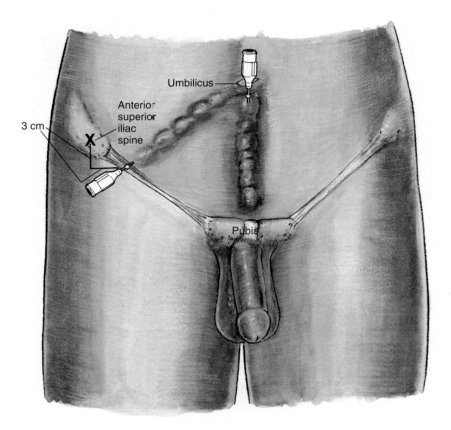

Figure 38-5. Inguinal block: infiltration technique.

Paravertebral Block 39

Ehab Farag

INDICATIONS

- Thoracic paravertebral catheter can be used in lieu of thoracic epidural analgesia for unilateral procedures like thoracotomies, nephrectomies (either partial or radical), rib fractures, and breast surgeries.
- This block is used in cases where epidural catheter is difficult or failed epidural analgesia for unilateral procedures.
- Bilateral paravertebral blocks, with or without catheter insertion, can be used for bilateral procedures with caution to avoid the development of bilateral pneumothoraces and local anesthetic overdose toxicity.

CONTRAINDICATIONS

- The same contraindications exist as with epidural catheter insertions regarding the use of anticoagulants and antiplatelet drugs.
- Pneumothorax is the main complication of thoracic paravertebral block, with or without catheter insertion. Therefore inexperience with performing regional anesthesia using ultrasound is considered a relative contraindication for thoracic paravertebral block.

SONOANATOMY

The thoracic paravertebral space lies adjacent to the thoracic spine bodies and contains the spinal nerves as they emerge from the intervertebral foramina, the anterior divisions (intercostal nerves), the posterior divisions, and the rami communicantes. The thoracic paravertebral space is sandwiched between the parietal pleura anteriorly and the superior costotransverse ligament posteriorly. The vertebral body, intervertebral disc, and intervertebral foramen form the medial boundary. The thoracic paravertebral space is connected to the level above and below, with the caudad limit being the origin of the psoas major at T12.

The thoracic paravertebral space can be scanned in both the transverse (intercostal) and paramedian approaches. In the transverse approach, the probe is aligned in the space between two adjacent ribs overlying the transverse process.

In this approach, the external intercostal muscle, internal intercostal membrane that binds medially with the costotransverse ligament, and the parietal pleura can be viewed. The landmarks in this scan are the bony reflections from the transverse process, with its dropout shadow, and the pleural reflection, which moves with respiration.

In the paramedian (longitudinal) approach, the probe lies in the paramedian plane of the transverse processes. The main landmarks in this approach are reflections and dropout from the tips of the transverse processes. The external intercostal muscle and costotransverse ligament lie between the transverse processes. The parietal pleura lie deep to these layers and can be recognized by their movement with respirations as evidenced by sliding sign and comet tails (Fig. 39-1).

TECHNIQUE

The linear ultrasound probe (50-mm footprint) is usually used for this block. In the transverse approach, the probe is aligned over the long axis of the rib; then it is moved medially to visualize the transverse process. By toggling (tilting) the probe, the external intercostal muscle, internal intercostal membrane that binds medially with the costotransverse ligament, and the parietal pleura can be identified. The needle is introduced in-plane at the lateral end of the probe from the lateral to medial direction. The needle tip should be positioned just deep to the costotransverse ligament in the paravertebral space. Local anesthetic spread should cause displacement of the pleura anteriorly.

In the paramedian (longitudinal) approach, the linear ultrasound probe (50-mm footprint) or curvilinear probe can be used for this approach. However, I prefer to use the linear probe for this block. First, the technician scans the spinous process and then moves the probe laterally to visualize the transverse process. The probe then will be rotated through 90 degrees to lie 2.5 cm lateral to the spine over the desired thoracic levels. The needle is introduced in-plane at the lower end of the probe. For better needle visualization, the probe can be rotated to lie oblique to the spine rather than parallel to it. As in the transverse approach, the needle tip should be positioned just deep to the costotransverse ligament in the paravertebral space. Injecting local anesthetics will displace the pleural anteriorly. In both techniques the catheter can be inserted via Tuohy needle (Figs 39-2, 39-3A and B, 39-4 and 39-5).

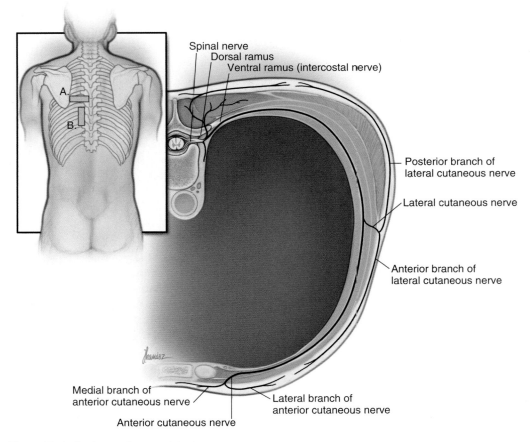

Spinal nerve
Dorsal ramus
Ventral ramus (intercostal nerve)

Posterior branch of
lateral cutaneous nerve

Lateral cutaneous nerve

Anterior branch of
lateral cutaneous nerve

Medial branch of
anterior cutaneous nerve

Lateral branch of
anterior cutaneous nerve

Anterior cutaneous nerve

Figure 39-1. Anatomy of paravertebral space.

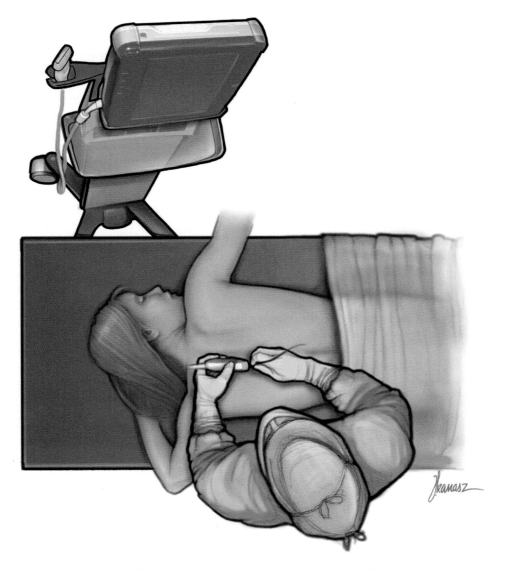

Figure 39-2. Patient positioned with ultrasound machine for paravertebral block.

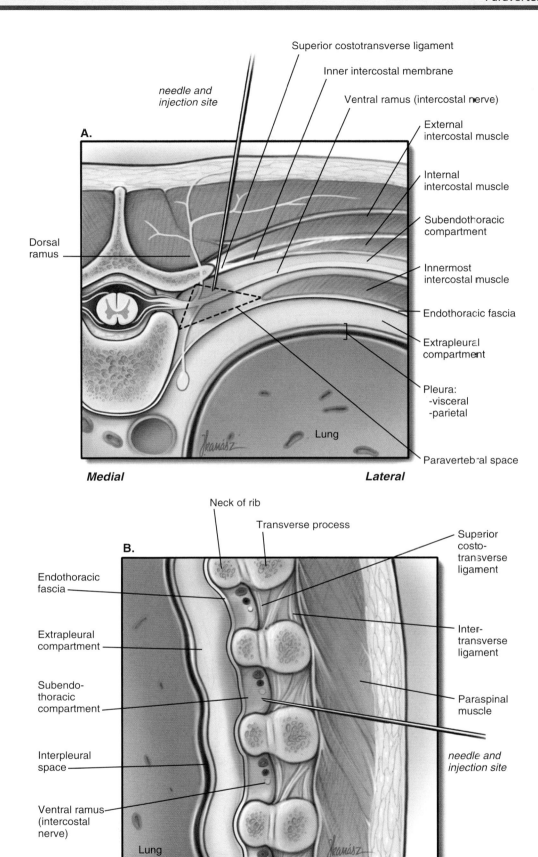

Superior costotransverse ligament

Inner intercostal membrane

Ventral ramus (intercostal nerve)

needle and injection site

A.

External intercostal muscle

Internal intercostal muscle

Subendothoracic compartment

Dorsal ramus

Innermost intercostal muscle

Endothoracic fascia

Extrapleural compartment

Pleura:
-visceral
-parietal

Lung

Paravertebral space

Medial   **Lateral**

Neck of rib

Transverse process

B.

Superior costo-transverse ligament

Endothoracic fascia

Inter-transverse ligament

Extrapleural compartment

Subendo-thoracic compartment

Paraspinal muscle

Interpleural space

Ventral ramus (intercostal nerve)

needle and injection site

Lung

Anterior   **Posterior**

Figure 39-3. A, Transverse intercostal technique for paravertebral block. Note the internal intercostal membrane binds medially with the costotransverse ligament. B, Paramedian (longitudinal) approach for paravertebral block.

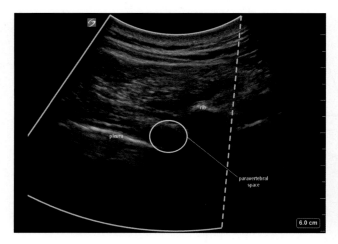

Figure 39-4. Ultrasound still of anatomy of paravertebral block.

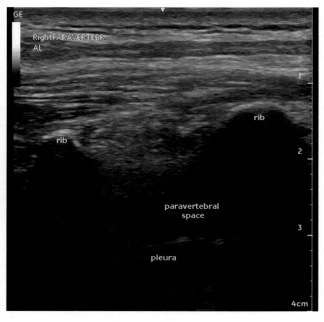

Figure 39-5. Ultrasound still of anatomy of paravertebral block.

PEARLS

- Patients may be positioned in the sitting, lateral decubitus (surgical side up), or prone position during the block.
- The parietal pleura appear as a glittering hyperechoic structure between the transverse processes.
- The presence of lung sliding, which is the to and fro movement of the lung caused by respiration, and comet tail signs rule out pneumothorax after thoracic paravertebral block.
- Patients with lung hyperventilation, as in chronic obstructive lung disease, are at higher risk of developing pneumothorax.
- The costotransverse ligament can be mistakenly identified as parietal pleura, and the injection of local anesthetics superficial to the ligament will result in block failure. Optimizing the image depth and gain will help with proper identification of the pleura and the costotransverse ligament. Furthermore, asking the patient to take a deep breath will identify the visceral and parietal pleura. The latter maneuver will cause a visible movement of the visceral and parietal pleura over each other (sliding sign).
- The paramedian approach is the preferred one for catheter insertion, as theoretically it decreases the

incidence of placing the catheter in the epidural space.
- The continuous thoracic paravertebral catheter infusion rate is 5 to 10 mL per hour of 0.2% ropivacaine. However, for paravertebral block without catheter insertion, 5 mL of 0.2% or 0.5% ropivacaine is injected at each level.
- Pneumothorax is the major complication of this block. Injections into the root canal and epidural or spinal blockade are other possible complications.

KEY POINTS

- The thoracic paravertebral block, with or without catheter, can be used in lieu of thoracic epidural catheter for unilateral procedures and for breast surgeries.
- Pneumothorax is the major complication of this block.
- When performing the block and the injection, make sure the needle tip always remains visible in the plane.

Transversus Abdominis Plane Block (Classic Approach)

40

Loran Mounir-Soliman

RELEVANT ANATOMY

The ventral rami of the lower six thoracic nerves (T7 to L1) emerge through the intervertebral foraminae to pass through the corresponding intercostal spaces and enter a fascial plane between the transversus abdominis and the internal oblique muscles of the abdominal muscular wall (known as the *transversus abdominis plane* [TAP]) accompanied by blood vessels. They follow the curvilinear course of this neurovascular plane to reach the anterior abdominal wall as far as the semilunar line at the lateral border of the rectus abdominis muscle (Fig. 40-1).

The abdominal wall consists of three muscle layers: the external oblique, the internal oblique, and the transversus abdominis muscles and their associated fascial sheaths. The three muscles, as well as the parietal peritoneum, are innervated by the ipsilateral ventral rami of T7 to L1. The external oblique and the anterior lamella of the internal oblique aponeurosis pass anteriorly to the rectus muscle, forming the anterior rectus sheath. The aponeuroses from the posterior lamella of the internal oblique muscle and the transversus abdominis muscle pass posteriorly to the rectus muscle, forming the posterior layer of the sheath. At this point, the ventral rami of the lower thoracic nerves are located between the posterior rectus sheath and the rectus muscle. They run medially within the sheath before perforating the muscle anteriorly, forming the anterior cutaneous branches. Along their course through the TAP, the lower thoracic spinal nerves give origin to the lateral cutaneous branches posterior to the midaxillary line. Within the TAP, the nerves communicate with each other, forming neural plexuses in close proximity to the vessels in this neurovascular plane.

TECHNIQUE

A linear, high-frequency probe (8 to 12 MHz) is usually used for optimal identification of the different muscle layers and their corresponding fascial sheaths. However, a curvilinear, lower-frequency probe (2 to 5 MHz) may be used in obese patients. The block can be performed in the supine position or lateral position with the side to be blocked upwards, with a wedge beneath the lower side in order to stretch the flank on the upper side. The lower costal margin and the iliac crest are identified, and the probe is placed in a transverse orientation between the two bony landmarks at the midaxillary line. The probe is moved both cephalad and caudad to get the best view of the three muscles. Scanning too medially may only show two muscle layers because the external oblique muscle forms an aponeurosis; also, scanning more posteriorly may encounter the large latissimus dorsi muscle, which may confuse the view of the muscles.

The fascial layers appear as hyperechoic structures under ultrasound, giving the muscles their characteristic multiple striations.

A blunt needle is introduced from the posterior edge of the probe with the in-plane technique (parallel to the ultrasound beam) and advanced in a medial anterior direction through the skin, subcutaneous fat, and external and internal oblique muscles to reach the interfascial layer between the internal oblique and transversus abdominis muscles (TAP). The endpoint of the needle should be superficial to the transversus abdominis muscle. Deeper to this muscle, there is a layer of preperitoneal fat separating it from the peritoneum and the bowels, which are often identified by its peristaltic movements. A blunt needle is preferred to appreciate the tactile "pop" when crossing each fascial layer. The intramuscular location of the needle within the internal oblique muscle is identified by retraction of the needle when it is released, as well as swelling of the muscle with injection instead of separation from the transversus abdominis.

INDICATIONS

- The TAP block can potentially provide unilateral analgesia to the skin, muscles, and parietal peritoneum of the anterior abdominal wall, although the extent of the block has been reported to be variable in different studies.
- Bilateral blocks have been used for midline and transverse incisions.
- Classical TAP has been reported to provide adequate analgesia following caesarian section, hysterectomy, hernia repair, kidney transplant, colostomy closure, and multiple other lower abdominal surgeries.
- Both single-shot and continuous catheters have been used successfully.
- The TAP block has been used for patients with chronic abdominal pain to identify somatic pain originating from the abdominal muscular wall and

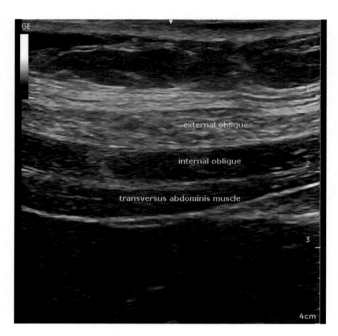

Figure 40-1. Ultrasound still of anatomy of TAP block.

the parietal peritoneum versus visceral pain, which is transmitted via sympathetic innervation instead.

KEY POINTS

- The TAP block is a tissue plane block depending on adequate spread of local anesthetics through the plane—accordingly a minimum volume of 20 mL is usually needed for effective block.

- Frequent, small incremental injections of saline while advancing the needle can identify the progress of the needle tip through the various tissue planes.
- When performed appropriately, the TAP block is very safe and devoid of major complications and can be placed safely in anesthetized patients.
- For midline incisions, bilateral blocks are needed; the rectus sheath block may be considered as an alternative.

PEARLS

- Placement of the needle as far posteriorly as possible (by the midaxillary line or behind) has the theoretical advantage of blocking the lateral cutaneous branches before they exit the TAP.
- The internal oblique muscle is usually identified as the largest muscle among the three abdominal muscles.
- The transversus abdominis muscle sometimes shows as a hypoechoic band that can be confused with the underlying preperitoneal fatty layer. The peristaltic movements of the bowels within the preperitoneal fatty layer can identify it from the muscular layer.
- An out-of-plane technique can be more suitable in obese patients when the needle path is not easily seen.

Subcostal Transversus Abdominal Plane Block

41

Ehab Farag

SONOANATOMY

There are four paired muscles of the anterolateral abdominal wall: the anterior rectus abdominis muscles and, from deep to superficial, the three lateral muscles: transversus abdominis, internal oblique, and external oblique muscles. It is only in the lateral abdomen that the three fleshy muscle bellies overlie one another because medially they become an aponeurosis. Under ultrasound the rectus abdominis can be easily identified, and by moving laterally, the transversus abdominis muscle will appear beneath the rectus abdominis muscle. The transversus abdominis has two key features on ultrasound imaging. It is usually darker (more hypoechoic) than other muscles, and it passes beneath the rectus abdominis muscle (Fig. 41-1).

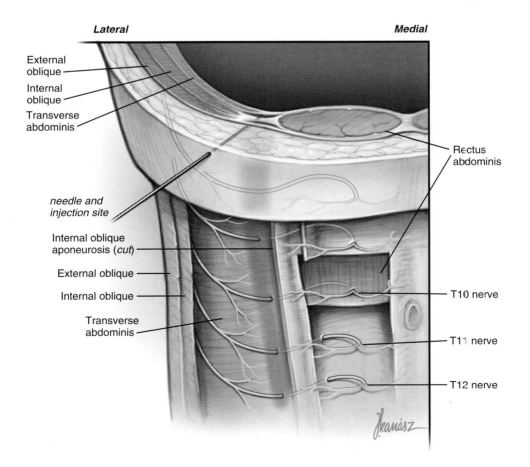

Figure 41-1. Anatomy of anterior abdominal wall.

TECHNIQUE

The linear ultrasound probe will be placed over the anterior abdominal wall immediately inferior and parallel to the costal margin. The rectus abdominis muscle will be identified medially, and then the probe will be moved laterally until the transversus abdominis muscles are identified as well. Further lateral movement of the ultrasound probe will demonstrate the lateral abdominal wall muscles (external and internal obliques and transverse abdominis muscles) to provide further confirmation of sonographic anatomy. Using the in-plane approach, the needle will be inserted from the posterolateral position and advanced anteromedially until its tip is in the fascial plane between the rectus abdominis and transverse abdominis muscles. In my practice, I usually inject 20 mL of ropivacaine 0.5% in each side of the bilateral block (Figs 41-2 through 41-4).

INDICATION

- Used in supraumbilical procedures.
- Bilateral continuous subcostal transversus abdominis plane (TAP) can be used in lieu of epidural analgesia for midline supraumbilical procedures.

KEY POINTS

- The subcostal TAP approach is very useful for supraumbilical procedures.
- The most cephalad sensory dermatomal spread is T8.
- The bilateral continuous catheter infusion can be used in the upper abdominal surgeries where epidural analgesia is contraindicated or failed.

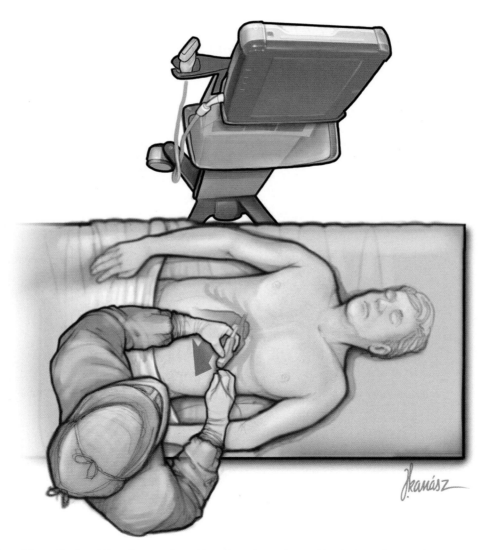

Figure 41-2. Position of the patient and the ultrasound machine. Note the probe position is immediately inferior and parallel to the costal margin. Moving the probe laterally will visualize the rectus abdominis and transverse abdominis muscles.

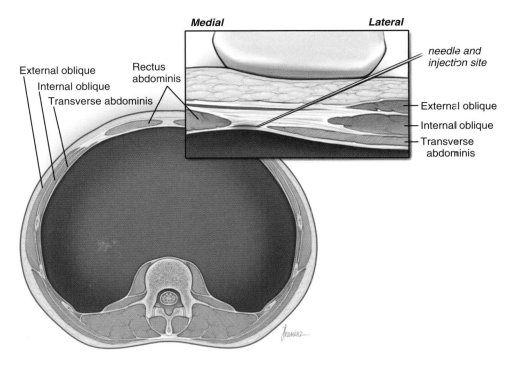

Medial   *Lateral*

External oblique
Internal oblique
Transverse abdominis

Rectus abdominis

needle and injection site

External oblique
Internal oblique
Transverse abdominis

Figure 41-3. In-plane technique for the subcostal TAP block. The needle direction is from lateral to medial.

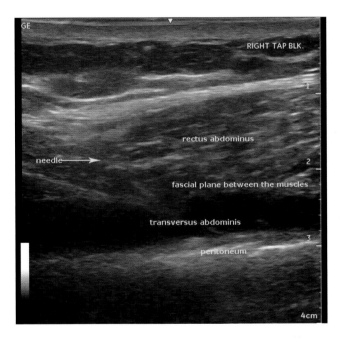

Figure 41-4. Ultrasound image of subcostal TAP block with needle.

• The key for the success of this technique is the proper identification of the fascial plane between the transversus abdominis and rectus abdominis muscles.

PEARLS

• When performing the procedure in the right side, care should be taken not to injure the liver, especially in patients with hepatomegaly or a thin patient.
• For the single-shot technique, I prefer to use 22-gauge needles; however, in the continuous catheter technique, I insert the catheter via a 17- to 18-gauge Tuohy needle.

Quadratus Lumborum Block 42

Ehab Farag

SONOANATOMY

When the ultrasound probe is placed in the posterior axillary line above the iliac crest, the transversus abdominis muscle first disappears, then the internal oblique and external oblique muscles form the aponeurosis of the quadratus lumborum (QL) muscle. Further, moving the probe posteriorly will show the QL muscle deeper to the serratus posterior inferior and latissimus dorsi muscles. Of note, the QL muscle is sandwiched between the superficial medial and deep layers of the thoracolumbar fascia (Figs 42-1 to 42-3).

TECHNIQUE

With the patient in the lateral position, the ultrasound linear probe is placed in the anterior axillary line above the iliac crest to visualize the typical triple abdominal layers, and then the probe is moved posteriorly into the posterior axillary line to visualize the aponeurosis of the QL muscle. Using the in-plane technique, the needle is inserted and its position confirmed by injecting saline. There are two types QL blocks: QL block type I, in which the injection is in the aponeurosis of the QL muscle, and type II, in which the injection is performed between the QL muscle and the

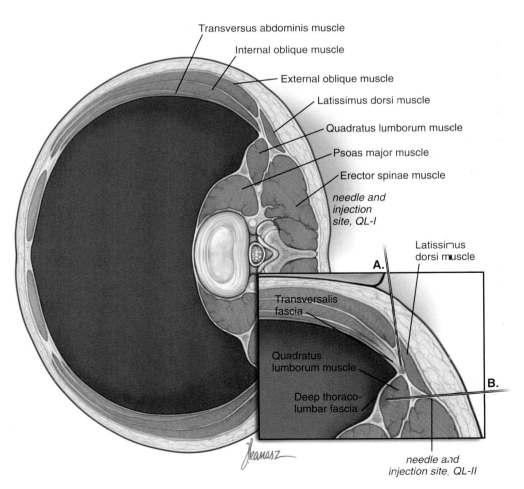

Figure 42-1. Sonoanatomy of QL block. Note the needle position for QL type I and type II

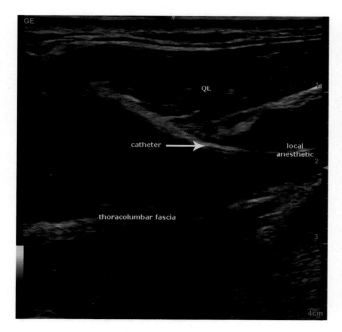

Figure 42-2. Ultrasound still of QL block procedure.

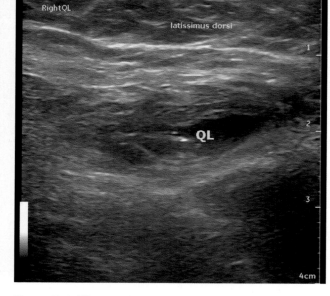

Figure 42-3. Ultrasound still of anatomy of QL block.

deep thoracolumbar fascia. For the catheter insertion technique in my practice, I visualize the QL muscle and the deep thoracolumbar fascia and insert the catheter using the in-plane technique in the space between (Fig. 42-4).

KEY POINTS

- A bilateral QL block can be used for postoperative pain relief after midline abdominal surgeries instead of epidurals.
- The sensory dermatomal coverage of the QL block can extend from T4 to L2.
- Visualizing the tapering of the abdominal muscles into the QL aponeurosis is the key to the successful block.
- The use of continuous QL block is very helpful to decrease the opioid requirement in the postoperative period.

PEARLS

- The analgesic effect of the QL block is mainly due to the accumulation of the local anesthetics in the anterior aspect of the QL and psoas muscles to lie in the paravertebral space.
- The usual initial dose is 0.3 mL/kg of ropivacaine 0.2%. However, higher doses up to 0.6 mL/kg can cover more dermatomes.
- Visualizing the peritoneum when performing this block is essential to avoid bowel injuries.
- I avoid performing this block at a higher level to avoid renal injury.

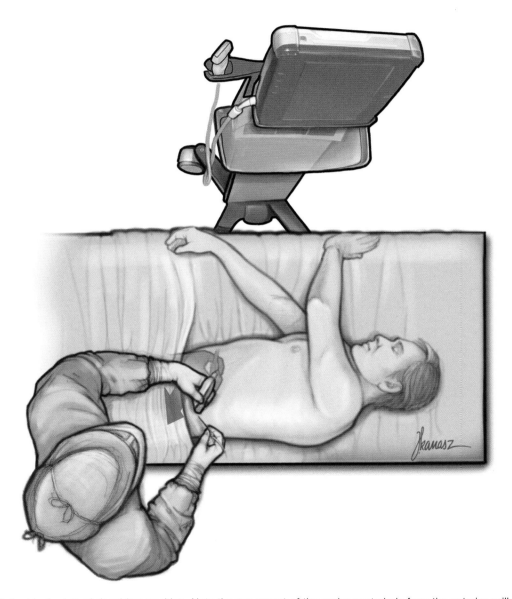

Figure 42-4. Patient in the lateral decubitus position. Note the movement of the probe posteriorly from the arterior axillary line to visualize the QL muscle.

SECTION VII

Neuraxial Blocks

Ultrasound-Assisted Neuraxial Blocks 43

Loran Mounir-Soliman

RELEVANT SONOANATOMY OF THE SPINE

There are a couple of challenges for ultrasound imaging of the spine and the neuraxial structures. The depth of the spine makes it less than optimal for the ultrasound beams to produce higher-resolution images. Also the osseous structure of the laminae and articular processes conceal the underlying neuraxial structures of interest to perform the blocks. Accordingly it is important to have a visual appreciation of the spine outline when scanning for neuraxial blocks.

In general, scanning the vertebrae demonstrates three hyperechoic levels: the spinous process, the lamina, and the articular facet joint with the transverse process.

The spinous processes reflect the most superficial hyperechoic shadow closest to the skin. Careful scanning cephalad and caudad to the spinous process reveals an acoustic window representing the interspinous space occupied with the less echogenic interspinous ligaments. Careful examination of the deeper layer of the ligamentous structure shows the ligamentum flavum as a slightly more hyperechoic layer separated from another hyperechoic layer—the posterior dura—by the epidural space. The spinal canal underneath represents the next anechoic layer deeper to the posterior dura. On the deeper side of the spinal canal (anterior), the anterior dura with the postlongitudinal ligament form a hyperechoic structure called the *anterior complex*.

With the aforementioned echogenic characteristics of the neuraxial structures in mind, scanning the different levels of the spine leads to different views. These views also depend on the scanning plane and orientation of the ultrasound beam. These are the main planes for scanning the spine:

- **Median sagittal plane:** A longitudinal scan along the midline where the beam of the ultrasound is parallel to the long axis of the spine on top of the spinous processes (unless the spine is scoliotic).
- **Paramedian sagittal plane:** A longitudinal scan parallel to the long axis of the spine but off the midline. The beams are usually on top of the transverse processes or the laminae, with the articular joints (facets) between the adjacent spines.

- **Paramedian sagittal oblique plane:** Another longitudinal plane that is similar to the paramedian sagittal plane with the probe tilted medially to direct the beams toward midline. The ultrasound beams usually travel across the laminae with the intervertebral foraminae in between. Access to the ligaments, dura, and spinal canal are usually accessed with the beam within the interlaminar windows.
- **Transverse axial view:** A transverse view where the beam of the ultrasound is perpendicular to the long axis of the spine. With this orientation, the ultrasound probe can be on top of the vertebra where the beams cross the spinous process, lamina, and transverse process. If the beam is steered cephalad or caudad by sliding the probe or tilting it, an interspinous (acoustic) window is obtained. The ligaments, epidural space, and spinal canal can be visualized through this window.

TECHNIQUE

Except for the caudal block, the neuraxial scanning requires a low-frequency (2 to 5 MHz) curvilinear probe to see the depth of the target structures. In addition to the ability to scan deeper structures, the curved probe provides a divergent beam, giving a wider field of vision and helping to scan the different anatomic structures in a single view compared with the limited field of vision produced by the linear probe. The disadvantage of the curved probe is a lack of spatial resolution at deeper levels, making viewing the needle a challenge when performing the block. Scanning the spine for procedures can be performed in sitting, lateral, and prone positions depending on the level of the procedure to be performed.

CAUDAL EPIDURAL BLOCK

Because the sacral hiatus is a relatively superficial structure, a high-frequency linear probe (6 to 13 MHz) is usually used for caudal scanning. The block is performed in the prone position with a pillow under the pelvis. The ultrasound probe is placed in a transverse orientation (axial scan) to scan the sacral cornua as two hyperechoic, reversed U-shaped structures. The sacrococcygeal ligament connecting both cornua, forming the superficial boundary of the sacral hiatus, appears as a hyperechoic band. The anterior boundary of the sacral canal is formed by the posterior surface of the sacrum, which appears as another hyperechoic linear structure anterior (deep) to the sacrococcygeal ligament. The sacral hiatus appears as a hypoechoic space between these two described hyperechoic lines. With this view, the needle can be introduced in the middle of the probe perpendicular to the ultrasound beams, out of the plane approach and targeting the sacral hiatus (Fig. 43-1).

With the sacral hiatus and the sacrococcygeal ligament identified, the ultrasound probe can be rotated 90 degrees to the median sagittal plane scan. A long-axis view of the sacrococcygeal ligament and the sacral bony surface are reidentified with the sacral hiatus between them. The

needle is introduced with an in-plane approach from the caudal end of the probe to be able to visualize the whole length of the needle. Crossing the tip of the needle into the sacrococcygeal membrane into the sacral canal is associated with a "pop" feeling, especially when using a blunt needle. The sacral bony structure impedes the ultrasound beams, making it hard to see the tip of the needle or the spread of the injection in the sacral canal (Figs 43-2, 43-3, and 43-4).

LUMBAR NEURAXIAL BLOCKS

The lumbar epidural space can be scanned in the sitting, lateral, or prone position. The author's preference is to perform the scan in the sitting position to allow for maximum flexion of the spine (similar to the familiar landmark technique). Identification of the desired level for the

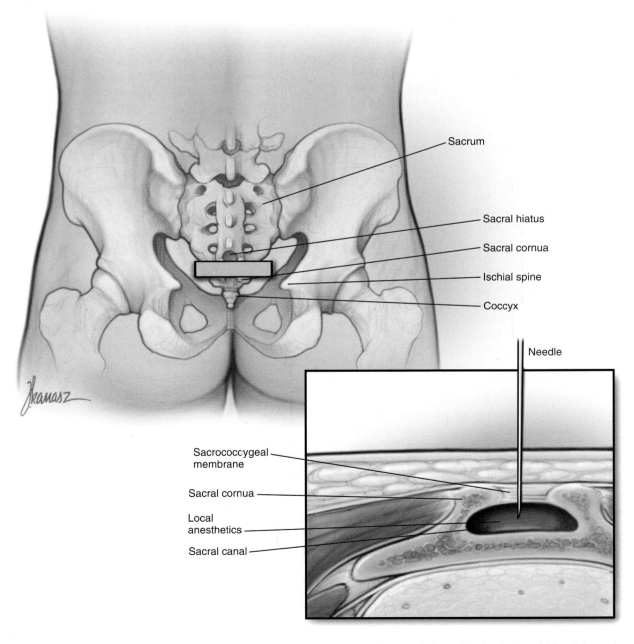

Figure 43-1. Transverse approach to the caudal block. The needle is introduced in out-of-plane direction in the middle of the probe targeting the sacral hiatus.

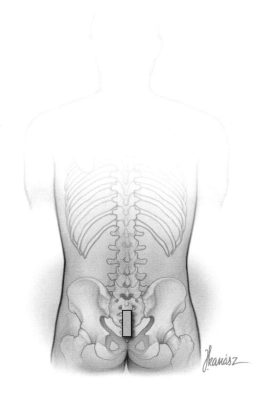

Figure 43-2. Median approach of caudal block. Note the probe is in long-axis view of the sacrococcygeal ligament.

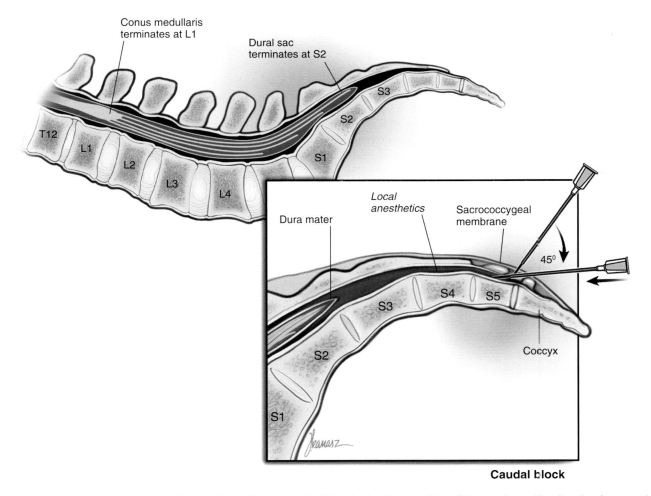

Caudal block

Figure 43-3. Anatomy of the caudal block with median approach. Note the in-plane position of the needle and its direction from caudal to cephalad position.

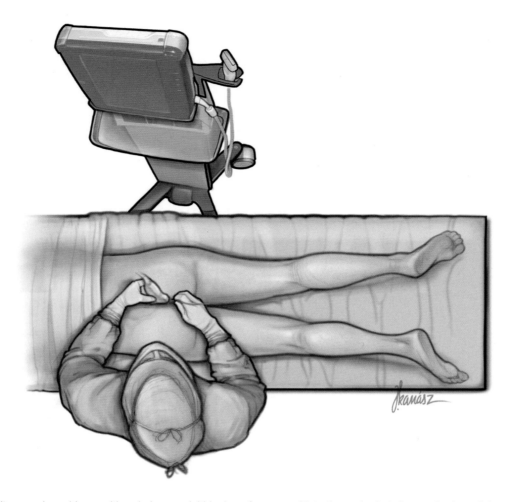

Figure 43-4. Ultrasound machine position during caudal block performance. Note the probe is in long-axis view of the spine.

procedure starts by placing the ultrasound probe parallel to the long axis of the sacrum in the midline to identify its flat surface. The probe is moved cephalad slowly to identify the intervertebral space between L5 and S1 as an interruption of the continuity of the sacral line. The ultrasound probe can be advanced longitudinally cephalad along this midline plane or turned 90 degrees to obtain a transverse view of the L5 to S1 interspinous space and then advanced cephalad, keeping the transverse orientation of the probe. Counting the spinous processes (hyperechoic shadows) and the interspinous spaces (hypoechoic windows) will help identify the desired level for the block.

Transverse Axial View

The ligamentous structure on the interspinous space is identified at the desired level by its characteristic echogenic appearance (as discussed previously), as well as the ability to see the deeper spinal canal. The needle is usually advanced from lateral to medial parallel to the ultrasound beam (in-plane approach) until the tip of the needle is engaged in the ligamentum flavum. The epidural space is usually identified by the traditional loss of resistance technique by putting the ultrasound probe down (single operator) or through a second operator.

Tip: The lateral edge of the ultrasound probe can be lifted off the skin to obtain a needle insertion point closer to the midline (Figs 43-5 and 43-6).

Paramedian Sagittal Oblique View

After identifying the appropriate level (as described earlier), the probe is oriented in a paramedian sagittal oblique view (discussed earlier) to allow identification of the epidural space through the interlaminar acoustic window. The epidural space shows as a hypoechoic space between two hyperechoic lines: the ligamentum flavum (posteriorly) and posterior dura (anteriorly). The spinal canal (intrathecal space) can be seen as an anechoic space anterior to the posterior dura, separating it from the anterior complex that appears as a hyperechoic structure.

The needle can be approached through either an in-plane technique from the caudad side of the probe or an out-of-plane technique from the medial side (midline) of the middle of the probe (Fig. 43-7).

THORACIC NEURAXIAL BLOCKS

The same concepts and ultrasound techniques are used for scanning the thoracic spine. However, due to the acute angulation and narrower interspinous and interlaminar spaces, the echogenic windows are more challenging to identify and the neuraxial structures are less visible. Paramedian scanning is the only relevant technique for approaching the thoracic epidural space (especially the midthoracic segments with the maximum angulation).

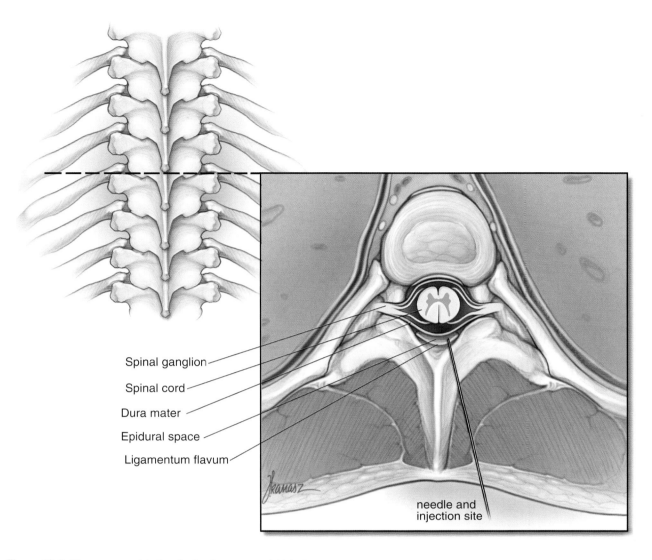

Spinal ganglion

Spinal cord

Dura mater

Epidural space

Ligamentum flavum

needle and
injection site

Figure 43-5. Transverse axial view for lumbar neuroaxial block.

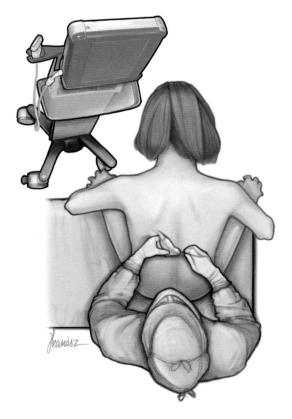

Figure 43-6. Patient and ultrasound machine position for lumbar neuroaxial block using the transverse axial view.

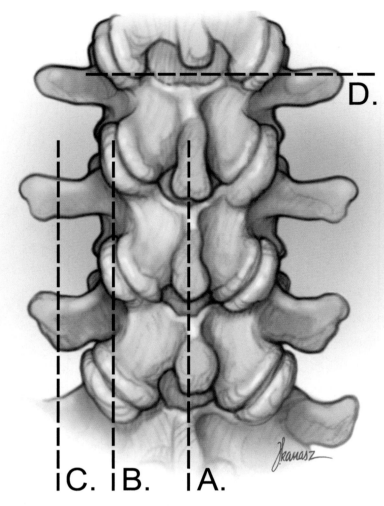

Figure 43-7. Paramedian sagittal oblique view for lumbar neuroaxial block.

Usually, the ultrasound is used to guide the needle to the upper edge of the corresponding lamina, and loss of resistance is used to guide the needle through the ligamentum flavum and epidural space.

KEY POINTS

- Prepuncture ultrasound scanning is helpful to determine the midline, the depth from the skin, the desired level, and rotation of the spine.
- There are limited outcome data on the real-time guidance with ultrasound for neuraxial blocks.
- The available evidence suggests that the use of ultrasound may improve the success rate from the first attempt, reduce the number of attempts, and improve patient comfort.
- The use of ultrasound for epidural access is a technically advanced procedure. It requires adequate experience with ultrasound scanning and ultrasound guidance of the needle at deep levels with a less-than-optimal angle of incidence.
- Thorough understanding of the neuraxial anatomy and conceptual visualization of the different

echogenic structures are necessary for ultrasound scanning of the epidural space.

PEARLS

- Echogenic Tuohy needles can be helpful to identify the tip of the needle.
- Usually, loss of resistance is needed to confirm the position of the needle tip within the epidural space.
- In pediatric patients and thin patients, some changes can be identified with loss of resistance to saline, a characteristic of correct needle placement, mainly:
  - Widening of the epidural space with anterior displacement of the posterior dura.
  - Compression of the thecal sac can be occasionally seen.
  - Doppler flow of the injected fluid (mainly in small children).
- Spring-loaded syringes have been recently introduced to the market. They make it possible to perform real-time ultrasound-guided access to the epidural space with loss of resistance confirmed by a single operator.

Spinal Block

44

David L. Brown

PERSPECTIVE

Spinal anesthesia is unparalleled in that a small mass of drug, virtually devoid of systemic pharmacologic effect, can produce profound, reproducible surgical anesthesia. Further, by altering the small mass of drug, very different types of spinal anesthesia can be produced. Low spinal anesthesia, a block below T10, has a different physiologic impact than does a block performed to produce higher spinal anesthesia (above T5). The block is unexcelled for lower abdominal or lower extremity surgical procedures. However, for operations in the mid abdomen to upper abdomen, light general anesthesia may have to supplement the spinal block because stimulation of the diaphragm during upper abdominal procedures often causes some discomfort. This area is difficult to block completely through high spinal anesthesia because to do so requires blockade of the phrenic nerve.

Patient Selection. Patient selection for spinal anesthesia often places too much emphasis on a side effect of the technique—namely, spinal headache—than on the applicability of the technique in a given patient. It is clear that the incidence of spinal headache increases with decreasing age and female sex; however, with proper technique and selection of needle size and tip configuration, the incidence of headache should not preclude the use of spinal anesthesia in young, healthy patients if the block has advantages over epidural anesthesia. Almost any patient who is to have a lower extremity operation is a candidate for spinal anesthesia, as are most patients scheduled for lower abdominal surgery, such as inguinal herniorrhaphy and gynecologic, urologic, and obstetric procedures.

Pharmacologic Choice. In the United States, three local anesthetics are commonly used to produce spinal anesthesia: lidocaine, tetracaine, and bupivacaine. Lidocaine is a short-acting to intermediate-acting spinal drug; tetracaine and bupivacaine provide intermediate- to long-acting block. Lidocaine, without epinephrine, is often chosen for procedures that can be completed in 1 hour or less. It is likely that the lidocaine mixture most commonly used is still a 5% solution in 7.5% dextrose, although increasingly anesthesiologists are using 1.5% to 2% concentrations of lidocaine without dextrose as alternatives. When epinephrine (0.2 mg) is added to lidocaine, the useful length of clinical anesthesia in the lower abdomen and lower extremities is approximately 90 minutes. Tetracaine is packaged

both as niphanoid crystals (20 mg) and as a 1% solution (2 mL total). When dextrose is added to make tetracaine hyperbaric, the drug generally produces effective clinical anesthesia for procedures of up to 1.5 to 2 hours in the plain form, for up to 2 to 3 hours when epinephrine (0.2 mg) is added, and for up to 5 hours for lower extremity procedures when phenylephrine (5 mg) is added as a vasoconstrictor. Bupivacaine spinal anesthesia is commonly carried out with 0.5% or 0.75% solution, either plain or in 8.25% dextrose. My impression is that the clinical difference between 0.5% tetracaine and 0.75% bupivacaine as a hyperbaric solution is minimal. Bupivacaine is appropriate for procedures lasting up to 2 or 3 hours.

In addition, local anesthetics can be mixed to produce hypobaric spinal anesthesia. A common method of formulating a hypobaric solution is to mix tetracaine in a 0.1% to 0.33% solution with sterile water. Also, lidocaine can be mixed to provide useful hypobaric spinal anesthesia. This drug is diluted from a 2% solution with sterile water to make a 0.5% solution, using a total of 30 to 40 mg.

Many anesthesiologists avoid vasoconstrictors for fear of somehow increasing the risk with spinal anesthesia. These anesthesiologists believe that phenylephrine or epinephrine has such potent vasoconstrictive action that it puts the blood supply of the spinal cord at risk. There are no human data supporting this theory. In fact, because most local anesthetics are vasodilators, the addition of these vasoconstrictors does little more than maintain spinal cord blood flow at a basal level. Commonly used doses of vasoconstrictors are 0.2 to 0.3 mg of epinephrine and 5 mg of phenylephrine added to the spinal anesthetic.

PLACEMENT

Anatomy. As outlined in Chapter 43, Neuraxial Block Anatomy, the spinous processes of the lumbar vertebrae have an almost horizontal orientation in relation to the long axis of their respective vertebral bodies (Fig. 44-1). When a midline needle is inserted between the lumbar vertebral spinous processes, it is most effective if it is placed almost perpendicularly in relation to the long axis of the back. To facilitate spinal anesthesia, the anesthesiologist must constantly keep in mind the midline of the patient's body and the neuraxis in relation to the needle. As illustrated in Figure 44-1, as a midline needle is inserted into the cerebrospinal fluid (CSF), it logically must puncture

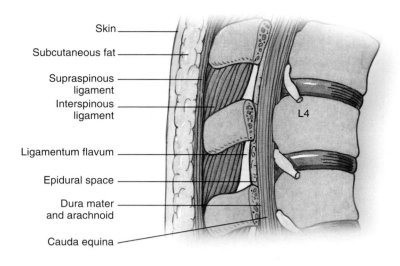

Figure 44-1. Spinal block: functional lumbar anatomy.

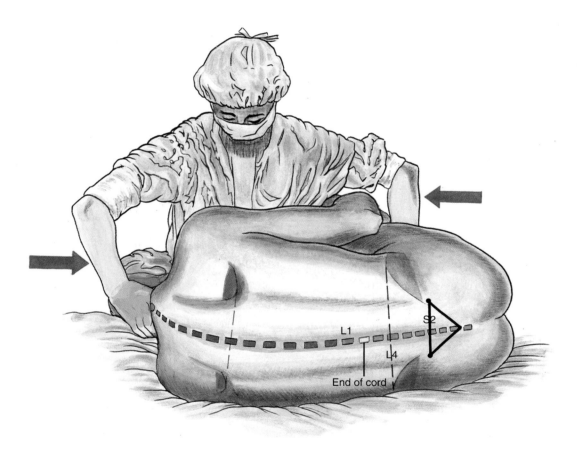

Figure 44-2. Spinal block: lateral decubitus position.

the skin, subcutaneous tissue, supraspinous ligament, interspinous ligament, ligamentum flavum, epidural space, and finally the dura mater and arachnoid mater to reach the CSF.

Position. Spinal anesthesia is carried out in three principal positions: lateral decubitus (Fig. 44-2), sitting (Fig. 44-3), and prone jackknife (Fig. 44-4). In both the lateral decubitus and sitting positions, a well-trained assistant is essential if the block is to be easily and efficiently administered by the anesthesiologist. As illustrated in Figure 44-2,

the assistant can help the patient assume the position of legs flexed on the abdomen and chin flexed on the chest. This is most easily accomplished by having the assistant pull the head toward the chest, place an arm behind the patient's knees, and push the head and knees together. The position can also be facilitated by using an appropriate amount of sedation that allows the patient to be relaxed yet cooperative.

In some patients, the sitting position can facilitate location of the midline, especially in obese patients or in those with some scoliosis that makes midline identification more difficult. As illustrated in Figure 44-3A, the patient should assume a comfortable sitting position, with the legs placed over the edge of the operating table and the feet supported by a stool. A pillow should be placed in the patient's lap and the patient's arms allowed to drape over the pillow, resting on the flexed lower extremities. The assistant should be positioned immediately in front of the patient, supporting the shoulders and allowing the patient to minimize lumbar lordosis while ensuring that the vertebral midline remains in a vertical position (see Fig. 44-3B).

Sometimes it is more efficient to place the patient in a prone jackknife position before administering the spinal anesthetic (see Fig. 44-4). An assistant is not as essential for this technique as for the lateral decubitus and sitting positions, although to make the most efficient use of operating room block time, it is often helpful for the assistant

to position the patient in the prone jackknife position while the anesthesiologist readies the spinal anesthesia tray and drugs.

In all three positions, the goal is to place the patient so that the midline is readily identifiable and lumbar lordosis is reduced. Figure 44-5 shows what the lumbar anatomy looks like when the patient's lumbar lordosis has been ineffectively reduced by poor positioning. As illustrated, the intralaminar space is small and difficult to enter with a needle in the midline. In contrast, Figure 44-6 illustrates how effective positioning can open the intralaminar space to allow easy access for subarachnoid puncture.

Needle Puncture.   One of the first decisions to be made in considering spinal anesthesia is what kind of needle to use. Although there are many eponyms for spinal needles, they fall into two main categories: those that cut the dura sharply and those that disrupt the dural fibers by spreading with a

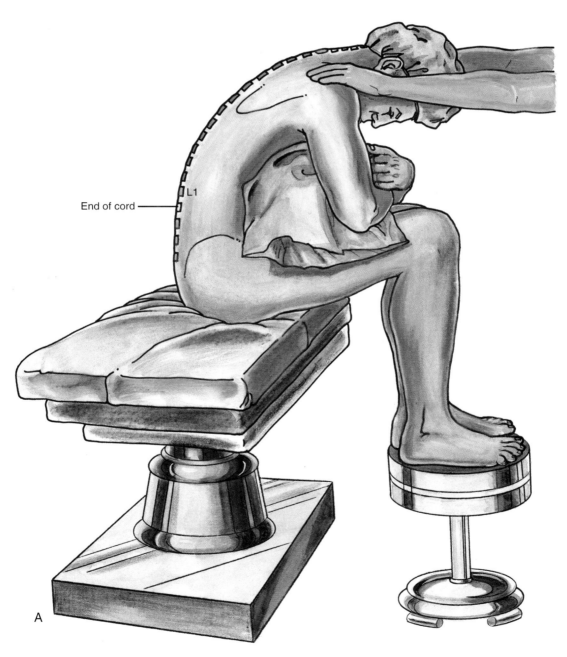

End of cord — L1

A

Figure 44-3. Spinal block: sitting position. A, Lateral view.

Continued

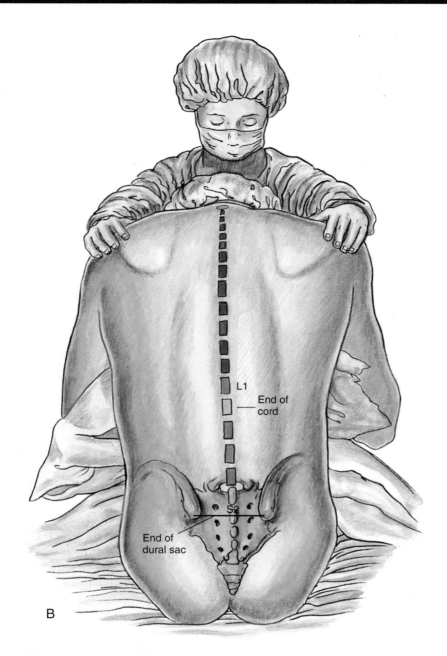

L1 —— End of cord

S2

End of dural sac

B

Figure 44-3, cont'd B, Posterior view.

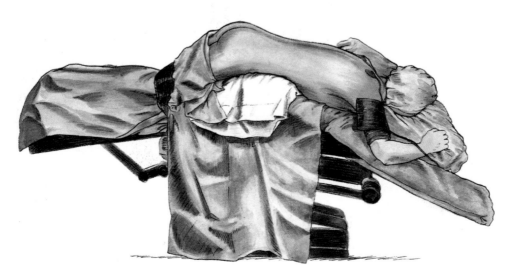

Figure 44-4. Spinal block: prone jackknife position.

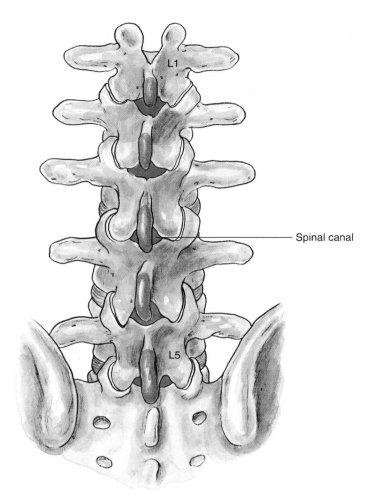

L1

Spinal canal

L5

Figure 44-5. Spinal block: lumbar vertebra. Lumbar lordosis is present because the positioning is inadequate.

cone-shaped tip. The former category includes the traditional disposable spinal needle, the Quincke–Babcock needle; the latter category comprises the Greene, Whitacre, and Sprotte needles. If a continuous spinal technique is chosen, the use of a Tuohy or other thin-walled, curve-tipped needle will facilitate passage of the catheter. To make a logical choice of a spinal needle, the risks and benefits of each must be understood. The use of small needles reduces the incidence of post–dural puncture headache; the use of larger needles improves the tactile sense of needle placement, thus increasing operator confidence.

Probably the risk–benefit calculation is not as simple as this. For example, the use of a small needle, such as a 27-gauge needle, will not decrease the incidence of headache in younger patients if a number of "passes" through the dura are required before CSF flow is recognized. Likewise, a larger needle, such as a 22-gauge Whitacre needle, may result in a lower incidence of post–dural puncture headache if the subarachnoid needle location is recognized on the first pass. Different needle tip designs result in differences in the incidence of post–dural puncture headache even when needle sizes are comparable.

With the patient in the proper position, the anesthesiologist uses the palpating hand to clearly identify the patient's intervertebral space and midline. As illustrated in Figure 44-7, *Step 1*, the anesthesiologist can effectively carry

out this important maneuver by moving the fingers of the palpating hand alternately cephalocaudad and rolling them from side to side. When the appropriate intervertebral space has been clearly identified, a skin wheal is raised over the space. Next, an introducer is inserted into the substance of the interspinous ligament, taking care to firmly seat it in the midline (Fig. 44-7, *Step 2*). The introducer is grasped with the palpating fingers and steadied while the other hand holds the spinal needle, somewhat like a dart, as illustrated in Figure 44-7, *Step 3*. With the fifth finger of the needle hand used as a tripod against the patient's back, the needle, with bevel (if present) parallel to the long axis of the spine, is advanced slowly to heighten the sense of tissue planes traversed, as well as to avoid skewing the nerve roots, until a characteristic change in resistance is noted as the needle passes through the ligamentum flavum and dura. The stylet is then removed, and CSF should appear at the needle hub. If it does not, the needle is rotated in 90-degree increments until CSF appears. If CSF does not appear in any quadrant, the needle should be advanced a few millimeters and rechecked in all four quadrants. If CSF still has not appeared and the needle is at a depth appropriate for the patient, the needle and introducer should be withdrawn and the insertion steps repeated because the most common reason for lack of CSF return is that the needle was inserted off the midline. Another common error

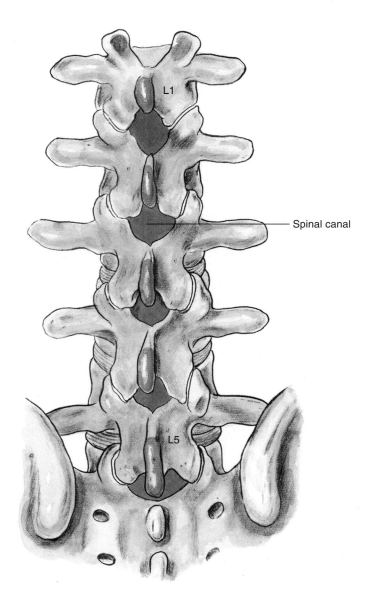

L1

Spinal canal

L5

Figure 44-6. Spinal block: lumbar vertebra. Lumbar lordosis is reversed with ideal spiral positioning.

preventing subarachnoid placement is insertion of the needle with too great a cephalad angle on the initial insertion (Fig. 44-8).

Once CSF is freely obtained, the dorsum of the anesthesiologist's nondominant hand steadies the spinal needle against the patient's back while the syringe containing the therapeutic dose is attached to the needle. CSF is again freely aspirated into the syringe, and the dose is injected. Sometimes, when the syringe has been attached to a needle from which CSF was clearly previously dripping, aspiration of additional CSF becomes impossible. As illustrated in Figure 44-9, one technique that can be used to facilitate CSF aspiration is to "unscrew" the syringe plunger (see Fig. 44-9A) rather than providing constant steady pressure (see Fig. 44-9B).

After the local anesthetic has been injected, the patient and the operating table should be placed in the position appropriate for the surgical procedure and the drugs being used. The midline approach to subarachnoid block is the technique of first choice because it requires anatomic projection in only two planes, and the needle insertion plane is a relatively avascular one. When difficulties with needle insertion are encountered with the midline approach, an option is to use the paramedian route, which does not require the same level of patient cooperation or reversal of lumbar lordosis to be successful. As illustrated in Figure 44-10, the paramedian approach exploits the larger "subarachnoid target" that exists if a needle is inserted slightly lateral to the midline. In the paramedian approach, the palpating fingers should identify the caudal edge of the cephalad spinous process of the intervertebral space chosen, and a skin wheal should be raised 1 cm lateral and 1 cm caudal to this point. A longer needle, such as a 4-cm, 22-gauge, short-beveled needle, is then used to infiltrate the deeper tissues in a cephalomedial plane. The spinal introducer and needle are then inserted 10 to 15 degrees off the sagittal plane in a cephalomedial plane, as noted in Figure 44-10. As with the midline approach, the most common error made with this technique is to angle the needle too far cephalad in its initial insertion. Once the needle contacts bone with this approach, it is redirected in slightly cephalad. If bone is again contacted after the

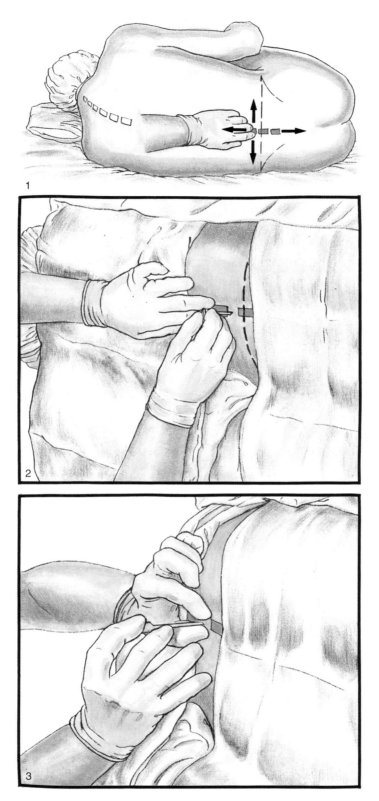

Figure 44-7. Spinal block: technique.

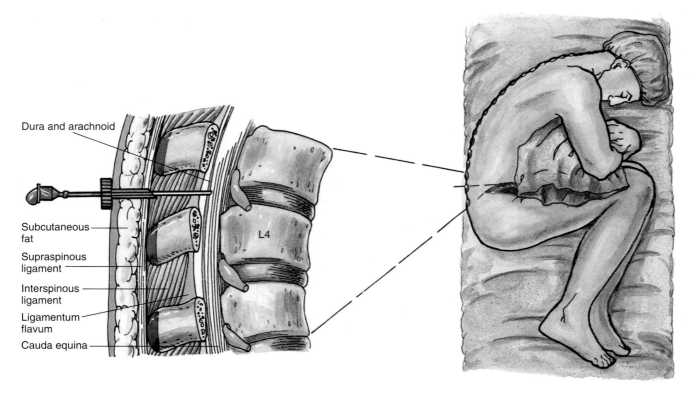

Dura and arachnoid

Subcutaneous fat

Supraspinous ligament

Interspinous ligament

Ligamentum flavum

Cauda equina

L4

Figure 44-8. Spinal block: avoiding too large a cephalad angle on insertion.

needle has been redirected, but at a deeper level, this needle redirection is continued because it is likely that the needle is being "walked up" the lamina toward the intervertebral space. After CSF is obtained, the block continues in the same way as that described for the midline approach.

A variation of the paramedian approach is the lumbosacral approach of Taylor. The technique is carried out at the L5 to S1 interspace, the largest interlaminar interspace of the vertebral column. As illustrated in Figure 44-11, the skin insertion site is 1 cm medial and 1 cm caudal to the ipsilateral posterosuperior iliac spine. Through this point, a 12- to 15-cm spinal needle is inserted in a cephalomedial direction toward the midline. If bone is encountered on the first needle insertion, the needle is "walked off" the sacrum into the subarachnoid space, as in the method used for a lumbar paramedian approach. Once CSF is obtained, the steps are similar to those previously outlined.

POTENTIAL PROBLEMS

The complication most feared by patients and many anesthesiologists after spinal anesthesia is neurologic injury. However, the risk–benefit calculation of neurologic injury after anesthesia must include those cases that are possible after general anesthesia. These comparisons may show that the incidence of neurologic injury after spinal anesthesia is in fact lower than that after general anesthesia. However, this statement must remain speculative.

In patients in whom the spinal block level has to be precisely controlled or in whom the operation is expected to outlast the usual duration of the anesthetic drugs, a continuous spinal catheter may be used. However, when using a continuous spinal technique, one should be cautious about repeating local anesthetic injections if the block height does not reach the predicted levels. Neurotoxicity (cauda equina syndrome) is hypothetically possible when the spinal catheter position allows local anesthetic concentrations to reach higher-than-expected levels.

A more common complication of spinal anesthesia is postoperative headache. Factors that influence the incidence of post–dural puncture headache are age (more frequent in younger patients), sex (more likely in female patients), needle size (more frequent with larger needles), needle bevel orientation (increased incidence when dural fibers are cut transversely), pregnancy (incidence increased), and number of dural punctures necessary to obtain CSF (more likely with multiple punctures). Perhaps more important to physicians than knowing the factors resulting in an increased incidence of post–dural puncture headache is the knowledge of how and when to carry out definitive therapy—that is, an epidural blood patch. To use spinal anesthesia effectively, epidural blood patching, when indicated, must be used early. The success rate from a single epidural blood patch should be in the 90% to 95% range and, if a second patch is required, a similar percentage should be obtainable.

One other common side effect of spinal anesthesia is the appearance of a backache in approximately 25% of patients. Patients often blame "the spinal" for backache, but, when looked at systematically, it appears that just as many patients have backaches after general anesthesia as after spinal anesthesia. Thus backache after neuraxial block should not be attributed immediately to "needling" of the back.

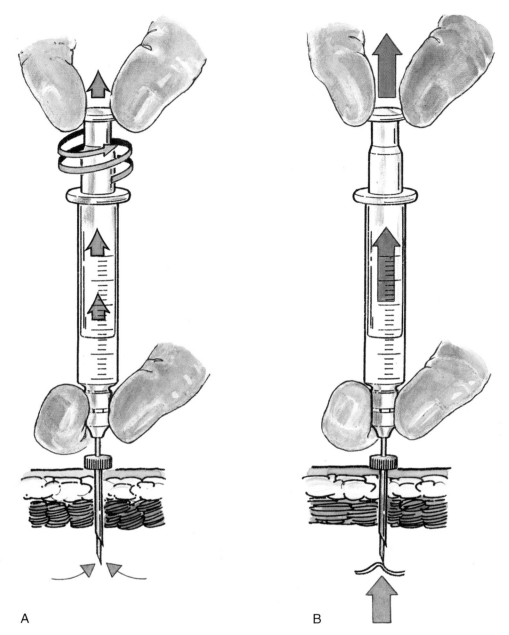

A   B

Figure 44-9. Spinal block: syringe technique to facilitate aspiration of cerebrospinal fluid.

PEARLS

Probably the most important factor contributing to success with spinal anesthesia in the day-to-day life of an anesthesiologist is the efficiency of the technique. If nurses and surgeons are to be advocates of spinal anesthesia, its use cannot measurably add time to the surgical day. Thus one should plan ahead to maximize efficiency. Often overlooked in this maxim is the fact that patient preparation for operation can begin almost as soon as the block is administered if the patient is properly sedated.

Intraoperatively during high spinal anesthesia (often during cesarean section) patients occasionally complain of dyspnea. This often appears to be a result of loss of chest wall sensation rather than of significantly decreased inspiratory capacity. The loss of chest wall sensation does not allow the patient to experience the reassurance of a deep breath. This impediment to patient acceptance can often be overcome simply by asking the patient to raise a hand in front of his or her mouth and exhale forcefully. The tactile appreciation of a deep exhalation often seems to provide the needed reassurance.

If spinal anesthesia has been used and a neurologic complication is noted after surgery, it is essential to obtain neurologic consultation early. In this way, an unbiased consultant can examine the patient and determine whether the "new" neurologic finding preexisted, is related to a peripheral neuropathy, or, more rarely, is potentially related to the spinal anesthetic. Latent electromyographic alterations associated with denervation due to neurologic injury take time to develop in the lower extremities (14 to 21 days). Therefore after a potentially spinal anesthesia–related lesion has been identified, electromyographic studies should be obtained early to establish a preblock baseline and allow serial comparison.

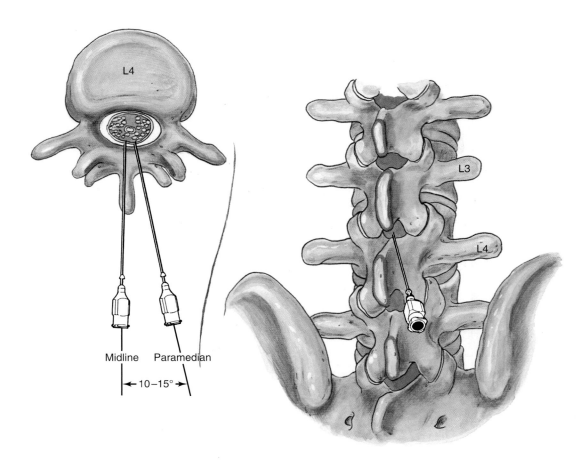

Figure 44-10. Spinal block: paramedian technique.

It is also useful to consider adding fentanyl (15 to 25 μg) rather than epinephrine to some shorter-acting spinal local anesthetic mixtures (e.g., lidocaine) because it prolongs the effective sensory block without measurably prolonging the motor block or the time to voiding. This is especially useful in selected surgical outpatients.

Another way to titrate spinal anesthesia for outpatients, or any surgical procedure in which the length of surgery is difficult to predict, is to use a combined spinal–epidural technique. In this technique an epidural needle is placed in the epidural space in a standard fashion, and then a small-gauge spinal needle is advanced through the epidural needle into the CSF. A spinal local anesthetic mixture is then injected and matched to the projected length of the shortest surgical procedure planned. After removal of the spinal needle, an epidural catheter is inserted into the epidural space. At this point, if the surgical procedure lasts longer than anticipated, the epidural catheter can be injected with a local anesthetic appropriate for the anticipated surgical needs. This combined spinal–epidural technique provides the flexibility for both spinal and epidural anesthesia in selected patients.

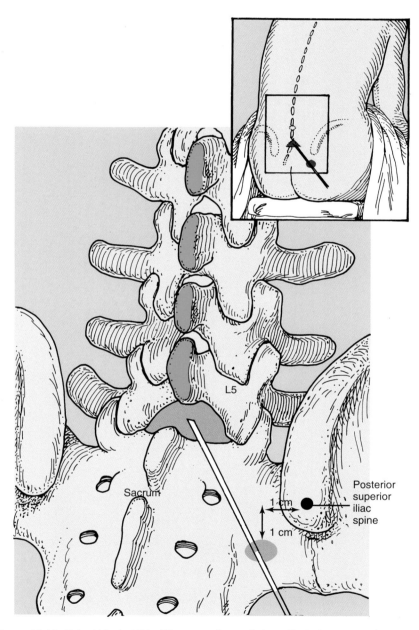

Figure 44-11. Spinal block: L5 to S1 paramedian technique (Taylor's approach).

Epidural Block

David L. Brown

45

PERSPECTIVE

Epidural anesthesia is the second primary method of neuraxial block. In contrast to spinal anesthesia, epidural block requires pharmacologic doses of local anesthetics, making systemic toxicity a concern. In skilled hands, the incidence of post–dural puncture headache should be lower with epidural anesthesia than with spinal anesthesia. Nevertheless, as outlined in Chapter 44, Spinal Block, I do not believe this should be the major differentiating point between the two techniques. Spinal anesthesia is typically a single-shot technique, whereas frequently intermittent injections are given through an epidural catheter, thus allowing reinjection and prolongation of epidural block. Another difference is that epidural block allows production of segmental anesthesia. Thus if a thoracic injection is made and an appropriate amount of local anesthetic is injected, a band of anesthesia that does not block the lower extremities can be produced.

Patient Selection. Epidural block is appropriate for virtually the same patients who are candidates for spinal anesthesia, except that epidural anesthesia can be used in the cervical and thoracic areas as well—levels at which spinal anesthesia is not advised. As with spinal anesthesia, if epidural block is to be used for intraabdominal procedures involving the upper abdomen, it is advisable to combine this technique with a light general anesthetic because diaphragmatic irritation can make the patient, surgeon, and anesthesiologist uncomfortable. Other candidates for epidural anesthesia are patients in whom a continuous technique has increasingly been found to be helpful in providing epidural local anesthesia or opioid analgesia after major surgical procedures. This clinical application likely explains the increased interest in epidural block over the last 20 years.

Pharmacologic Choice. To use epidural local anesthetics effectively, one must combine an understanding of the potency and duration of local anesthetics with estimates of the length of the operation and the postoperative analgesia requirements. Drugs available for epidural use can be categorized as short-acting, intermediate-acting, and long-acting agents; with the addition of epinephrine to these agents, surgical anesthesia ranging from 45 to 240 minutes after a single injection is possible.

Chloroprocaine, an amino ester local anesthetic, is a short-acting agent that allows efficient matching of the length of the surgical procedure and the duration of epidural analgesia, even in outpatients. 2-Chloroprocaine is available in 2% and 3% concentrations; the latter is preferable for surgical anesthesia and the former for techniques not requiring muscle relaxation.

Lidocaine is the prototypical amino amide local anesthetic and is used in 1.5% and 2% concentrations epidurally. Concentrations of mepivacaine necessary for epidural anesthesia are similar to those of lidocaine; however, mepivacaine lasts from 15 to 30 minutes longer at equivalent dosages. Epinephrine significantly prolongs (i.e., by approximately 50%) the duration of surgical anesthesia with 2-chloroprocaine and either lidocaine and mepivacaine. Plain lidocaine produces surgical anesthesia that lasts from 60 to 100 minutes.

Bupivacaine, an amino amide, is a widely used long-acting local anesthetic for epidural anesthesia. It is used in 0.5% and 0.75% concentrations, but analgesic techniques can be performed with concentrations ranging from 0.125% to 0.25%. Its duration of action is not prolonged as consistently by the addition of epinephrine, although up to 240 minutes of surgical anesthesia can be obtained when epinephrine is added.

Ropivacaine, another long-acting amino amide, is also used for regional and epidural anesthesia. For surgical anesthesia, it is used in 0.5%, 0.75%, and 1% concentrations. Analgesia can be obtained with concentrations of 0.2%. Its duration of action is slightly less than that of bupivacaine in the epidural technique, and it appears to produce slightly less motor blockade than a comparable concentration of bupivacaine.

In addition to the use of epinephrine as an epidural additive, some anesthesiologists recommend modifying epidural local anesthetic solutions to increase both the speed of onset and the quality of the block produced. One recommendation is to alkalinize the local anesthetic solution by adding bicarbonate to it to achieve both these purposes. Nevertheless, the clinical advisability of routinely adding bicarbonate to local anesthetic solutions should be determined by local practice protocols.

PLACEMENT

Anatomy. As with spinal anesthesia, the key to carrying out successful epidural anesthesia is understanding the three-dimensional midline neuraxial anatomy that underlies the palpating fingers (Fig. 45-1). When a lumbar approach to the epidural space is used in adults, the depth

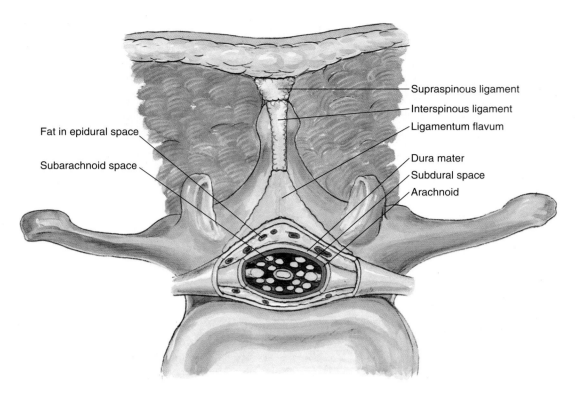

Figure 45-1. Epidural block: cross-sectional anatomy.

from the skin to the ligamentum flavum is commonly near 4 cm; in 80% of patients the epidural space is cannulated at a distance of 3.5 to 6 cm from the skin. In a small number of patients the lumbar epidural space is as near as 2 cm from the skin. In the lumbar region, the ligamentum flavum is 5 to 6 mm thick in the midline, whereas in the thoracic region it is 3 to 5 mm thick. In the thoracic region, the depth from the skin to the epidural space depends on the degree of cephalad angulation used for the paramedian approach, as well as the body habitus of the patient (Fig. 45-2). In the cervical region the depth to the ligamentum flavum is approximately the same as that in the lumbar region, 4 to 6 cm.

The ligamentum flavum will be perceived as a thicker ligament if the needle is kept in the midline than if the needle is inserted off the midline and enters the lateral extension of the ligamentum flavum. Figure 45-3 illustrates how important it is to maintain the midline position of the epidural needle (*needle A*) during lumbar epidural techniques. If an oblique approach is taken, a "false release" can be produced (*needle C*) or the perception of a thin ligament can be reinforced (*needle B*).

Position. Patient positioning for epidural anesthesia is similar to that for spinal anesthesia, with lateral decubitus, sitting, and prone jackknife positions all applicable. The lateral decubitus position is applicable for both lumbar and thoracic epidural techniques, and the sitting position allows the administration of lumbar, thoracic, and cervical epidural anesthetics. The prone jackknife position allows access to the caudal epidural space.

Needle Puncture: Lumbar Epidural. A technique similar to that used for spinal anesthesia should be carried out to identify the midline structures, and the bony landmarks should be used to determine the vertebral level appropriate

for needle insertion (Fig. 45-4). When choosing a needle for epidural anesthesia, one must decide whether a continuous or single-shot technique is desired. This is the principal determinant of needle selection. If a single-shot epidural technique is chosen, a Crawford needle is appropriate; if a continuous catheter technique is indicated, a Tuohy or other needle with a lateral-facing opening is chosen.

The midline approach is most often indicated for a lumbar epidural procedure. The needle is inserted into the midline in the same way as for spinal anesthesia. In the epidural technique, the needle is slowly advanced until the change in tissue resistance is noted as the needle abuts the ligamentum flavum. At this point, a 3- to 5-mL glass syringe is filled with 2 mL of saline solution, and a small (0.25 mL) air bubble is added. The syringe is attached to the needle, and if the needle tip is in the substance of the ligamentum flavum, the air bubble will be compressible (Fig. 45-5A). If the ligamentum flavum has not yet been reached, pressure on the syringe plunger will not compress the air bubble (Fig. 45-5B). Once compression of the air bubble has been achieved, the needle is grasped with the nondominant hand and pulled toward the epidural space, while the dominant hand (thumb) applies constant steady pressure on the syringe plunger, thus compressing the air bubble. When the epidural space is entered, the pressure applied to the syringe plunger will allow the solution to flow without resistance into the epidural space. An alternative technique, although one that I believe has a less precise endpoint, is the hanging-drop technique for identifying entry into the epidural space. In this technique, when the needle is placed in the ligamentum flavum, a drop of solution is introduced into the hub of the needle (Fig. 45-6A). No syringe is attached, and when the needle is advanced

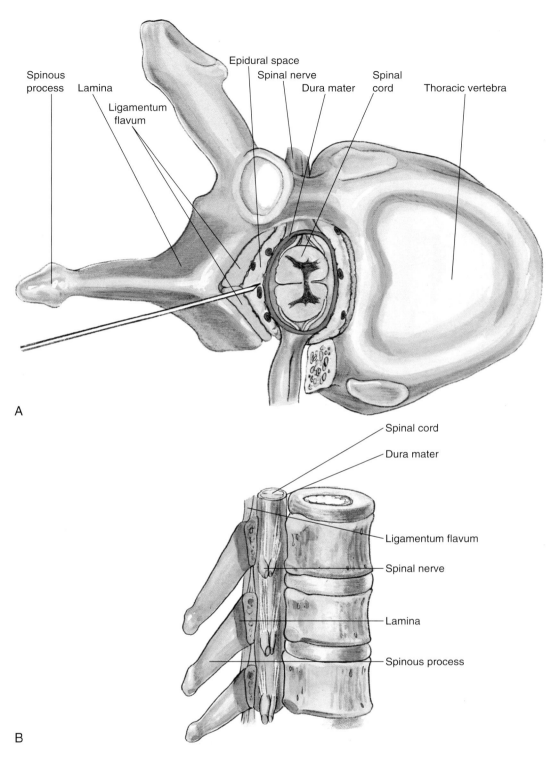

Figure 45-2. Thoracic epidural block anatomy: overlapping of midthoracic spinous processes requires a paramedian technique. A, Cross-section, superior view. B, Lateral view, paramedian section.

into the epidural space, the solution should be "sucked into" the space (Fig. 45-6B).

No matter what method is chosen for needle insertion, when the epidural space is cannulated with a catheter, success may be increased by advancing the needle 1 to 2 mm farther once the space has been identified. In addition, the incidence of unintentional intravenous cannulation with an epidural catheter may be decreased by injecting 5 to 10 mL of solution before threading the catheter. If a catheter is inserted, it should be inserted only 2 to 3 cm

into the epidural space because threading it farther may increase the likelihood of catheter malposition. Obstetric patients require catheters to be inserted to 3 to 5 cm into the epidural space to minimize dislodgement during labor analgesia.

Needle Puncture: Thoracic Epidural.   As with lumbar epidural anesthesia, patients are usually placed into a lateral decubitus position for needle insertion into the thoracic epidural space (Fig. 45-7). In this technique, the paramedian approach is preferred because it allows easier access to

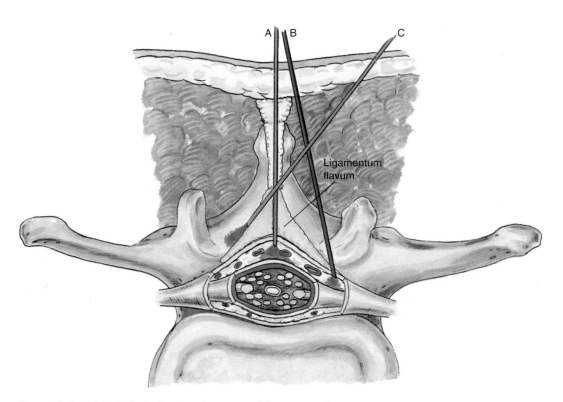

Figure 45-3. Epidural block: functional anatomy of ligamentum flavum.

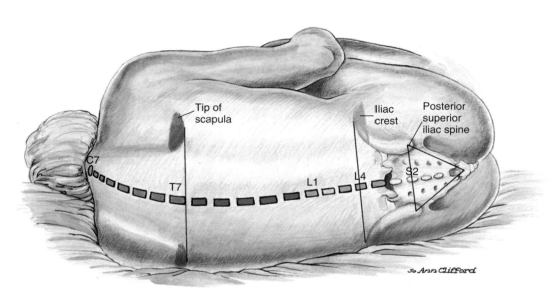

Figure 45-4. Neuraxial anatomy: surface relationships.

the epidural space. This is because the spinous processes in the midthoracic region overlap each other from cephalad to caudad (Fig. 45-8). The paramedian approach is carried out in a manner similar to that used for the lumbar epidural space, although in almost every instance the initial needle insertion will result in contact with the thoracic vertebral lamina by the epidural needle (Fig. 45-9). When this occurs, the needle is withdrawn slightly and the tip redirected cephalad in small incremental steps until the needle is firmly seated in the ligamentum flavum. At this point, the loss-of-resistance technique and insertion of the catheter are carried out in a manner identical to that used for lumbar epidural block. Again, the hanging-drop tech-

nique is an alternative method of identifying the thoracic epidural space, although the classic Bromage needle–syringe grip is my first choice for the thoracic epidural block (Fig. 45-10).

Needle Puncture: Cervical Epidural.   In the cervical epidural technique, the patient is typically in a sitting position with the head bent forward and supported on a table (Fig. 45-11). A comparison of the cervical epidural block with the lumbar epidural block reveals many similarities. The spinous processes of the cervical vertebrae are nearly perpendicular to the long axis of the vertebral column; thus a midline technique is applicable for the cervical epidural block. The most prominent vertebral spinous processes,

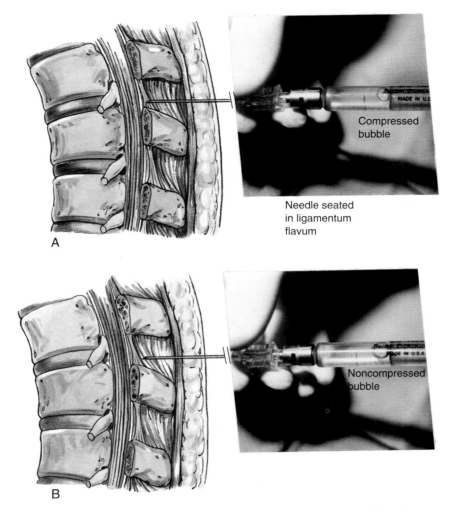

Figure 45-5. A and B, Epidural block: loss-of-resistance technique showing bubble compression (A) and noncompression (B).

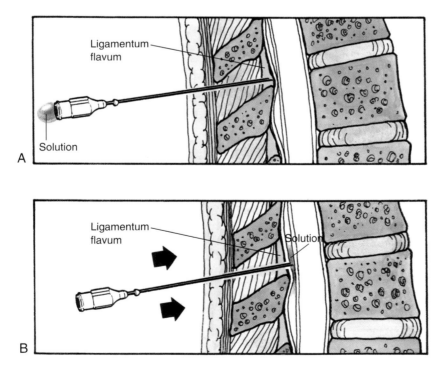

Figure 45-6. Epidural block: hanging-drop technique.

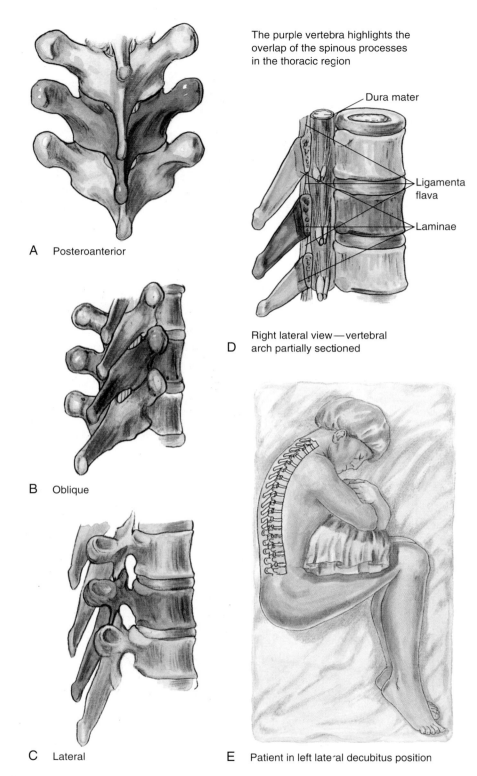

The purple vertebra highlights the overlap of the spinous processes in the thoracic region

A Posteroanterior

B Oblique

C Lateral

D Right lateral view—vertebral arch partially sectioned

Dura mater

Ligamenta flava

Laminae

E Patient in left lateral decubitus position

Figure 45-7. Thoracic epidural block anatomy: midthoracic spine. A, Posteroanterior view. B, Oblique view. C, Lateral view. D, Lateral view after removal of right vertebral arch. E, Patient in left lateral decubitus position for thoracic epidural anesthesia.

those of C7 and T1, are identified with the neck flexed (Fig. 45-12). The second (index) and third fingers of the palpating hand straddle the space between C7 and T1, and the epidural needle is slowly inserted in a plane approximately parallel to the floor (or parallel to the long axis of the cervical vertebral spinous processes). Abutment of the needle onto the ligamentum flavum will be appreciated at a depth similar to that seen in the lumbar epidural block (i.e., 3.5 to 5.5 cm), and needle placement is then performed using

the loss-of-resistance technique as in the other epidural methods. The hanging-drop method is also an option for identification of the cervical epidural space.

POTENTIAL PROBLEMS

One of the most feared complications of epidural anesthesia is systemic toxicity resulting from intravenous injection

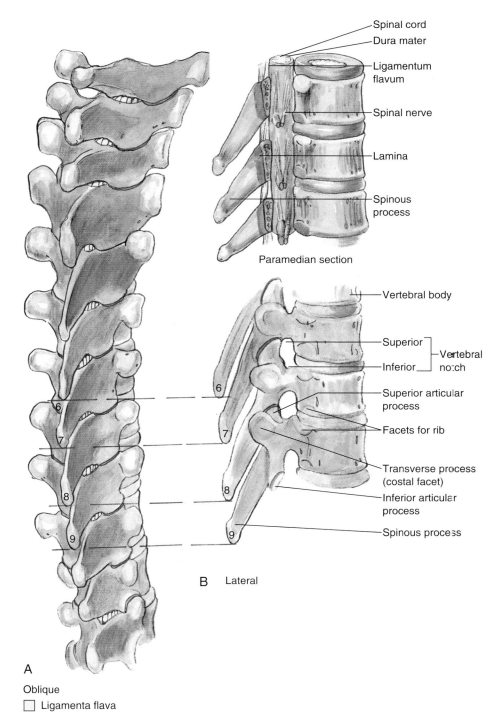

Figure 45-8. Thoracic vertebral anatomy: degree of spinous process overlap changes from high thoracic to midthoracic to low thoracic. A, Oblique view. B, Lateral view and paramedian section.

of the intended epidural anesthetic (Fig. 45-13). This can occur with either catheter or needle injection. One way to minimize intravenous injection of the pharmacologic doses of local anesthetic needed for epidural anesthesia is to verify needle or catheter placement by administering a test dose before the definitive epidural anesthetic injection. The current recommendation for the test dose is 3 mL of local anesthetic solution containing 1:200,000 epinephrine (15 µg of epinephrine). Even if the test dose is negative, the anesthesiologist should inject the epidural solution incrementally, be vigilant for unintentional intravascular injection, and have all necessary equipment and drugs available to treat local anesthetic–induced systemic toxicity.

Another problem that can occur with epidural anesthesia is the unintentional administration of an epidural dose into the spinal fluid. In this event, as when any neuraxial block reaches high sensory levels, blood pressure and heart rate should be supported pharmacologically and ventilation should be assisted as indicated. Usually atropine and ephedrine will suffice to manage this situation, or at least will provide time to administer more potent catecholamines. If the entire dose (20 to 25 mL) of local anesthetic is administered into the cerebrospinal fluid, tracheal intubation and mechanical ventilation are indicated because it will be approximately 1 to 2 hours before the patient can consistently maintain adequate spontaneous ventilation.

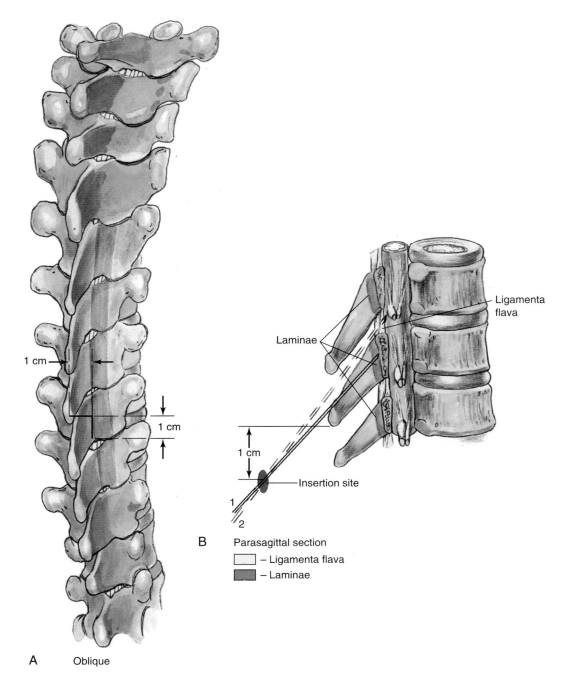

Figure 45-9. Thoracic epidural block technique. A, Using the paramedian approach, needle insertion site is 1 cm caudad and 1 cm lateral to the tip of the more cephalad spinous process, similar to the needle insertion used in the lumbar paramedian technique. B, Parasagittal view of needle insertion and initial contact with lamina *(blue shading)*.

When epidural anesthesia is performed and a higher-than-expected block develops after a delay of only 15 to 30 minutes, subdural placement of the local anesthetic must be considered. Treatment is symptomatic, with the most difficult part involving recognition that a subdural injection is possible.

As with spinal anesthesia, if neurologic injury occurs after epidural anesthesia, a systematic approach to the problem is necessary. No particular local anesthetic, use of needle versus catheter technique, addition or omission of epinephrine, or location of epidural puncture seems to be associated with an increased incidence of neurologic injury. Despite this observation, the performance of cervical or thoracic epidural techniques demands special care

with hand and needle control because the spinal cord is immediately deep to the site of both these epidural blocks.

An additional problem with epidural anesthesia is the fear of creating an epidural hematoma with the needles or catheters. This probably happens less frequently than severe neurologic injury after general anesthesia. Concern about epidural hematoma formation is greater in patients who have been taking antiplatelet drugs such as aspirin or who have been receiving preoperative anticoagulants. The magnitude of an acceptable level of preoperative anticoagulation and the risk–benefit calculation of performing epidural anesthesia in the anticoagulated patient remain indeterminate at this time. The use of epidural techniques in patients

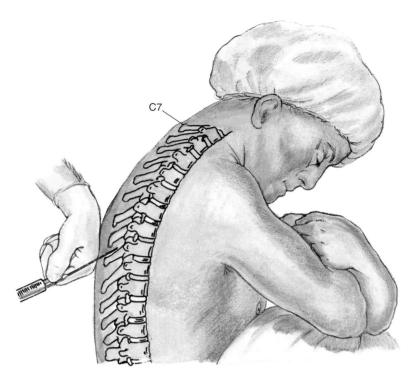

Figure 45-10. Thoracic epidural block technique: Bromage grip for loss-of-resistance technique in thoracic block.

receiving subcutaneous heparin therapy is probably acceptable if the block can be performed atraumatically, although the risk–benefit ratio of the technique must be weighed for each patient. Perioperative anticoagulant regimens that demand special consideration are the use of low-molecular-weight heparin (LMWH) or potent antiplatelet drugs concurrently with epidural block. Low-molecular-weight heparin is used for prophylaxis of deep venous thrombosis and produces more profound effects than other intermittently dosed heparin products. It is currently recommended that no procedure, including withdrawal or manipulation of an epidural catheter, should occur within 12 hours after a dose of LMWH, and the next dose of LMWH should be delayed for at least 2 hours after atraumatic epidural needle or catheter insertion or manipulation. The antiplatelet drugs (e.g., ticlopidine, clopidogrel, and platelet glycoprotein IIb/IIIa receptor antagonists) are sometimes combined with aspirin and other anticoagulants. Expert guidelines need to be consulted when using regional blocks in the increasing number of patients on antiplatelet compounds.

As in spinal anesthesia, post–dural puncture headache can result from epidural anesthesia when unintentional subarachnoid puncture accompanies the technique. When using the larger-diameter epidural needles (18 and 19 gauge), it can be expected that at least 50% of patients experiencing unintentional dural puncture will have a postoperative headache.

PEARLS

Avoiding catheters during epidural anesthesia—that is, by selecting an appropriate local anesthetic—can avoid a potential source of difficulty with the technique. Epidural

catheters can be malpositioned in a number of ways. If a catheter is inserted too far into the epidural space, it can be routed out of foramina, resulting in patchy epidural block. The catheter can also be inserted into the subdural or subarachnoid space or into an epidural vein. Similarly, the use of epidural catheters may be complicated by a prominent dorsomedian connective tissue band (epidural septum or fat pad), which is found in some patients.

Another means of facilitating the success of epidural anesthesia is to allow the block enough "soak time" before beginning the surgical procedure. This is most effectively accomplished if the block is carried out in an induction room separate from the operating room. There appears to be a plateau effect in the doses of epidural local anesthetics; that is, once a certain quantity of local anesthetic has been injected, more of the same agent does not significantly increase the block height, but rather may make the block denser, perhaps improving quality.

One observation about epidural anesthesia through a catheter that needs to be emphasized is the often faulty clinical logic that, by giving incremental doses through a catheter, the level of sensory anesthesia can be slowly developed, thereby allowing frail and physiologically compromised patients to undergo epidural anesthesia. However, when this approach is taken, anesthesiologists usually do not allow enough time between injections because of the reality of time pressures in the normal operating room. They inject small doses through the catheter but then do not allow sufficient time to pass before performing the next incremental injection. Often the clinical result is high block levels in just those patients in whom lower levels were the goal. Furthermore, this approach to epidural anesthesia unnecessarily delays preparing the patient for the operation and makes surgical and nursing colleagues less accepting of the technique.

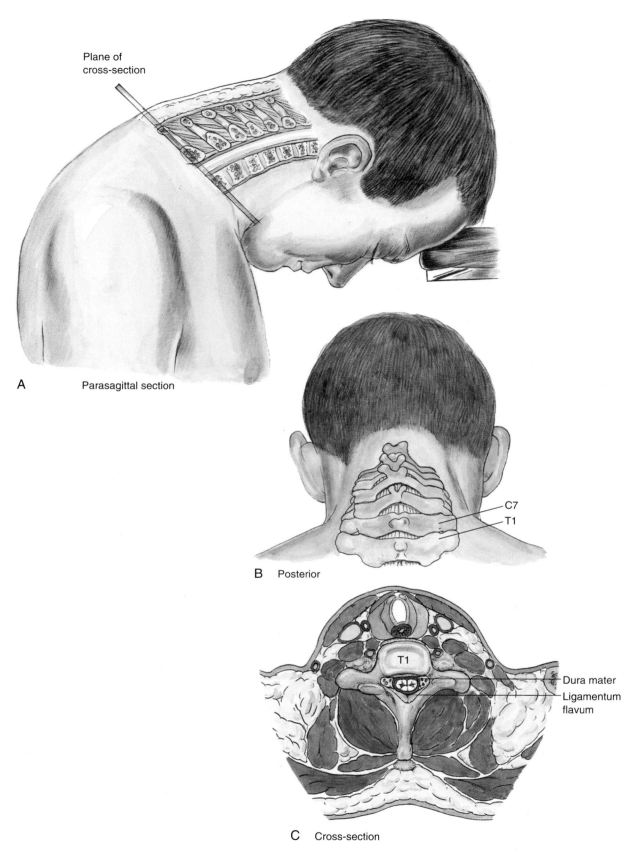

A   Parasagittal section

B   Posterior

C   Cross-section

Plane of
cross-section

C7
T1

T1

Dura mater

Ligamentum
flavum

Figure 45-11. Cervical epidural anatomy. A, Patient sitting with head supported by table, and plane of vertebral cross-section. B, Posterior view. C, Vertebral cross-section at C7 to T1.

Epidural catheters are indicated in many situations, especially when the technique is used for postoperative analgesia. To place a known length of catheter into the epidural space, either the catheter and needle must have distance markers or a way must be found to maintain the catheter position once the needle has been withdrawn over the catheter. Because some epidural needles do not have distance markers, a method of maintaining catheter position while the needle is withdrawn over the catheter is required. One technique of positioning the catheter is

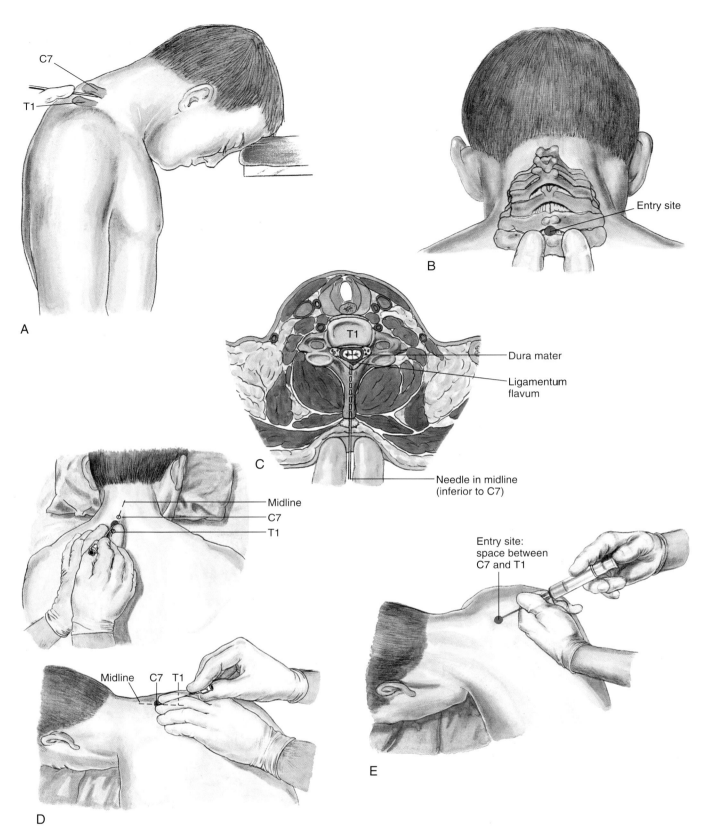

Figure 45-12. Cervical epidural technique. A, Patient sitting with head supported by table with needle oriented parallel to floor. B, Application of fingers to posterior neck to facilitate cervical epidural block. C, Insertion of needle into ligamentum flavum. D, Insertion of needle during palpation. E, Bromage grip during needle advancement.

illustrated in Figure 45-14. An object of known length, such as a syringe or the anesthesiologist's finger, is selected, and that object is placed next to the needle–catheter assembly after the catheter has been inserted 3 cm (or other known distance) into the epidural space. Because the cath-

eter is marked, a known point on the catheter can be related to a known point on either the finger or the syringe. As shown in Figure 45-14A, the 15-cm mark is opposite the plunger on the syringe or the anesthesiologist's knuckle. Once this relationship has been noted, the needle is

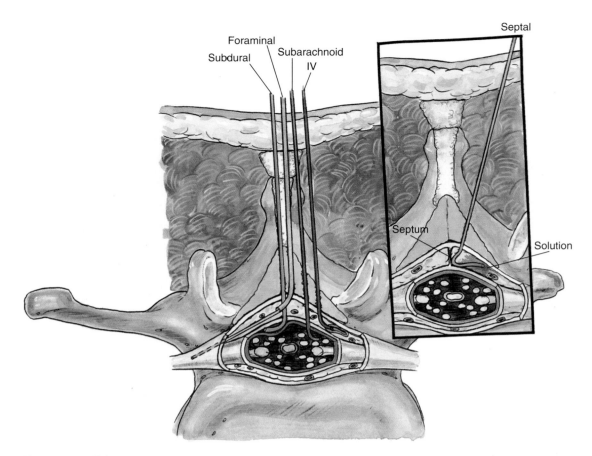

Figure 45-13. Epidural block: cross-sectional anatomy, showing potential incorrect injection sites. IV, intravenous.

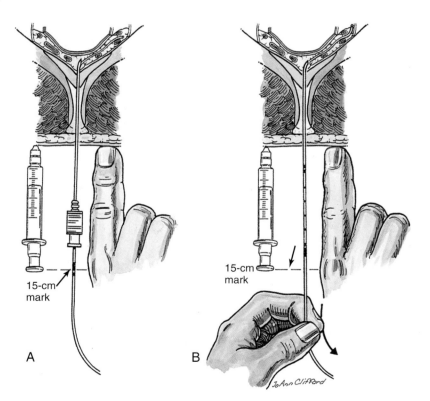

Figure 45-14. A and B, Epidural block: catheter measurement technique.

removed while the catheter position is maintained. The measurement object is then placed next to the catheter, as illustrated in Figure 45-14B, and the catheter is withdrawn to the point at which the distance marker on the catheter relates to the previously identified point. In this example, the 15-cm mark on the catheter is placed opposite the plunger of the syringe or the anesthesiologist's knuckle. By using this technique, the epidural catheter can be accurately placed without the need for either a marked needle or a ruler.

Caudal Block 46

David L. Brown

David L. Brown

PERSPECTIVE

With advances in lumbar epidural anesthesia, caudal anesthesia has become an infrequently used and taught technique. Nevertheless, caudal anesthesia can be effectively used for anorectal and perineal procedures, as well as some lower extremity operations.

Patient Selection. Patient selection for caudal anesthesia should be determined by examining the anatomy of the sacral hiatus. In approximately 5% of adult patients, the sacral hiatus is nearly impossible to cannulate with needle or catheter; thus in 1 of 20 patients the technique is clinically unusable. Likewise, there are patients in whom the tissue mass overlying the sacrum makes the technique difficult, and if another technique is applicable, caudal anesthesia should be avoided. Probably more so than for any other block, experience and confidence on the anesthesiologist's part are necessary to carry out the technique effectively.

Pharmacologic Choice. When choosing local anesthetics for caudal anesthesia, the same considerations as those applied to epidural anesthesia are needed. Volumes of local anesthetic in the 25- to 35-mL range are necessary to predictably provide a sensory level of T12 to T10 with caudal injection for adults.

PLACEMENT

Anatomy. Anatomy pertinent to caudal anesthesia centers on the sacral hiatus (Fig. 46-1). This can be most effectively localized by finding the posterosuperior iliac spines bilaterally, drawing a line to join them, and then completing an equilateral triangle caudad. The tip of the equilateral triangle will overlie the sacral hiatus (Fig. 46-2). The

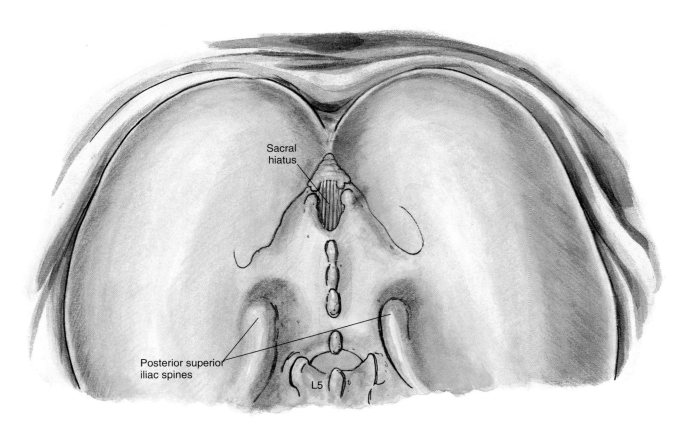

Sacral
hiatus

Posterior superior
iliac spines

L5

Figure 46-1. Caudal block: surface anatomy.

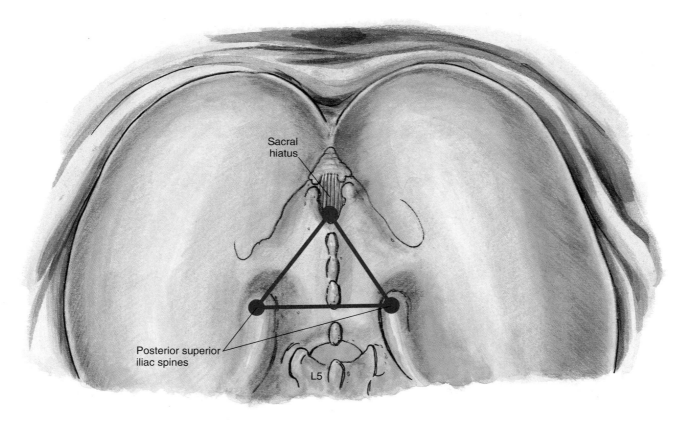

Figure 46-2. Caudal block: surface anatomy showing sacral hiatus localization.

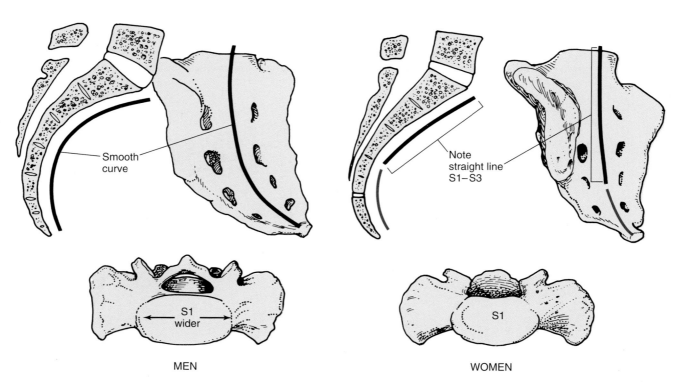

Figure 46-3. Caudal block: relationship of sacral anatomy to sex.

caudal tip of the triangle will rest near the sacral cornua, which are unfused remnants of the spinous processes of the fifth sacral vertebra. Overlying the sacral hiatus is a fibroelastic membrane, which is the functional counterpart of the ligamentum flavum. Perhaps more than with any other sex difference found in regional anesthesia, the sacrum is distinctly different in men and women. In men,

the cavity of the sacrum has a smooth curve from S1 to S5. Conversely, in women, the sacrum is quite flat from S1 to S3, with a more pronounced curve in the S4 to S5 region (Fig. 46-3).

Position. Caudal block can be carried out in a lateral decubitus position or a prone position. In adults, I find the prone position with a pillow placed beneath the lower

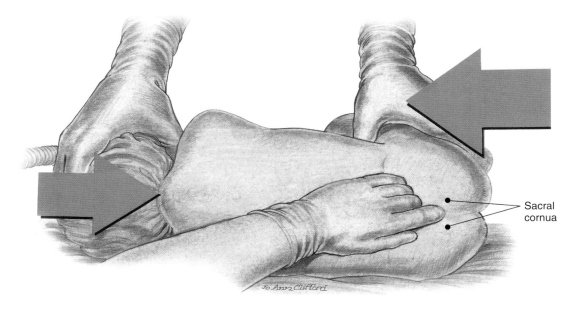

Figure 46-4. Caudal block: pediatric position.

abdomen most effective. In this position, patients can be sufficiently sedated to make the block comfortable, and it makes the midline more easily identifiable than in the lateral position. As illustrated in Figure 46-4, pediatric caudal anesthesia is commonly carried out with the child in the lateral decubitus position. Because most pediatric caudal blocks are performed after induction with general anesthesia, the lateral position is almost mandatory. Identification of the midline and performance of the block are less complicated in the pediatric patient, thus making the lateral position clinically practical. To optimize identification of the sacral hiatus, the prone patient should have the legs abducted to a 20-degree angle with the toes rotated inward and the heels outward. This helps relax the gluteal muscles, making it easier to identify the sacral hiatus (Fig. 46-5).

Needle Puncture. As with lumbar epidural anesthesia, caudal anesthesia requires a decision about the use of a single-injection or a catheter technique. If a single-shot caudal block is to be performed, almost any needle of sufficient length to reach the caudal canal is acceptable. In adults, a needle of at least 22 gauge is recommended because it is large enough to allow sufficiently rapid injection of solution to help detect misplaced local anesthetic injections. If a catheter is to be used, a needle that is large enough to allow passage of the catheter is required. As illustrated in Figure 46-6, after the sacral hiatus is identified, the index and middle fingers of the palpating hand are each placed on the sacral cornua, and the caudal needle is inserted at an angle of approximately 45 degrees to the sacrum. As the anesthesiologist advances the needle, he or she will become aware of a decrease in resistance as the needle enters the caudal canal (*needle position 1*). The needle is then advanced until it contacts bone; this should be the dorsal aspect of the ventral plate of the sacrum. The needle is then withdrawn slightly and redirected so that the angle of insertion relative to the skin surface is decreased. In male patients, this angle will be almost parallel with the

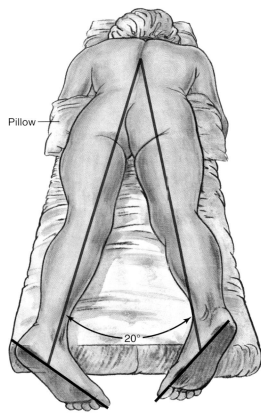

Figure 46-5. Caudal block: prone position.

tabletop, whereas in female patients, a slightly steeper angle will be necessary (*needle position 2*).

During the redirection of the needle and after noting loss of resistance, the needle should be advanced approximately 1 to 1.5 cm into the caudal canal. Further advance is not advised because dural puncture and unintentional

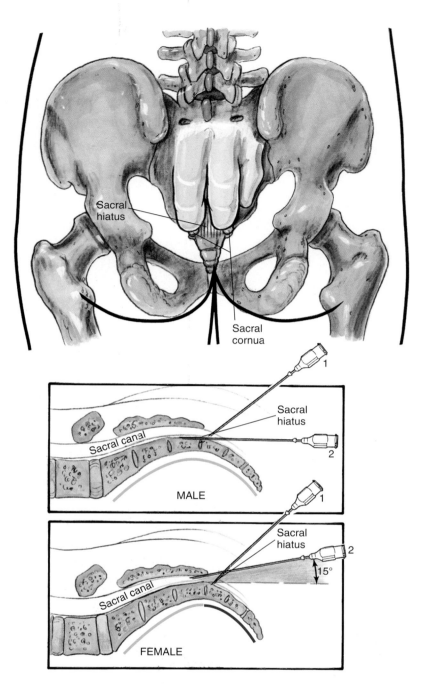

Figure 46-6. Caudal block: technique.

intravascular cannulation become more likely. Before the injection of the therapeutic dose of local anesthetic, aspiration should be performed and a test dose administered because a vein or the subarachnoid space can be entered unintentionally, as is the case in lumbar epidural anesthesia.

POTENTIAL PROBLEMS

Caudal anesthesia entails most of the same complications that can accompany lumbar epidural anesthesia, although there are some differences. The frequency of local anesthetic toxicity after caudal anesthesia appears to be higher than it is with lumbar epidural block. Another distinct dif-

ference is that the incidence of subarachnoid puncture is exceedingly low with the caudal technique. The dural sac ends at approximately the level of S2; thus unless a needle is inserted deeply within the caudal canal, subarachnoid puncture is unlikely. In children, the dural sac is more distally placed in the caudal canal, and this should be considered when carrying out pediatric caudal anesthesia.

Perhaps the most frequent problem with caudal anesthesia is ineffective blockade, which results from the considerable variation in the anatomy of the sacral hiatus. If anesthesiologists are unfamiliar with the caudal technique and the needle passes anterior to the ventral plate of the sacrum, puncture of the rectum or, in obstetric anesthesia, of fetal parts is possible. As illustrated in Figure 46-7, the area surrounding the sacral hiatus can be imagined as a

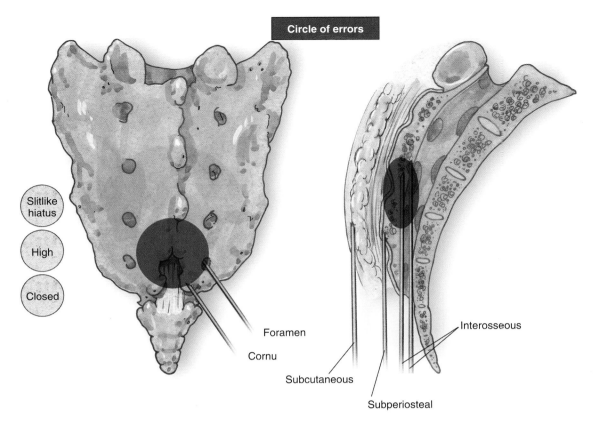

Figure 46-7. Caudal block: circle of errors.

potential "circle of errors." The practitioner may be faced with a slitlike hiatus that does not allow easy needle insertion; the hiatus may be located more cephalad than anticipated or, in fact, may be closed. Likewise, loss of resistance may be encountered as the needle is inserted into one of the sacral foramina rather than the hiatus. In the lateral view, it is obvious that needles may be misdirected into subcutaneous or periosteal locations as well as into the marrow of sacral bones.

PEARLS

To produce effective caudal anesthesia, anesthesiologists should be selective about the patients in whom it is attempted. It makes no sense to use the technique in a patient whose anatomy is unfavorable. Because of the anatomic variations in the area around the sacral hiatus, this block seems to require more operator experience and a longer time to attain proficiency than many other regional blocks. As a result, anesthesiologists should develop their technique in patients whose anatomy is favorable.

One helpful hint that will confirm needle location when carrying out caudal anesthesia is illustrated in Figure 46-8. Once the needle has entered what is thought to be the caudal canal, the anesthesiologist should place a palpating hand across the sacral region dorsally. Then 5 mL of saline solution should be rapidly injected through the caudal needle. By placing the hand as shown, the anesthesiologist should be immediately aware of the subcutaneous needle position overlying the sacrum. If the needle is mispositioned subcutaneously, a bulge during injection will develop in the midline. If the needle is correctly positioned in the caudal canal, no midline bulge should be palpable. In thin individuals, accurate needle placement in the caudal canal and rapid injection of solution may allow the anesthesiologist to feel small pressure waves more laterally overlying the sacral foramina. These smaller pressure waves should not be confused with those associated with a misplaced subcutaneous needle.

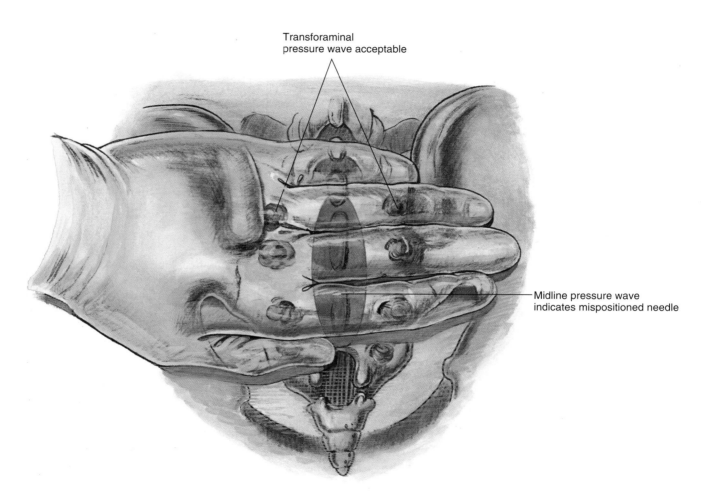

Transforaminal
pressure wave acceptable

Midline pressure wave
indicates mispositioned needle

Figure 46-8. Caudal block: palpation technique.

SECTION VIII

Chronic Pain Blocks

Chronic and Cancer Pain Care: An Introduction and Perspective

47

David L. Brown

Chronic pain and cancer pain invoke many images to physicians, patients, and families. For too long, chronic pain and cancer pain have been undertreated and neglected parts of our society's medical care delivery system. Those of us involved in pain medicine, as physicians and patients, know that these pain states are very real and often poorly managed by colleagues and patients.

Many have considered short-term approaches to pain care as the ideal, using nerve blocks to the exclusion of other therapies. Other colleagues have vigorously and actively avoided any use of regional analgesia techniques in the patient with chronic pain or cancer pain. As a physician with a practice of pain medicine spanning nearly three decades, I believe that the polar ends of this conceptual continuum (Fig. 47-1) represent incomplete and inappropriate approaches to pain medicine. Over the long years of my practice treating a wide selection of patients, increasingly fewer of my patients receive recommendations for an

exclusive regional analgesic/anesthetic approach to their pain control or rehabilitation regimen. In fact, many of my patients receive oral analgesia options with a physical rehabilitation and activity regimen, without any regional techniques as part of their therapy. These practices do not suggest that regional analgesic/anesthetic/neuromodulation regimens are not indicated in our patients. In fact, they are indicated in many patients, but they should be used with a clear indication for how they help in diagnosis or in the pain control and rehabilitation regimen in the patient with chronic pain. Their use should be incorporated into a chronic rehabilitation and cancer pain control regimen that focuses on return of function, always keeping in mind our charge as physicians to balance risk and benefit for each individual patient.

I ask that each of us use the techniques described in the following chapters on chronic pain medicine without seeking to establish positions at either polar end of the

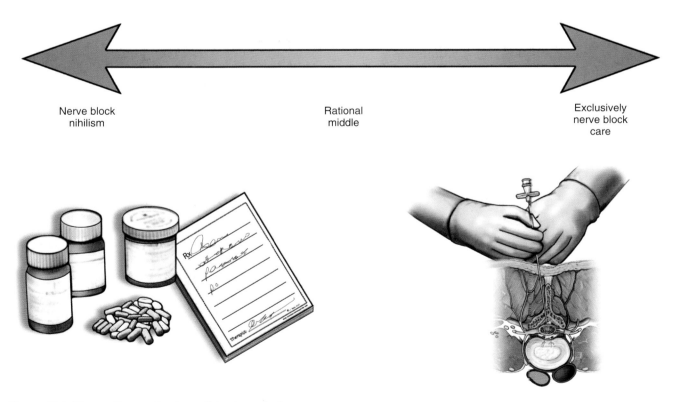

Nerve block
nihilism

Rational
middle

Exclusively
nerve block
care

Figure 47-1. The continuum of pain medicine for patient care.

regional anesthesia technique continuum, represented by *nerve block nihilism* and *exclusively nerve block care.* Our patients will be best cared for by a mature and logical application of the rehabilitation and palliation options so well outlined in the following chapters.

The techniques outlined represent a select group of techniques in pain medicine practice. The list is not exhaustive, but rather a group that my contributors and I have found helpful in our own pain medicine practices. Most important in the use of any of these techniques is to approach each patient as an individual with unique needs, while always thinking first like a physician and holding that age-old tenet of "first do no harm" close to our decision making.

Facet Block 48

David L. Brown

Facet blocks are used to diagnose and treat subsets of patients with chronic low-back and neck pain. Difficulties may arise in interpreting the results of facet blocks because the innervation of facet joints is diffuse, and radiographic changes in facet joints may or may not be linked to a specific patient's pain. Despite the caveats, the pain relief attained with facet injection seems convincing, although in contrast to many other pain management techniques, extra care must be taken in balancing the patient, the pain syndrome, and the treatment regimen with the individual clinical setting.

Patient Selection. Facet-related pain remains a diagnosis of exclusion, supported by reproduction of the pain during arthrography and relief of pain after diagnostic facet injection. In patients with lumbar pain syndromes, facet-related pain is often located in the low back and is described as a deep, dull ache that is difficult to localize. It may be referred to the buttocks or to the posterior leg, and infrequently it extends more distally into the lower leg. The pain is often made worse by lumbar extension, especially with lateral flexion to the affected side because this maneuver opposes the facet joints more forcefully. In cervical facet pain syndromes, the pain remains deep and aching, and the level of the facet involvement dictates the referral pattern of the pain. There are distinct upper, lower, and pancervical neck facet pain syndromes.

Pharmacologic Choice. Diagnostic blocks are most often performed with 1 to 2 mL of local anesthetic, either 1% to 1.5% lidocaine, 0.25% to 0.5% bupivacaine, or 0.2% to 0.5% ropivacaine. Lidocaine is chosen if immediate interpretation is sought, whereas bupivacaine or ropivacaine is used if diagnostic information is sought over a longer interval. For therapeutic injection, the total volume of solution is kept at 1.5 to 2.0 mL, although 20 mg of methylprednisolone is added to the local anesthetic (most often a longer-acting agent for a therapeutic injection). For either diagnostic or therapeutic injection, the needle position is confirmed with 0.25 to 0.5 mL of a radiocontrast agent, Hypaque-M 60% (Sanofi Winthrop, Irving, Tex).

Anatomy. The 33 vertebrae that make up the spinal column are linked by intervertebral disks and longitudinal ligaments anteriorly and through facet joints posteriorly. The posterior facet joints allow flexion, extension, and rotation of the vertebral column while providing a means for the axial nerves to exit the vertebral column on their way to becoming peripheral nerves. The facet joints are synovial joints formed by the inferior articular processes of one vertebra and the superior articular processes of the adjacent caudad vertebra. These articular processes are projections, two superior and two inferior, from the junction of the pedicles and the laminae. In the cervical and lumbar portions of the vertebral column, the facet joints are posterior to the transverse processes, whereas in the thoracic region, the facet joints are anterior to the transverse processes (Fig. 48-1). In the cervical vertebrae, the joint surfaces are midway between a coronal and an axial plane, whereas in the lumbar region, the joints (at least the posterior portion) assume an orientation approximately 30 degrees oblique to the sagittal plane (Fig. 48-2).

The capsule of a facet joint varies by location relative to the joint. A tough fibrous capsule is present on the posterolateral aspect of the joint, whereas on the anteromedial aspect of the joint, the facet synovial membrane is in direct contact with the ligamentum flavum.

The facet joints are innervated through the segmental sensory nerves that overlap the vertebral levels. Each joint has a dual innervation from the segmental nerve at its vertebral level, as well as from the nerve at the level caudad to it. In the lumbar region, the posterior and anterior primary rami of a segmental nerve diverge at the intervertebral foramen (Fig. 48-3A). The posterior ramus, also known as the *sinuvertebral nerve of Luschka,* passes dorsally and caudally to enter the spine through a foramen in the intertransverse ligament. Almost immediately it divides into medial, lateral, and intermediate branches. The medial branch supplies the lower pole of the facet joint at its own level and the upper pole of the facet joint caudad to it. Each medial branch of the lumbar posterior ramus also supplies paraspinous muscles, such as the multifidus and interspinalis, as well as ligaments and the periosteum of the neural arch (Fig. 48-3B). In the cervical region, the medial branch innervates primarily the facet joint and not the paraspinous musculature. Further, in the cervical region, the nerves of Luschka wrap around the waists of their respective articular pillars and are bound to the periosteum by an investing fascia and held against the articular pillars by tendons of the semispinalis capitis muscle (Fig. 48-4).

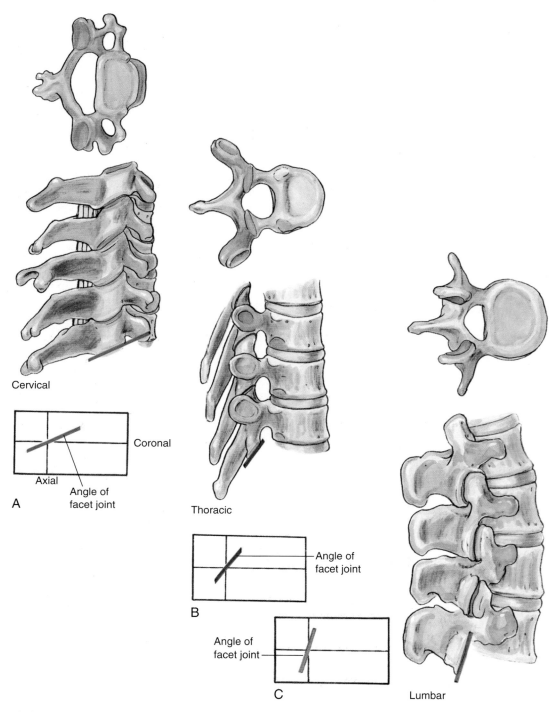

Cervical

Coronal

Axial

Angle of
facet joint

A

Thoracic

Angle of
facet joint

B

Angle of
facet joint

C

Lumbar

Figure 48-1. Superior and lateral views of cervical (A), thoracic (B), and lumbar (C) facet joints. Angle of the facet joints in the sagittal plane is indicated in the *insets*. Transverse processes are highlighted in *purple* in each image.

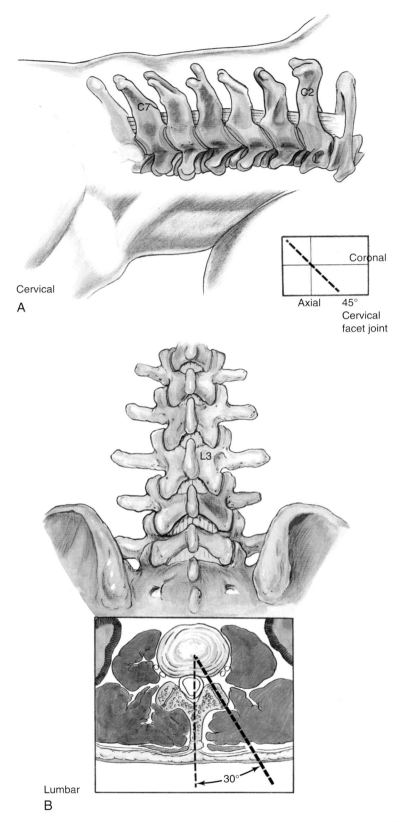

C7
C2

Coronal

Axial   45°

Cervical
A

Cervical
facet joint

L3

Lumbar
B

30°

Figure 48-2. Facet joint orientation. A, Cervical facet joint orientation is midway between axial and coronal. B Lumbar facet joint orientation is 30 degrees oblique to the parasagittal plane.

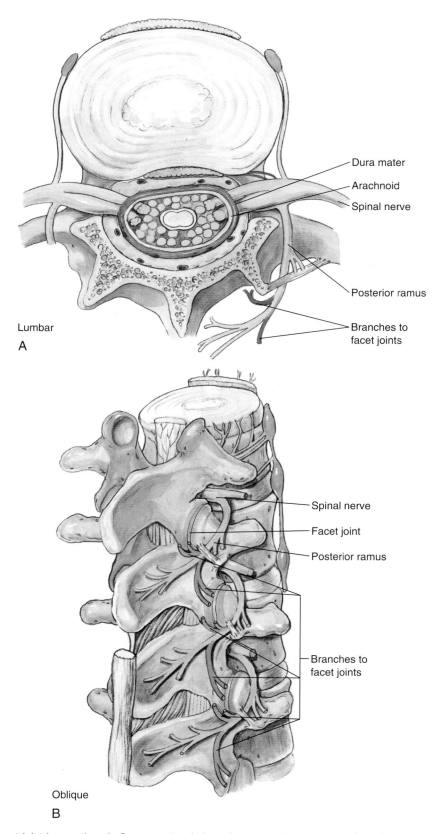

Dura mater

Arachnoid

Spinal nerve

Posterior ramus

Branches to
facet joints

Lumbar

A

Spinal nerve

Facet joint

Posterior ramus

Branches to
facet joints

Oblique

B

Figure 48-3. Lumbar facet joint innervation. A, Cross-sectional view of segmental nerve innervation of facet joint. B, Oblique parasagittal view of overlapping segmental innervation of facet joint.

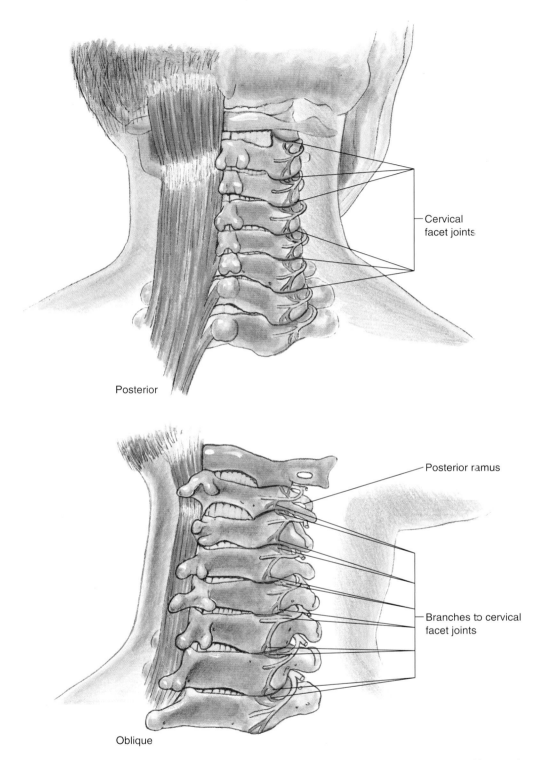

Figure 48-4. Cervical facet joint innervation. Posterior and oblique parasagittal views of overlapping segmental innervation of facet joint.

Position. Lumbar facet blocks are performed with the patient prone on an imaging table with the hips and lower abdomen supported by a pillow. After the level of the facet joint is identified, the fluoroscopy unit is angled approximately 30 degrees off the parasagittal plane to obtain optimum visualization of the lumbar facet joint (Fig. 48-5). Cervical facet blocks are also performed with the patient prone on an imaging table with the forehead and chest supported by pillows or individual silicone pads (Fig. 48-6A). Again, fluoroscopy is used to identify the facet

joint, and after its position has been marked, the fluoroscopy unit is rotated to produce a lateral image of the cervical spine.

Needle Puncture. The facet joint is often located at the cephalocaudad level of the inferior extent of the more cephalad spinous process of the vertebra contributing to the facet joint. For example, the inferior extent of the spinous process of L3 corresponds to the L3 to L4 facet joint. After the level of the facet joint has been marked, the fluoroscopy unit is angled approximately 30 degrees off the

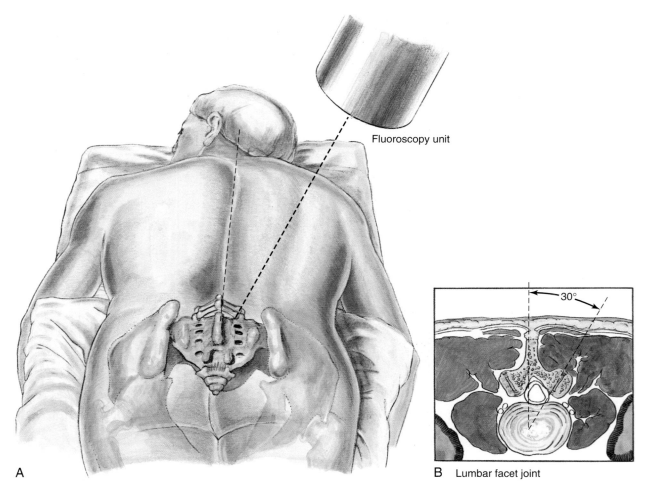

Fluoroscopy unit

30°

A   B Lumbar facet joint

Figure 48-5. Lumbar facet joint. A, Position of patient and fluoroscopic imaging unit for optimal visualization of lumbar facet joint. B, Cross-sectional image of lumbar facet joint.

parasagittal plane, as described previously (see Fig. 48-5). A mark is then made 5 cm lateral to the vertebral midline at the previously identified facet joint level. After aseptic skin preparation, a 22-gauge, 6- to 10-cm needle is inserted at a slightly medial parasagittal angle. Under fluoroscopic guidance, the needle tip is placed in the facet joint (Fig. 48-7). Then a radiocontrast agent is injected to verify the position of the needle tip (see Fig. 48-6B). Once the needle position is confirmed, the therapeutic or diagnostic injection is performed.

Cervical facet blocks are also performed with the patient prone on an imaging table, as described earlier. Fluoroscopy is used to identify the facet joint to be blocked, and its cephalocaudad vertebral level is marked. After the paravertebral cephalocaudad and mediolateral positions of the facet joint have been marked, the fluoroscopy unit is rotated to produce a lateral image of the cervical spine. This allows optimum visualization of the cervical facet joint during needle placement. A needle entry skin mark is made 3 to 4 cm caudad to the facet joint previously identified and approximately 3 cm lateral to the vertebral midline (Fig. 48-8A). After the skin has been aseptically prepared, a 22-gauge, 6- to 8-cm needle is inserted in a cephaloanterior direction and guided with fluoroscopic assistance into the previously identified cervical facet joint (Fig. 48-8B). Radiocontrast medium is then injected to verify the posi-

tion of the needle tip (Fig. 48-8C). Once the needle position has been confirmed, the therapeutic or diagnostic injection is performed.

POTENTIAL PROBLEMS

As in any other regional block, facet injections should be avoided if the patient has a coagulopathy or infection at the site of the injection. Because these injections are administered near the neuraxis, epidural or intrathecal effects are possible, as is injection of the vertebral artery in the cervical region.

PEARLS

The most important word of advice about facet blocks is that they should be used selectively after a thorough history and physical examination directed at the patient's pain complaints. The radiographic and neurodiagnostic studies are integrated with the patient's signs and symptoms. Heeding this advice allows the anesthesiologist to be more precise in performing facet blocks and minimizes frustration over any lack of diagnostic or therapeutic results. Also, to use facet blocks effectively, it is important to understand the innervation of both the lumbar and the cervical facet

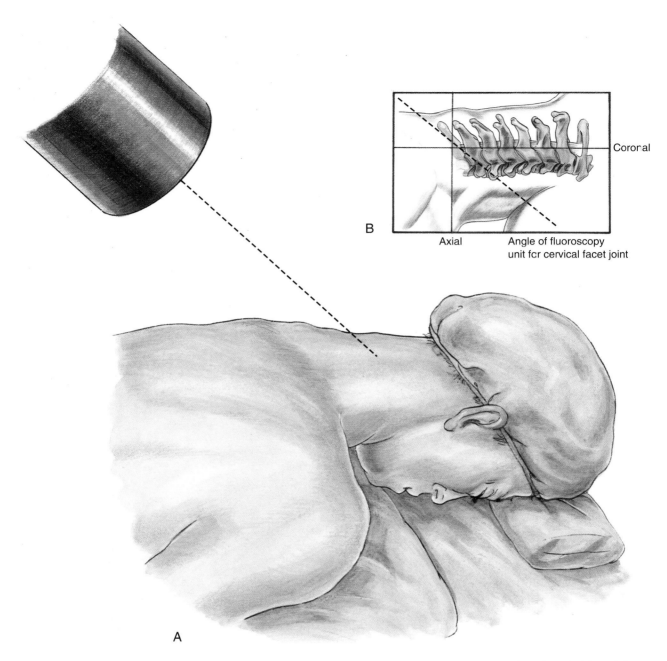

Coronal

B

Axial   Angle of fluoroscopy
               unit for cervical facet joint

Figure 48-6. Cervical facet joint. A, Position of patient and fluoroscopic imaging unit for optimal visualization of cervical facet joint. B, Oblique posteroanterior image of cervical facet joints, showing cephalad angulation of fluoroscopic unit.

joints. Such an understanding helps minimize diagnostic confusion.

Another help in minimizing diagnostic confusion is to become comfortable with radiocontrast agents and their use near the neuraxis; Hypaque-M 60% is currently the preferred agent. It is also important to constantly remind oneself and one's colleagues that radiographic changes in the facet joints have never been effectively linked to specific facet pain states. If larger volumes (4 to 5 mL) of therapeutic solutions are injected at the lumbar facet joints, the results may be difficult to interpret because the solution will not be contained within the facet joint but will spread to the segmental nerves and the paraspinous muscles. Finally, I believe it is important to warn patients that neuraxial block effects are possible (although rare) after facet injections; thus the blocks should be performed only when complete stabilization or resuscitation of unintentional postinjection effects is possible.

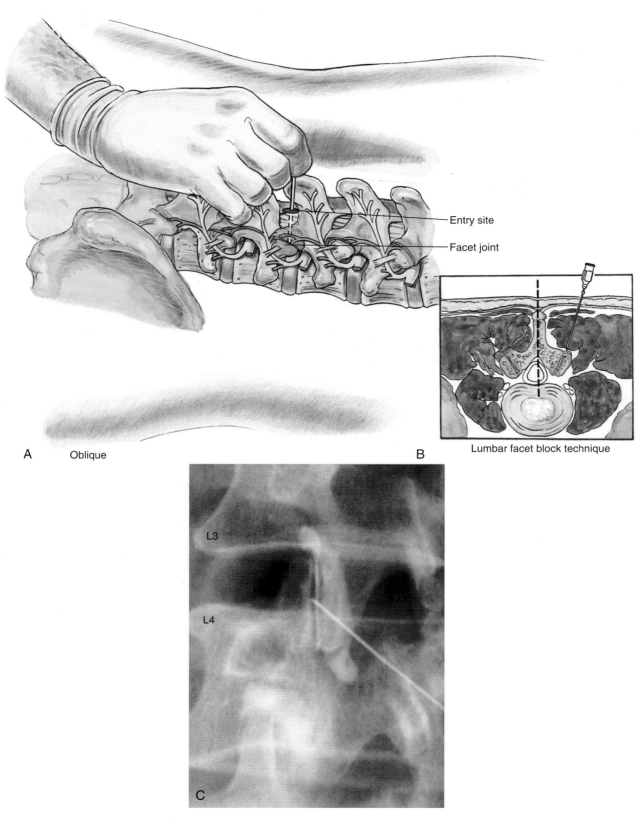

A   Oblique

Entry site

Facet joint

B   Lumbar facet block technique

L3

L4

C

Figure 48-7. Lumbar facet joint injection. Oblique (A) and cross-sectional (B) views of lumbar facet block technique. C, Radiographic image of injection of 1.5 mL of contrast into lumbar facet joint.

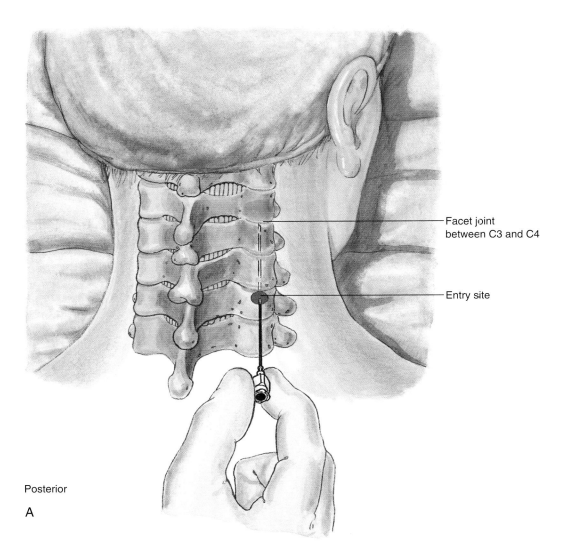

Facet joint
between C3 and C4

Entry site

Posterior

A

Figure 48-8. Cervical facet joint injection. A, Posteroanterior view of needle insertion for a cervical facet block.

Continued

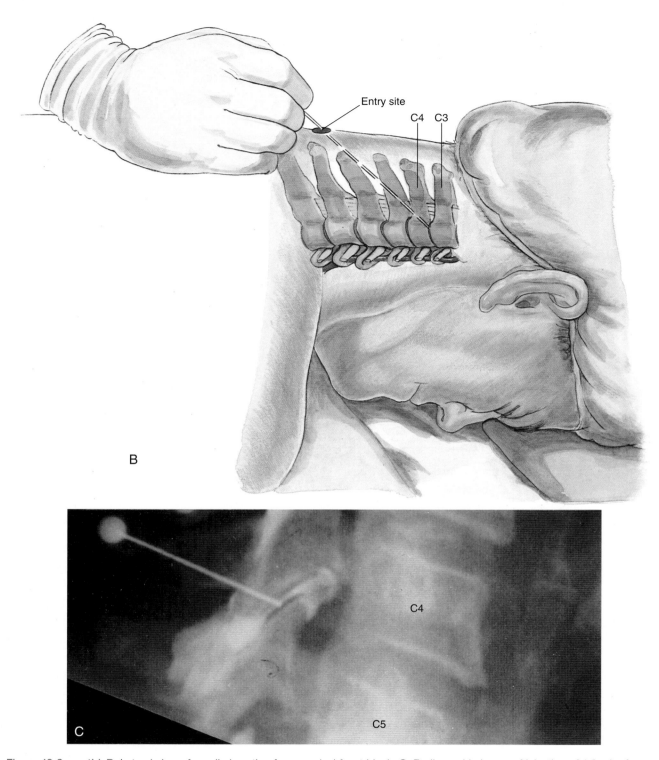

Figure 48-8, cont'd B, Lateral view of needle insertion for a cervical facet block. C, Radiographic image of injection of 1.0 mL of contrast into C4 to C5 cervical facet joint.

Sacroiliac Block 49

David L. Brown

PERSPECTIVE

The sacroiliac block is most often used for patients with chronic low-back pain, both diagnostically and therapeutically. Patients with low-back pain treated at chronic pain centers often experience relief of their pain after a sacroiliac block. Pain secondary to sacroiliac arthropathy is a cause of low-back pain that is often overlooked by physicians infrequently involved in comprehensive pain programs.

Patient Selection. Patients undergoing evaluation for low-back pain should be examined clinically for sacroiliac pain. These patients typically complain of unilateral low-

back pain, which often radiates into the ipsilateral buttock, groin, or leg. Often these patients have symptoms similar to those characteristic of facet joint syndromes. During the clinical examination, an increase in pain with pressure over the sacroiliac joint suggests sacroiliac pain. If such pain is present, provocative maneuvers that increase sacroiliac joint motion should be performed, such as Gaenslen's test and the flamingo test (Fig. 49-1).

Pharmacologic Choice. During fluoroscopically guided provocative diagnostic sacroiliac joint injection, 1 to 2 mL of radiocontrast solution (e.g., Isovue-300 [Bracco Diagnostics, Princeton, NJ] mixed with an equal volume of isotonic saline solution) should be used. This injection

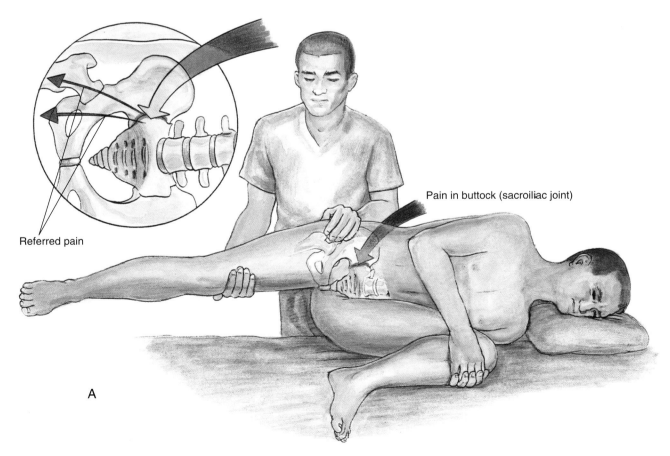

Referred pain

Pain in buttock (sacroiliac joint)

A

Figure 49-1. Sacroiliac joint provocative testing. A, Gaenslen's test: examiner stands behind the patient and hyperextends the leg of the sacroiliac joint being tested while stabilizing the pelvis. Pain with this maneuver may indicate sacroiliac joint involvement, but may also indicate a hip lesion or lumbar root problem.

Continued

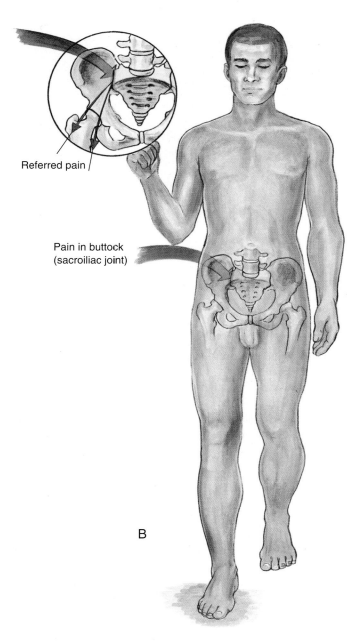

Referred pain

Pain in buttock
(sacroiliac joint)

B

Figure 49-1, cont'd B, Flamingo test: the patient is asked to stand on the involved leg alone and then hop. Pain in the region of the sacroiliac joint is a positive test result.

often provokes pain similar to that experienced by the patient with activity. After sacroiliac joint involvement has been confirmed, a therapeutic injection of 5 to 10 mL of 1% lidocaine mixed with 20 to 40 mg of methylprednisolone can be performed. If fluoroscopy is unavailable and a combined diagnostic–therapeutic injection is performed empirically, 5 to 10 mL of 1% lidocaine, 0.25% bupivacaine, or 0.2% ropivacaine mixed with 20 to 40 mg of methylprednisolone is used.

PLACEMENT

Anatomy. The sacroiliac joint has a well-developed joint space lined a by synovial membrane with typical hyaline articular cartilage on the sacral side of the joint and a thinner layer of fibrocartilage on the iliac side. Anteriorly,

the joint capsule is well developed, forming the thin anterior sacroiliac ligament. There is no joint capsule posteriorly, and the joint space is in continuity with the interosseous sacroiliac ligament. Immediately posterior to the interosseous sacroiliac ligament is the large and strong posterior sacroiliac ligament (Fig. 49-2A). The joint surfaces can rotate 3 to 5 degrees in younger, symptom-free patients, and the joint provides elasticity to the pelvic rim and serves as a buffer between the lumbosacral joint and the hip joint.

Position. Patient position depends on whether fluoroscopy is used to confirm the position of the needle. When fluoroscopy is used, the patient is placed prone with the contralateral hip raised slightly on a pillow (approximately 20 degrees off the horizontal). This position allows the anterior and posterior orifices of the lower third of the joint to be superimposed, maximizing visualization of the joint. If fluoroscopy is not used, a pillow can simply be placed beneath the pelvis and lower abdomen with the patient prone (Fig. 49-2B).

The anesthesiologist can approach the technique in one of two ways. He or she can stand on the side of the sacroiliac joint undergoing injection. This allows palpation of the sacroiliac joint with the fingers of the dominant hand from a lateral position and frees more space medially for joint injection (Fig. 49-3A). Conversely, the anesthesiologist can stand opposite the sacroiliac joint to be blocked, allowing needle insertion with the dominant hand (Fig. 49-3B).

Needle Puncture. When fluoroscopy is used for needle guidance, the patient is placed in the slightly oblique position described in the section "Position." Fluoroscopy is used to superimpose the lower third of the anterior and posterior orifices of the sacroiliac joint, which should appear as a Y-shaped image (Fig. 49-4). After aseptic skin preparation and skin infiltration with local anesthetic, a 22-gauge, 7- to 9-cm needle is advanced into the lower third of the joint, and its position is confirmed with radio-contrast injection. If inadequate spread of contrast medium is noted, the needle can be repositioned under fluoroscopic

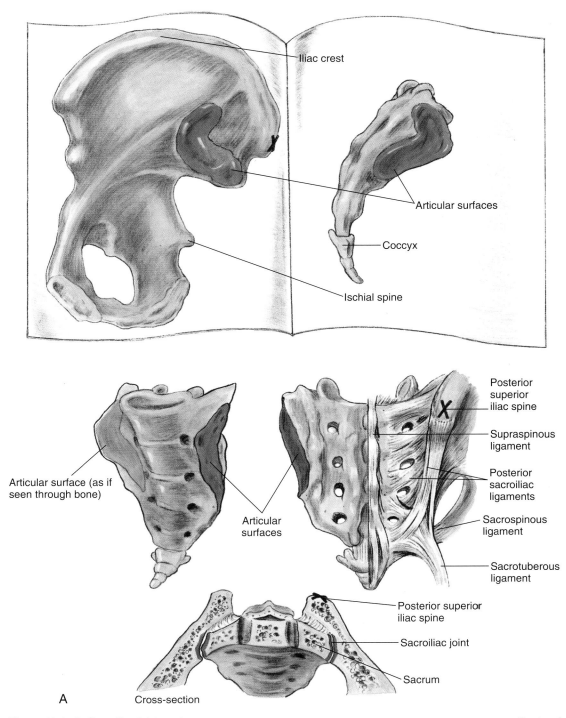

Figure 49-2. A, Sacroiliac joint anatomy.

Continued

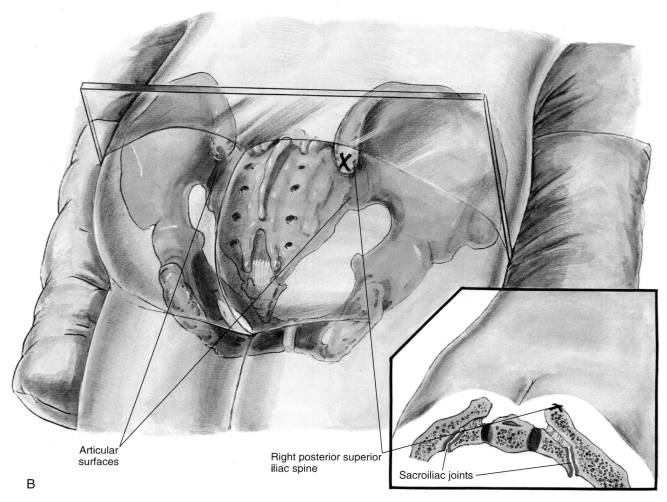

Articular
surfaces

Right posterior superior
iliac spine

Sacroiliac joints

B

Figure 49-2, cont'd B, Clinical cross-sectional sacroiliac joint anatomy in a position similar to that used during block technique.

guidance and the cycle repeated. If no fluoroscopic needle guidance is planned, after aseptic skin preparation and local anesthetic skin infiltration, a 22-gauge, 7- to 9-cm needle on a 10-mL, three-ring control syringe is inserted in an anterolateral direction into the region between the posterosuperior and the posteroinferior iliac spines. The needle may be repositioned along an arc extending between the posterosuperior and the posteroinferior iliac spines, and the solution can be reinjected incrementally (see Fig. 49-3B). Again, it is typical to use approximately 5 to 10 mL of solution during these injections. In the nonfluoroscopic needle insertion, the local anesthetic–steroid solution is directed primarily at and deep to the posterior sacroiliac ligament, and some of the solution may find its way into the joint. Verification of joint injection is possible only through fluoroscopy.

POTENTIAL PROBLEMS

Like any block performed near the sacrum, sciatic or sacral root block is a possible outcome, especially if larger volumes of local anesthetic are used. Misdiagnosis is also possible when fluoroscopy is not used to guide needle placement

and the patient reports no pain relief. In this situation, it may simply be that the drug did not reach the sacroiliac joint.

PEARLS

Sacroiliac block appears to be an underused diagnostic and therapeutic pain control technique. One of the first requirements in using this block effectively is to consider the possibility that sacroiliac joint pain is a source of the patient's low-back pain. In addition, a logical, prospectively planned sequence of fluoroscopically guided sacroiliac block injections should be developed. Although radiographic guidance validates correct injection, it is not used in all cases. An underappreciated symptom of sacroiliac joint pain is referral of pain to the ipsilateral groin. Relief of groin pain after sacroiliac block seems to be linked to the sacroiliac joint as a real source of low-back pain. Finally, before performing a sacroiliac block, it is helpful to warn the patient that a small percentage of patients experience a temporarily numb ipsilateral leg. Advance comment about this phenomenon seems to smooth clinical care even if the procedure results in a lower extremity block.

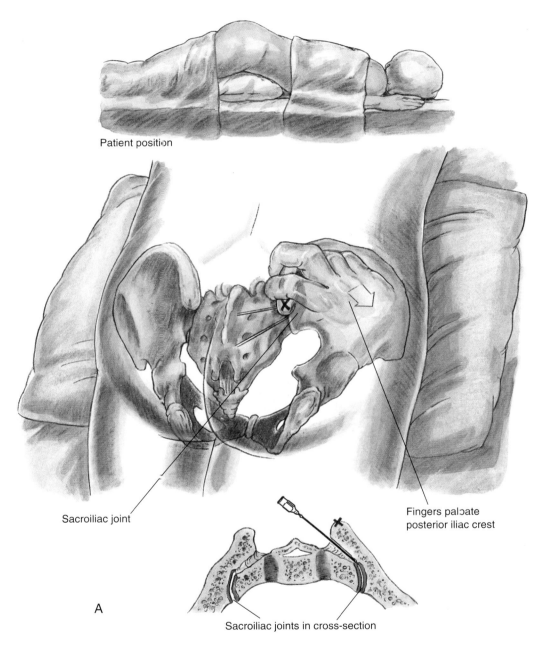

Patient position

Sacroiliac joint

Fingers palpate
posterior iliac crest

A

Sacroiliac joints in cross-section

Figure 49-3. Sacroiliac block technique. A, Palpation of ipsilateral sacroiliac joint when anesthesiologist is positioned on the side being blocked.

Continued

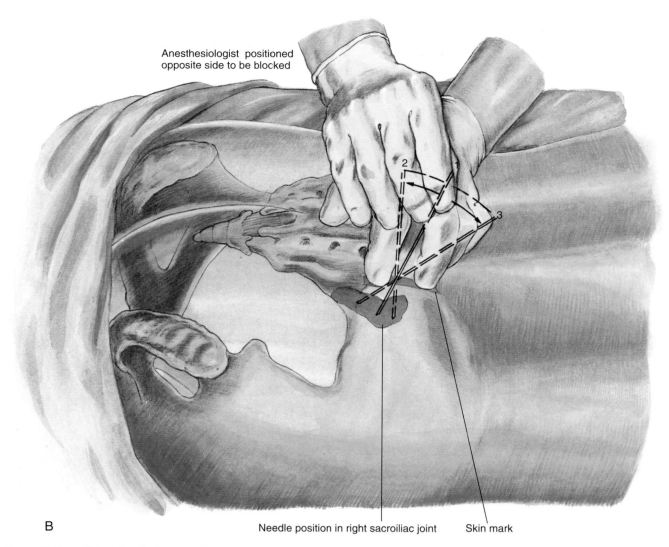

Anesthesiologist positioned
opposite side to be blocked

B

Needle position in right sacroiliac joint   Skin mark

Figure 49-3, cont'd B, Needle insertion for block when anesthesiologist is positioned opposite the side being blocked.

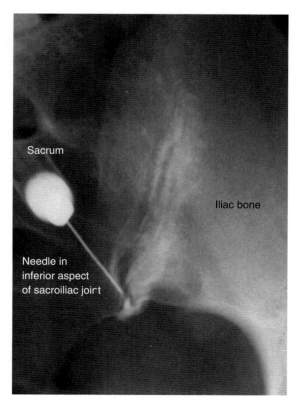

Figure 49-4. Sacroiliac joint fluoroscopic anatomy. The needle is in the inferior aspect of the sacroiliac joint; a small amount of contrast material is seen outlining the joint and spilling out inferiorly.

Lumbar Sympathetic Block

50

David L. Brown

PERSPECTIVE

Lumbar sympathetic blocks are typically carried out to improve blood flow to the lower extremities or provide pain relief to the lower extremities.

Patient Selection.   Patients requiring lumbar sympathetic block can be divided into two primary groups: (1) those requiring sympathetic block because of ischemic vascular disease to the lower extremities (these patients are often older); and (2) patients requiring the block for diagnosis or treatment of complex regional pain syndromes of the lower extremities (these patients have a much wider age range).

Pharmacologic Choice.   Block of the sympathetic nervous system can be performed with lower concentrations of local anesthetics than almost any other regional block. For example, 0.5% lidocaine, 0.125% or 0.25% bupivacaine, or 0.1% or 0.2% ropivacaine are appropriate choices.

PLACEMENT

Anatomy.   The lumbar sympathetic chain, with its accompanying ganglia, is located in the fascial plane immediately anterolateral to the lumbar vertebral bodies (Fig. 50-1). The sympathetic chain is separated from the somatic nerves by the psoas muscle and fascia. The lumbar regions L1, L2, and sometimes L3 provide white rami communicantes to the sympathetic chain, and all five lumbar vertebrae are associated with gray rami communicantes. These rami are longer in the lumbar region than in the thoracic region. This is anatomically important because it allows needle placement nearer the anterolateral border of the vertebral body in the lumbar region. Conceptually, the anatomy important to anesthesiologists performing lumbar sympathetic nerve block is also the anatomy important for celiac plexus nerve block.

Position.   My experience suggests that lumbar sympathetic nerve block is most effectively carried out in a manner similar to that used for celiac plexus block (see Chapter 51, Celiac Plexus Block). The patient should be prone with a pillow under the midabdomen to help reduce lumbar lordosis. (Despite this recommendation, many clinicians continue to use the lateral position successfully.)

Needle Puncture.   Most experienced anesthesiologists now carry out this block through a single needle. This is possible because placing the needle tip at the anterolateral border of the second or third lumbar vertebral body allows

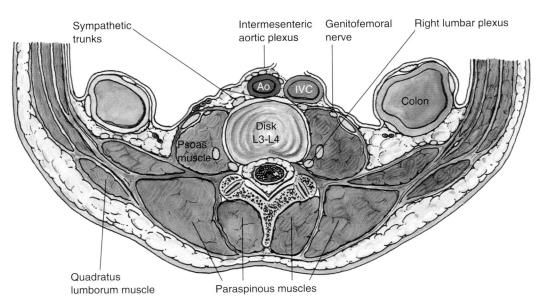

Figure 50-1. Lumbar sympathetic block: cross-sectional anatomy. Ao, aorta; IVC, inferior vena cava.

the local anesthetic solution to spread along the fascial plane, enveloping the sympathetic chain. As an example, the second lumbar vertebral spine is identified, and a mark is made lateral to it in the horizontal plane 7 to 9 cm from the midline, as illustrated in Figure 50-2. A skin wheal is raised, and a 15-cm, 20- or 22-gauge needle is directed in the horizontal plane at an angle of 30 to 45 degrees from a vertical plane through the patient's midline. It is inserted until it contacts the lateral aspect of the L2 vertebral body. If it comes into contact with the vertebral transverse process at a more superficial level (at only 3 to 5 cm), the needle can simply be redirected cephalad or caudad to avoid the transverse process. The vertebral body is usually located at a depth of 7 to 12 cm.

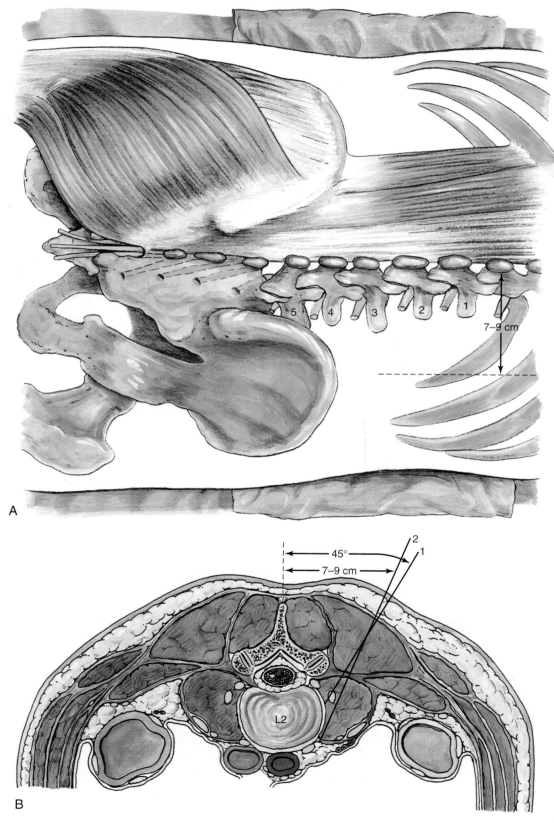

Figure 50-2. Lumbar sympathetic block: surface (A) and cross-sectional (B) technique.

Once the needle's position on the lateral aspect of the vertebral body is certain, the needle is withdrawn and redirected at a steeper angle until it slides off the anterolateral surface of L2. This needle insertion and redirection process is almost identical to that described for the celiac plexus block. For the lumbar sympathetic block, once the needle is in position, approximately 15 to 20 mL of local anesthetic solution is injected. With proper needle tip position, this volume will allow spread along the axis of the sympathetic chain (Fig. 50-3).

POTENTIAL PROBLEMS

As illustrated in Figure 50-4, a potential problem with the lumbar sympathetic block is puncture of the aorta. Most often this results in no sequelae. Nevertheless, anesthesiologists should be aware that the position of the aorta relative to the vertebral body ranges from an anterolateral position to a midline position. Because the needle is directed toward the neuraxial structures, both epidural and spinal block can result from an errantly placed needle. Thus development of a postural headache after a lumbar sympathetic block should lead the anesthesiologist to think of unrecognized dural puncture. Also, when using neurolytic agents, one should be aware that spillover onto lumbar roots is a possibility, although it happens rarely.

PEARLS

Few regional blocks are as similar as the lumbar sympathetic block and celiac plexus block. Thus it is easy to translate the anatomic understanding of one technique into successful performance of the other. Adequate sedation for placing the needle against the lateral portion of the second lumbar vertebra is also essential for patient—and thus anesthesiologist—satisfaction.

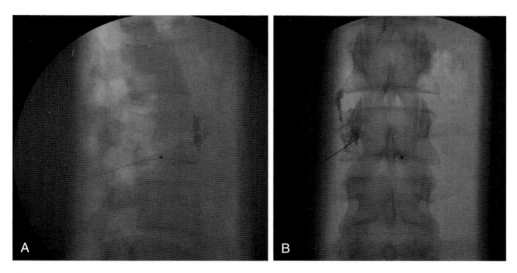

Figure 50-3. Lumbar sympathetic block: fluoroscopic spread of contrast in typical lumbar sympathetic block. Needle placement anterolateral to L3 and spread of 1.5 mL of contrast. A, Posteroanterior view. B, Lateral view.

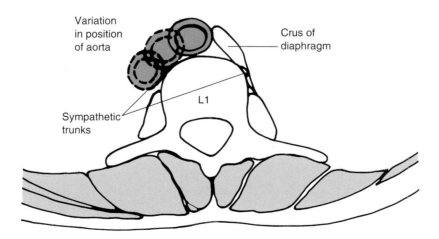

Figure 50-4. Lumbar sympathetic block: variable aortic position.

Celiac Plexus Block

David L. Brown

PERSPECTIVE

Celiac plexus block can be used for many types of intraabdominal visceral pain syndromes. Its most frequent application is to relieve pain associated with intraabdominal cancer using a neurolytic solution. Visceral analgesia can also be provided for patients undergoing upper abdominal surgery; combining celiac plexus block with intercostal nerve block provides an unrivaled quality of immediate postoperative analgesia.

Patient Selection. Most celiac plexus blocks are carried out for cancer pain therapy, and the majority of blocks used for cancer pain are related to gastric or pancreatic malignancies. The celiac plexus provides innervation to most of the gut from the lower esophagus to the level of the splenic flexure of the colon. Therefore celiac plexus block may be applicable to a wide variety of patients with intraabdominal malignancy.

Pharmacologic Choice. The celiac plexus is primarily a sympathetic ganglion; thus low concentrations of local anesthetics are successful in blocking the celiac plexus. For example, 0.5% lidocaine, 0.125% or 0.25% bupivacaine, or 0.1% or 0.2% ropivacaine is adequate. If celiac plexus neurolysis is sought, my choice is 50% alcohol, which is formulated by combining equal volumes of 100% alcohol with 0.25% bupivacaine or 0.2% ropivacaine to a total of 50 mL.

PLACEMENT

Anatomy. The celiac plexus has also been called the *solar plexus*, the *celiac ganglion*, and the *splanchnic plexus* (Fig. 51-1). It is the largest of the three great plexuses of the sympathetic nervous system in the chest and abdomen: the cardiac plexus innervates the thoracic structures, the celiac plexus innervates the abdominal organs, and the hypogastric plexus supplies the pelvic organs. All three of these plexuses contain visceral afferent and efferent fibers. In addition, they contain some parasympathetic fibers that pass through after originating in cranial or sacral areas of the parasympathetic nervous system.

The celiac plexus innervates most of the abdominal viscera, including the stomach, liver, biliary tract, pancreas, spleen, kidneys, adrenals, omentum, small bowel, and large bowel, to the level of the splenic flexure. The celiac plexus receives its primary innervation from the greater, lesser, and least splanchnic nerves, which arise from T5 through T12. The splanchnic nerves innervate the celiac plexus after traversing the posterior mediastinum and entering the abdomen through the crura of the diaphragm a variable distance above L1 (Figs. 51-2 and 51-3). The splanchnic nerves are preganglionic, and after they synapse in the celiac ganglion proper (or associated ganglia), their postganglionic fibers radiate to the abdominal viscera (Fig. 51-4). Autopsy examination has shown that the number of ganglia making up the celiac plexus ranges from one to five, with the size of ganglia ranging from 0.5 to 4.5 cm in diameter.

The celiac plexus is found anterolateral to the celiac artery. In addition, the vena cava is often anterolateral on the right, the aorta is posterior to the plexus in the midline, the kidneys are lateral, and the pancreas lies anteriorly (Figs. 51-5 and 51-6).

One point of anatomic clarification that is essential for understanding the celiac plexus block is that there are two basic methods of carrying out the block. In the longest-used method, the needles are inserted to perform a deep splanchnic block. This results in spread of the solution (*blue*, as illustrated in Fig. 51-7) cephalad and posterior to the diaphragmatic crura. The second method involves placing the needle through one crus of the diaphragm from a posterior approach, or through the anterior abdominal wall, to end up with the needle placed anterior to the aorta in the region of the celiac plexus. As illustrated in Figure 51-7, this results in spread of solution (*pink*) in the vicinity of the celiac artery anterior to the diaphragmatic crura.

Position. The patient should be positioned for the celiac plexus block in the prone position, with a pillow placed beneath the abdomen to reduce lumbar lordosis.

Needle Puncture: Method. The lumbar vertebral spinous processes, as well as the twelfth thoracic vertebral spinous process, should be identified and marked. Parallel lines

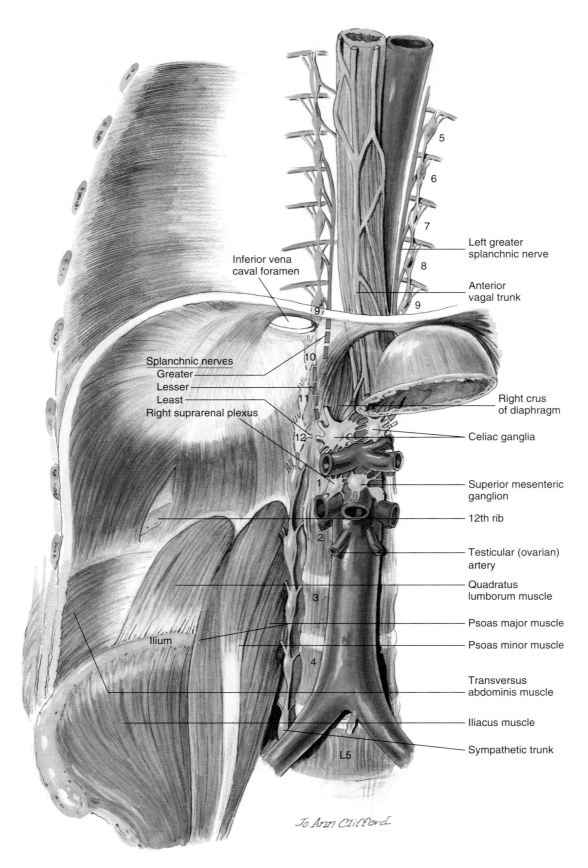

Inferior vena
caval foramen

Left greater
splanchnic nerve

Anterior
vagal trunk

Splanchnic nerves
Greater
Lesser
Least
Right suprarenal plexus

Right crus
of diaphragm

Celiac ganglia

Superior mesenteric
ganglion

12th rib

Testicular (ovarian)
artery

Quadratus
lumborum muscle

Psoas major muscle

Psoas minor muscle

Transversus
abdominis muscle

Iliacus muscle

Sympathetic trunk

Ilium

L5

Jo Ann Clifford

Figure 51-1. Celiac plexus block: anatomy.

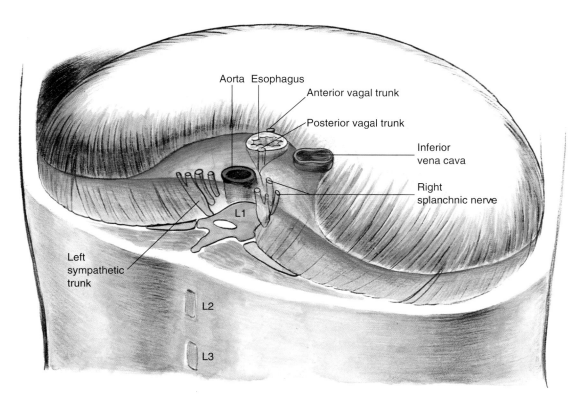

Figure 51-2. Celiac plexus block: cross-sectional anatomy.

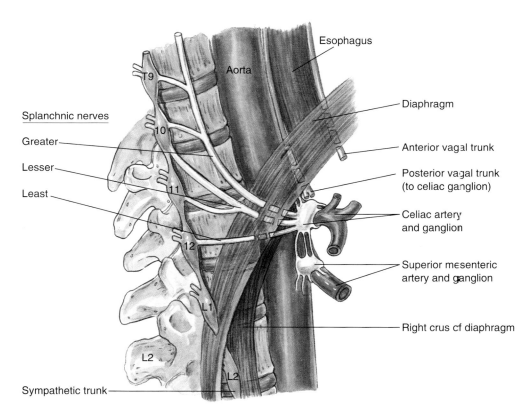

Figure 51-3. Celiac plexus block: parasagittal anatomy.

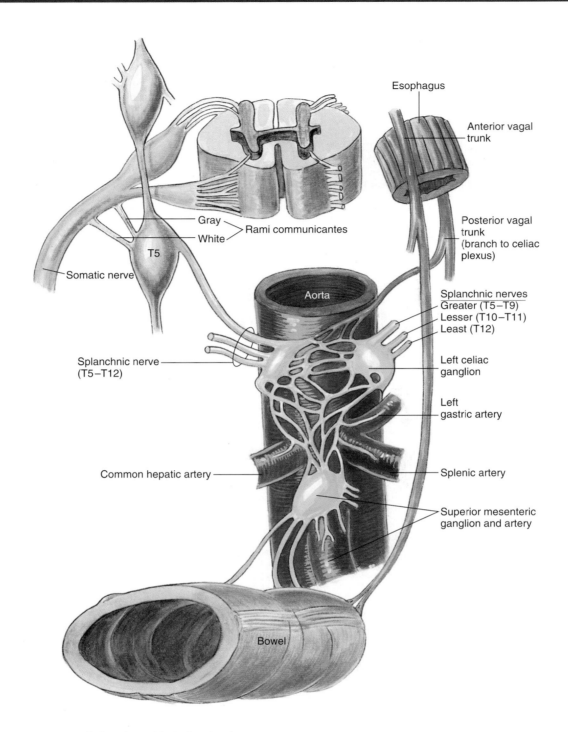

Figure 51-4. Celiac plexus block: functional anatomy.

should then be drawn 7 to 8 cm off the midline, as shown in Figure 51-8. The twelfth rib should be palpated and a mark placed where the paramedian lines cross the twelfth rib bilaterally. Another mark should be placed in the midline between the twelfth thoracic and first lumbar vertebral spinous processes. By drawing lines between the three marks, a flat isosceles triangle is created. The equal sides of this triangle (*A and B*) serve as directional guides for the bilaterally placed needles.

Skin wheals should then be raised on the marks immediately below the twelfth rib, and a 12- to 15-cm, 20- or 22-gauge needle is inserted without the syringe attached, as shown in Figure 51-9. The needle is inserted 45 degrees off the plane of the tabletop, directed at the space between

the T12 and the L1 vertebral spinous processes. This placement will allow contact with the L1 vertebral body at a depth of 7 to 9 cm. If bony contact is made at a more superficial level, it is likely that a vertebral transverse process has been contacted. In today's practice of pain care, most patients will have their celiac block performed with fluoroscopic guidance, simplifying needle insertion.

When the vertebral body is confidently identified, the needle is withdrawn to a subcutaneous level and the angle is increased to allow the tip to pass the lateral border of the vertebral body. On the left side (the side of the aorta), once the needle passes off the vertebral body, it should be inserted an additional 1.5 to 2 cm or until the aortic wall is identified by pulsations transmitted through the length

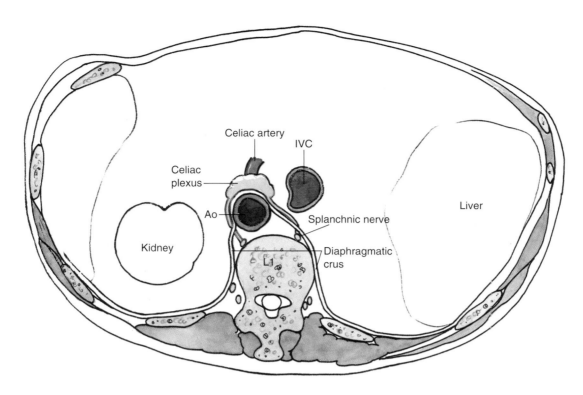

Figure 51-5. Celiac plexus block: interpretation of cross-sectional magnetic resonance imaging anatomy. Ao, aorta; IVC, inferior vena cava.

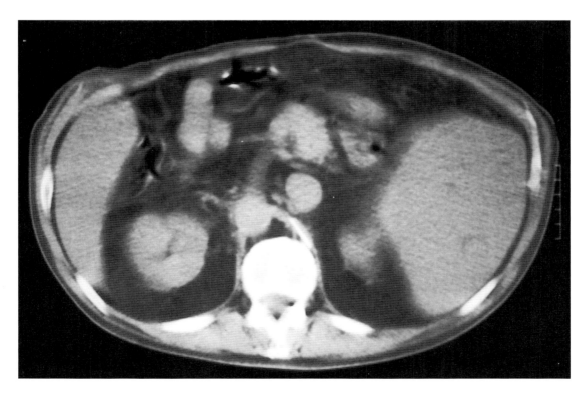

Figure 51-6. Celiac plexus block: anatomy on cross-sectional magnetic resonance imaging scar.

of the needle. On the right side, the needle can be inserted 2 to 3 cm after it "walks off" the vertebral body. It is helpful in inserting the needles to the proper depth to insert the left needle first because it can be advanced slowly until the operator's sensitive fingertips (Fig. 51-10) appreciate the aortic pulsations transmitted up the needle shaft. When this aortic depth is identified, the right needle can then be inserted and readily advanced to a slightly deeper level.

Before local anesthetic or neurolytic agent is injected, the needle should be carefully examined for leakage of blood, urine, or cerebrospinal fluid. If the needle is misplaced, leakage of these fluids should be spontaneous.

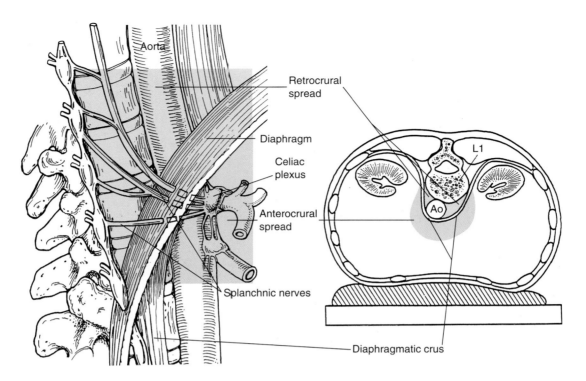

Figure 51-7. Celiac plexus block: retrocrural and anterocrural relationships. Ao, aorta.

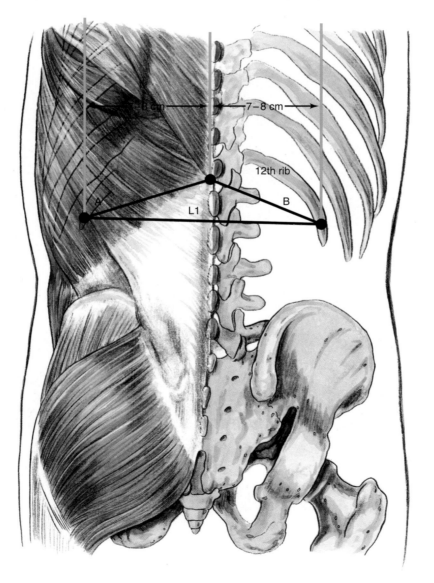

Figure 51-8. Celiac plexus block: surface anatomy and markings.

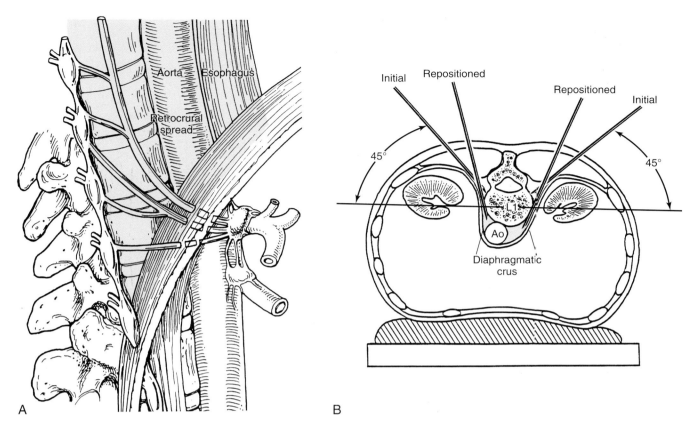

Figure 51-9. Celiac plexus block: retrocrural (deep splanchnic) technique. Ao, aorta.

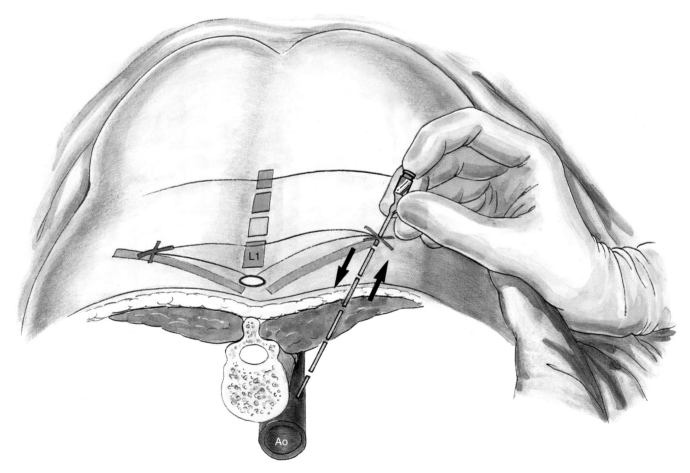

Figure 51-10. Celiac plexus block: technique of using finger as "pressure transducer." Ao, aorta.

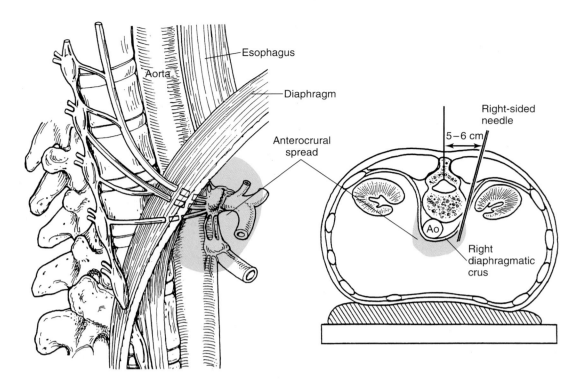

Figure 51-11. Celiac plexus block: anterocrural technique. Ao, aorta.

Injection of local anesthetic solution through the needle should be similar to when an epidural needle is properly placed. There should be very little resistance to injection if a 20- or 22-gauge needle is correctly placed in the retrocrural area.

Needle Puncture: Anterocrural Method. The second basic method of celiac plexus block is the anterocrural approach, which results in the needle tip's being placed anterior to the crus of the diaphragm on the right side, as illustrated in Figure 51-11. To carry out this block, all the foregoing steps are the same except that the paramedian line on the right is drawn 5 to 6 cm off the midline, rather than 7 to 8 cm as in the classic retrocrural approach. The needle is inserted to strike the vertebral body. Often an angle larger than 45 degrees is necessary to contact the vertebral body initially. When the vertebral body is contacted, the needle is withdrawn and redirected until it "walks off" the anterolateral edge of the vertebral body. To place an anterocrural needle properly, radiographic assistance is necessary. Commonly, the needle must be inserted 10 to 13 cm to place its tip anterior to the crus of the diaphragm. It is helpful to use a supplementary imaging technique for the transcrural approach because passage of the needle tip through the crus of the diaphragm is difficult to appreciate by palpation unless a transaortic method similar to the method of Ischia is used. Once the needle tip is in position anterior to the crus of the diaphragm, local anesthetic solution is injected through the single right-sided needle.

POTENTIAL PROBLEMS

Because of the location of the celiac plexus near the neuraxis, epidural or spinal anesthesia may develop with this technique. In addition, because of the close relationship of the celiac plexus to the aorta, aortic puncture occurs in approximately one-third of patients. Nevertheless, this rarely results in serious problems. As in lumbar sympathetic block, the placement of the needle tip for a celiac block may allow tracking of local anesthetic or neurolytic solution in the region of the lumbar roots, although this also appears to happen infrequently. An even less frequent neurologic injury after neurolytic celiac block, paraplegia, may result from drug-induced spasm of a major lumbar-feeding artery (artery of Adamkiewicz). This most likely hypothesis awaits clinical proof.

PEARLS

To understand the celiac plexus block fully, the anesthesiologist should be familiar with the concepts of retrocrural and anterocrural block, which help to develop a three-dimensional "feel" for the location of the needle tip. With the patient in the prone position, adequate sedation can also be administered, and this will go a long way toward making the anesthesiologist and the patient comfortable during the celiac plexus block.

Superior Hypogastric Plexus Block

52

David L. Brown

The superior hypogastric plexus block is conceptually patterned after the use of neurolysis of paravertebral neural plexuses to provide intraabdominal or lower extremity pain relief. Gynecologic surgeons have performed presacral neurectomy for many years to treat a variety of pelvic pain syndromes, and this surgical procedure is designed to interrupt the superior hypogastric plexus. The superior hypogastric plexus block is used for both diagnostic and therapeutic purposes in patients with both benign and cancer pain syndromes. Nevertheless, much of the focus remains on neurolysis to provide pain relief for patients with pelvic cancer pain syndromes who are otherwise difficult to treat.

Patient Selection. When superior hypogastric plexus block is used diagnostically in patients with chronic benign pelvic pain syndromes, it is designed to help define the source of the pain. It is used less frequently for this purpose than for neurolysis of the plexus to produce long-lasting pain relief in patients with pelvic cancers. Cancer pain syndromes that may be amenable to relief with a superior hypogastric plexus block include cervical, proximal vaginal, uterine, ovarian, testicular, prostatic, and rectal cancers. The technique has also been used to relieve pain in patients with distal colonic or rectal inflammatory bowel disease.

Pharmacologic Choice. During diagnostic blocks, the choice of local anesthetic should be determined by the desired duration of the block. Often, 0.25% bupivacaine or 0.2% ropivacaine with 1:200,000 epinephrine is used through bilaterally placed needles for a total dose of 20 to 30 mL. Shorter-acting local anesthetics such as 1% lidocaine, again often with 1:200,000 epinephrine, are also used effectively. When neurolysis is the goal, a radiocontrast agent, 2 to 4 mL through each needle, is used to ensure correct needle position; 8 to 10 mL of 10% aqueous phenol or 50% alcohol can be used as the neurolytic agent.

PLACEMENT

Anatomy. The superior hypogastric plexus is continuous with the intermesenteric plexus and is located retroperitoneally, caudad to the origin of the inferior mesenteric artery. It lies anterior to the lower part of the abdominal aorta, its bifurcation, and the middle sacral vessels; more specifically, it is anterior to the fourth and fifth lumbar vertebrae and the first sacral vertebra. The plexus is composed of a flattened band of intercommunicating nerve bundles that descend over the aortic bifurcation (Figs. 52-1 and 52-2). Broadening below, it divides into the right and left hypogastric nerves. In addition to its continuity with the intermesenteric plexus, the superior hypogastric plexus receives input from the lower two lumbar splanchnic nerves (Fig. 52-3). Figure 52-3 identifies with a *red triangle* a key concept in the superior hypogastric plexus nerve block. The red triangle highlights the anatomic window between the iliac crest, the L5 transverse process, and the L5 to S1 vertebral bodies, which allows successful needle insertion.

In addition to sympathetic fibers, the superior hypogastric plexus usually contains parasympathetic fibers that originate in the ventral roots of S2 to S4 and travel as slender nervi erigentes (pelvic splanchnic nerves) through the inferior hypogastric plexus.

The left and right hypogastric nerves descend laterally to the sigmoid colon and rectosigmoid junction to reach the two inferior hypogastric plexuses. The inferior hypogastric plexus is a bilateral structure situated on each side of the rectum, the lower portion of the bladder, and the prostate and seminal vesicles (in the male) or the uterine cervix and vaginal fornices (in the female). Because of its location and configuration, the inferior hypogastric plexus does not lend itself to neurolysis.

Position. Patients undergoing superior hypogastric plexus block are placed prone on a radiographic imaging table with a pillow beneath the lower abdomen to reduce lumbar lordosis (see Fig. 52-2A). Ideally, biplane fluoroscopy is available to assess needle placement, for which oblique posteroanterior and lateral images are needed.

Needle Puncture. The L4 to L5 interspace is identified fluoroscopically, and skin marks are placed 5 to 7 cm laterally to the midline at the level of the L4 to L5 interspace (Fig. 52-4). This preparation is needed for the insertion of the needles through the area of bony access (shown by the *red triangle* in Figs. 52-3 to 52-5) to the superior hypogastric plexus. After aseptic skin preparation, skin infiltration with local anesthetic is performed with a 30-gauge, 2-cm needle at the previously marked bilateral sites (Fig. 52-5). Local anesthetic infiltration is continued subcutaneously with a 22-gauge, 5- to 9-cm needle along the eventual caudomedial oblique needle path. The fluoroscopic beam is directed along the projected needle path to simplify needle insertion. The needle is then directed under fluoroscopic guidance to reach a point immediately anterior to the L5

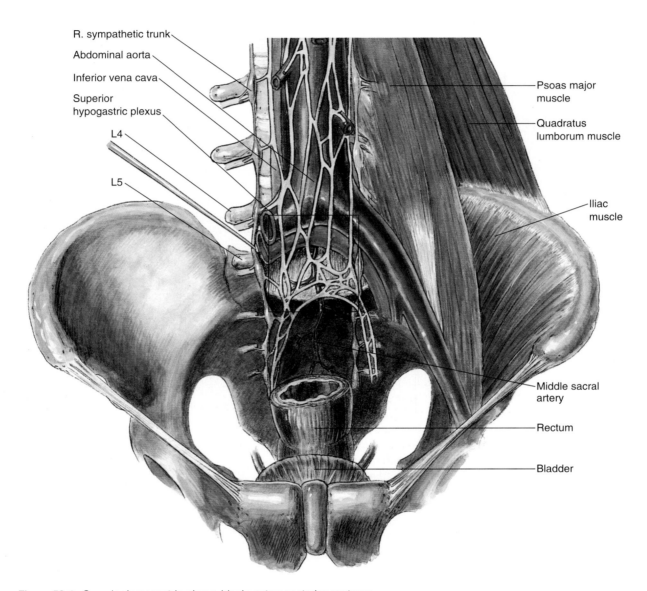

R. sympathetic trunk

Abdominal aorta

Inferior vena cava

Superior
hypogastric plexus

L4

L5

Psoas major
muscle

Quadratus
lumborum muscle

Iliac
muscle

Middle sacral
artery

Rectum

Bladder

Figure 52-1. Superior hypogastric plexus block: anteroposterior anatomy.

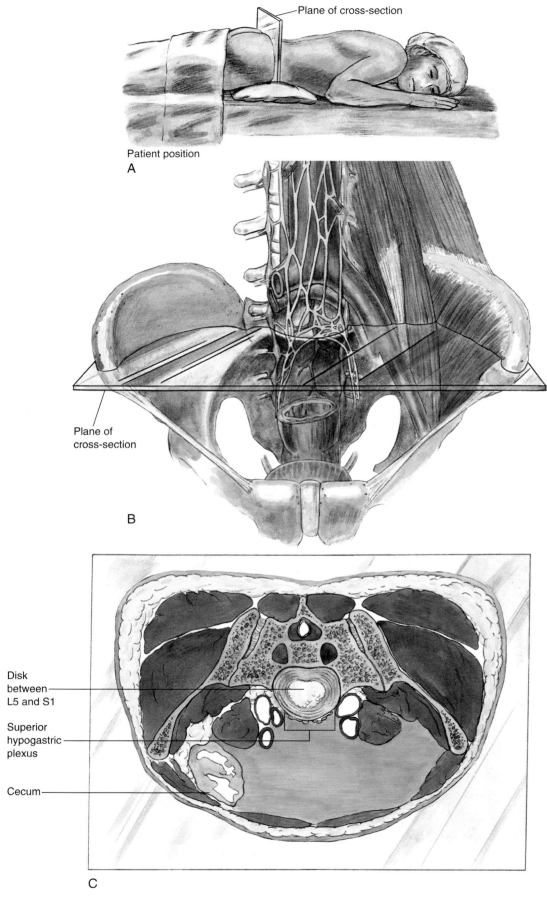

Plane of cross-section

Patient position

A

Plane of
cross-section

B

Disk
between
L5 and S1

Superior
hypogastric
plexus

Cecum

C

Figure 52-2. Superior hypogastric plexus block: cross-sectional anatomy.

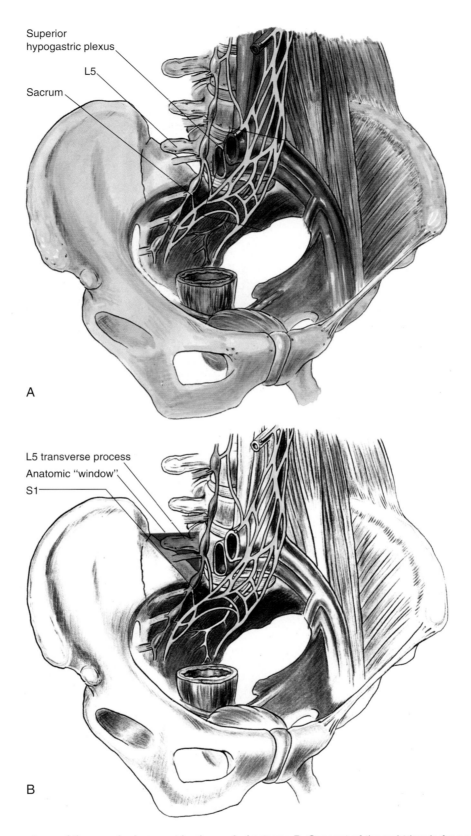

Superior
hypogastric plexus

L5

Sacrum

A

L5 transverse process
Anatomic "window"
S1

B

Figure 52-3. Oblique anatomy of the superior hypogastric plexus. A, Anatomy. B, Concept of the red triangle for access to the superior hypogastric plexus.

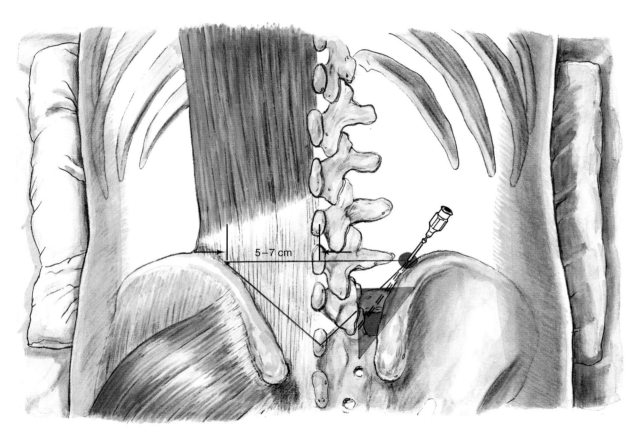

Figure 52-4. Surface anatomy and skin markings important for superior hypogastric plexus block: posteroanterior view.

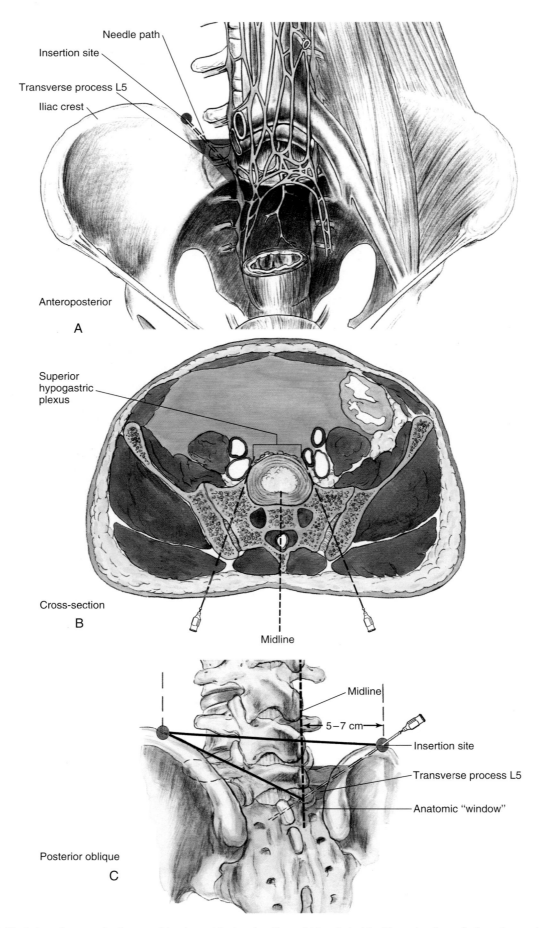

Figure 52-5. Technique for superior hypogastric plexus block using the red triangle to identify route of needle insertion and access to the superior hypogastric plexus. A, Anteroposterior view. B, Cross-section. C, Posterior oblique view.

to S1 vertebral junction; the fluoroscopic beam is directed to minimize the needle hub's radiographic size. If the fluoroscopic beam is directed properly, this approach should guide the needle tip to the correct position. The iliac crest and the L5 transverse process may obstruct passage of the needle; if this is the case, the needle is withdrawn and redirected in a cephalad or caudad angle to bypass the obstruction. As in the approach taken with either the celiac or lumbar sympathetic block, if the needle tip contacts the body of the vertebra (in this case, L5), the needle is simply redirected to "walk off" the body to its desired position immediately anterior to the L5 to S1 junction (the sacral prominence).

Once the needle tip is positioned adequately and the position has been confirmed with biplanar fluoroscopy, the contralateral needle is inserted in a similar manner. Once both needles are positioned, radiocontrast medium (2 to 4 mL of Hypaque-M 60 [Sanofi Winthrop, Irving, Tex]) is injected to verify adequate placement. The radiocontrast agent should spread in a band immediately anterior to the sacral promontory; its smooth posterior margin should identify needle tip placement anterior to the psoas fascia. The contrast should spread toward the midline from the bilaterally placed paramedian sites.

POTENTIAL PROBLEMS

Due to the proximity of the iliac vessels (arteries and veins) to the needle paths, care should be taken to minimize the potential for intravascular injection (Fig. 52-6). This anatomic relationship also makes hematoma formation possible. If the position of the needle tip is not accurately verified, both intramuscular and intraperitoneal injection is possible. Even when the needle is inserted correctly, paraspinous muscle spasm may result from needle-induced paraspinous muscle irritation. This usually lasts only a few days. Less frequent problems are lumbar or sacral somatic nerve injury and renal or ureteral puncture. It is advisable to caution the patient about the potential for bowel or bladder habit changes as well as decreases in sexual function after the neurolytic superior hypogastric plexus block, despite the rarity of these side effects.

PEARLS

When this block is used diagnostically for patients with pelvic pain syndromes, the anesthesiologist should emphasize that the block is being performed for diagnostic purposes, and no neurolytic block is planned. To use a superior hypogastric plexus block most effectively, the anesthesiologist must become comfortable with the anatomy, both bony and neurovascular. This block is not possible in my hands without fluoroscopy; thus another strong recommendation is to develop facility with fluoroscopic needle placement for this block. Lining up the needle path with the fluoroscopic beam is a radiographic guidance technique that simplifies placement of the needle.

Some subsets of patients with cancer who may be candidates for neurolysis have previously undergone extensive pelvic surgery, perhaps combined with radiation therapy of the pelvis. In these patients extra time should be spent to ensure that the pattern of radiocontrast spread appears typical. This recommendation stems from experience with patients in whom extensive prior surgery and radiation therapy has altered the typical neurovascular anatomy. As with celiac neurolysis, complete pain relief after this block is not frequent, but the block often increases patient comfort and minimizes the need for opioid therapy, which can improve the patient's quality of life during the remaining months of life.

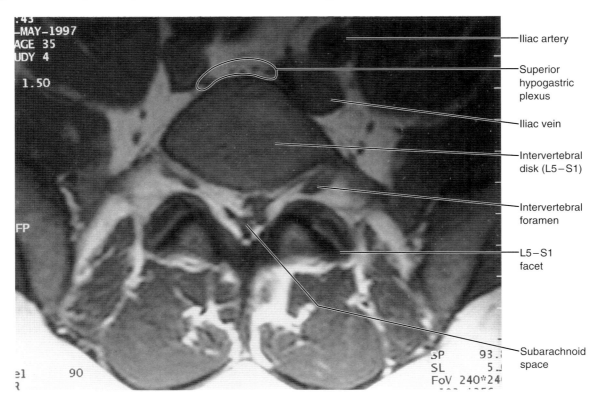

Figure 52-6. Anatomy on magnetic resonance imaging scan of the superior hypogastric plexus.

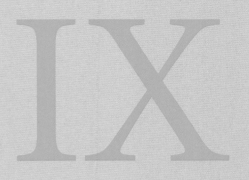

SECTION IX
Pediatric Regional Using Ultrasound

Caudal Block in Pediatrics 53

John Seif

POSITION

After induction with general anesthesia, the lateral decubitus position is the most optimum position for full exposure of the sacral hiatus. Flex both knees to the abdomen and identify the middle line above the gluteal crease, where the sacral hiatus can be palpated.

ANATOMY

Draw a triangle with the base line between the two posterosuperior iliac spines (PSIS) and the apex at the sacral hiatus. The caudal tip will lie between the two sacral cornua of the fifth sacral vertebrae. The sacrococcygeal ligament, which resembles the ligamentum flavum, lies between the two sacral cornua (Fig. 53-1).

SONOANATOMY

This technique becomes even more complex when considering variation in patient age, weight, and varying levels of bone ossification. Ultrasound guidance for this procedure is helpful in identifying the underlying anatomic structures. The ones most commonly of interest include the sacral hiatus, sacral cornua, coccyx, and sacrococcygeal ligament. Although probe orientation can be done using either a transverse or longitudinal view of the midline, it is typically best to orient and assess landmarks before performing the procedure. Placing the probe's transverse plane at the coccyx, the sacral cornua are viewed laterally as humps. The sacral hiatus is located between an upper hyperechoic line, representing the sacrococcygeal membrane or ligament, and an inferior hyperechoic line, representing the dorsum of the pelvic surface of the sacrum (Figs 53-2 and 53-3).

TECHNIQUE

If single-shot analgesia is required, a 22-gauge Angiocath is used, and if an epidural catheter is required, then a larger Angiocath—for example, 20- or 18-gauge—is the appropriate choice. After identifying the anatomy, palpate the sacral cornua with the index finger. Advance the needle at a 45-degree angle to the skin distal to the index finger. A doughy sensation is felt as the needle is advanced. Then the angle of the Angiocath is dropped to 15° and advanced until a loss of resistance is felt (a light "pop" in the pediatric population). Before injecting the local anesthetic, aspiration and a test dose should be performed.

KEY POINTS

- Checking the anatomy with ultrasound before and during the procedure assures success. Because the sacrum is not fully ossified, it can still be penetrated by the ultrasound beams.
- Loss of resistance is not significant when placing an epidural because the sacrococcygeal ligament is softer in the pediatric population.
- The needle may be misplaced in the subcutaneous periosteal location or in the dural sac.

PEARLS

- Check the block with normal saline first before injecting the local anesthetic, and palpate the sacrum for any subcutaneous injection.
- Patient selection and experience play a big role in the success of the block.

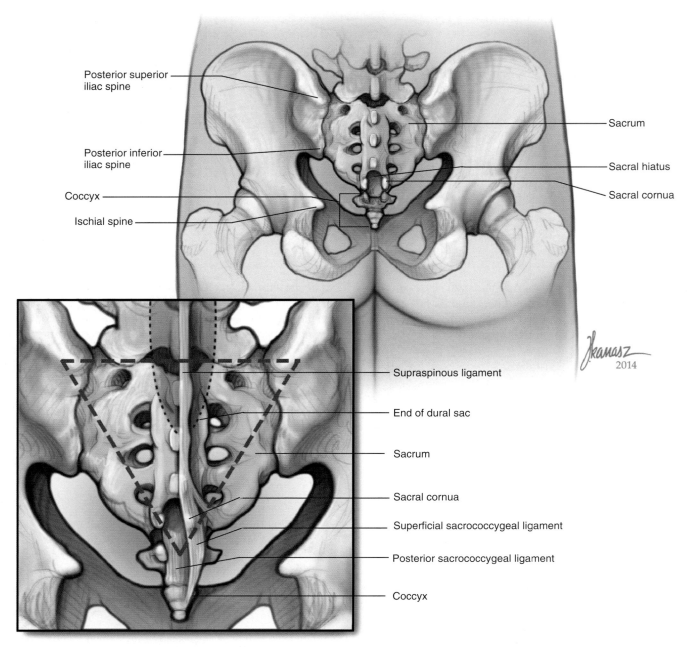

Figure 53-1. Surface anatomy of caudal space; PSIS and sacral hiatus.

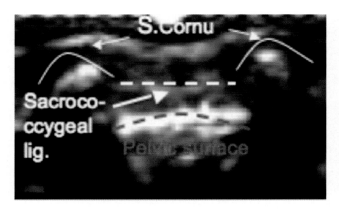

Figure 53-2. Ultrasound still of anatomy of caudal block in pediatrics.

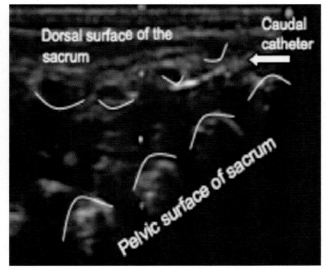

Figure 53-3. Ultrasound still of anatomy of caudal block in pediatrics.

Ilioinguinal and Iliohypogastric Block 54

John Seif

John Seif

POSITION

The patient is placed in the supine position with exposure of the abdominal and pelvic areas (Fig. 54-1).

ANATOMY

Identify the anterosuperior iliac spine (ASIS) and the umbilicus, and draw a line between these two points. Divide this line into three equal distances at the point where the outer one-third meets the inner two-thirds. This is the point of the needle entry. This point is about 2 cm medial and cephalad to the ASIS (Fig. 54-2).

The ilioinguinal and iliohypogastric nerves are formed by branches from T12 to L1, which pass between the internal oblique and transversalis muscles. Performing this block provides good analgesia for most operations of the inguinal regions.

SONOANATOMY AND TECHNIQUE

Place the ultrasound probe on the line connecting the umbilicus to the ASIS. A transverse longitudinal view will reveal the underlying muscles: the external oblique, internal oblique, and transversus abdominis muscle (Fig. 54-3). Advance the blunt injecting needle in plane with the ultrasound probe until two "pops" are felt. The first pop occurs between the external oblique and the internal oblique muscles. The second pop occurs between the internal oblique and the transversus abdominis muscle

(Fig. 54-4A)—this is where the local anesthetic is injected (Fig. 54-4B).

KEY POINTS

- Identifying the different layers of the muscles is crucial because the peritoneum is the shiniest layer under the transversus abdominis muscle. When the bowels are seen under the peritoneum under ultrasound, the sliding sign appears in response to breathing.
- Loss of resistance when penetrating the different muscle layers can be felt as a pop. Extra caution is needed because the needle could advance accidently into the peritoneum and perforate the bowel.
- Avoid puncturing the blood vessels, especially the inferior epigastric vessels, because they sometimes accompany the ilioinguinal and iliohypogastric nerves along their path. Ultrasound aids in visualizing these small vessels, especially if using Doppler mode.

PEARLS

- Visualizing the spread of local anesthetic in the plane between the internal oblique muscle and the transversus abdominis muscle can help ensure excellent results.
- Tenting the muscles is common when using the blunt needle, so a more perpendicular angle needle entrance technique is used.

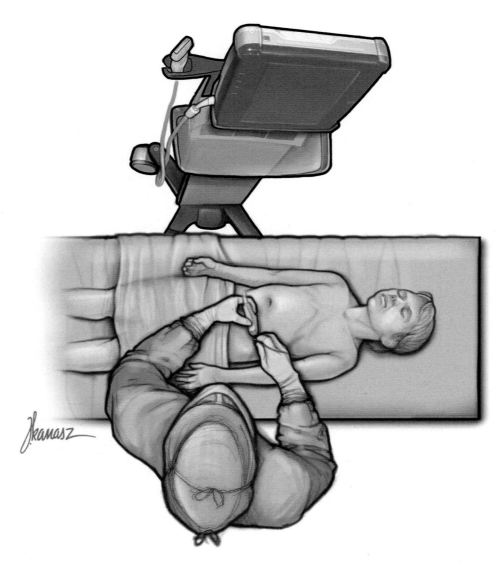

Figure 54-1. The inguinal and the abdominal areas are exposed and the ultrasound is on the opposite side of the block.

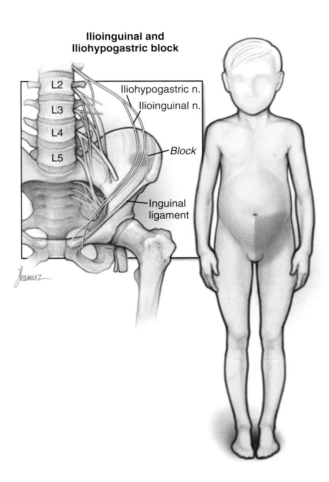

**Ilioinguinal and
Iliohypogastric block**

L2

L3

L4

L5

Iliohypogastric n.

Ilioinguinal n.

Block

Inguinal
ligament

Figure 54-2. Identify the ASIS and the umbilicus and draw a line connecting these two points. Apply the ultrasound probe on this line and the needle entrance point will be at the outer 1/3rd junction of the line.

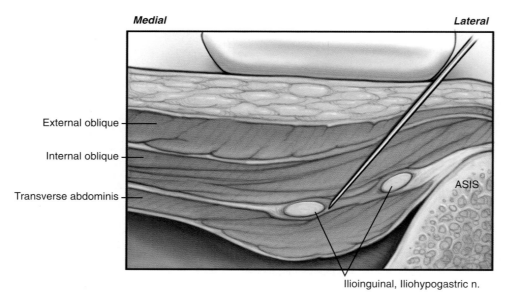

Medial   *Lateral*

External oblique —

Internal oblique —

Transverse abdominis —

ASIS

Ilioinguinal, Iliohypogastric n.

Figure 54-3. The needle is advanced under ultrasound in-plane approach, penetrating the external and internal oblique muscles targeting the ilioinguinal and iliohypogastric nerves lying in the plane between the Internal Oblique and the Transverse Abdominus muscles.

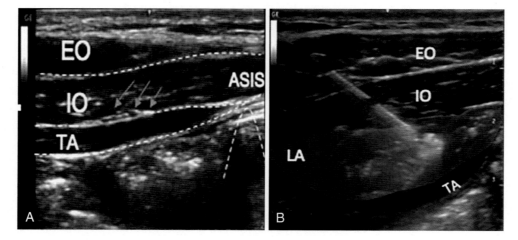

Figure 54-4. A The three muscles under ultrasound, visualizing the ilioinguinal and iliohypogastric nerves. B Local anesthetic spread between the Internal Oblique and Transverse Abdominus muscles as shown on the image.

Superficial Cervical Plexus Block

55

John Seif

POSITION

Place the patient in the supine position without a pillow. The head is turned to the opposite side of the one being blocked (Fig. 55-1).

ANATOMY AND TECHNIQUE

The superficial cervical plexus provides cutaneous innervation to the ventral rami of C1 to C4 (Fig. 55-2). It includes the lesser occipital, greater auricular, transverse cervical, and supraclavicular nerves (Fig. 55-3). At the midpoint on the posterior border of the sternocleidomastoid muscle is the point of needle entry. The needle is inserted, and local anesthetic is injected behind and along the posterior border of the clavicular head of the sternocleidomastoid muscle.

Under ultrasound, use the linear probe and place it in a transverse position at the needle entry point over the sternocleidomastoid muscle. The needle is aligned with the ultrasound probe in the in-plane position. Visualizing the local anesthetic spread on the posterior border of the sternocleidomastoid muscle is the key to a successful block (Fig. 55-4).

KEY POINTS

- Stabilize the neck position, and identify the sternocleidomastoid muscle.
- If not using the ultrasound, always feel for the infiltration with the other hand to avoid injecting the local anesthetic in any vascular structure.
- Infiltrate along the posterior border of the sternocleidomastoid muscle superior and inferior to the point of needle entry.

PEARLS

- If deep injection occurs, that could lead to deep cervical plexus block and partial phrenic nerve block. Hoarseness and an inability to clear secretions could occur.
- Superficial injection of local anesthetic with a 22-gauge needle is recommended.
- This block covers only cutaneous sensation and could be used in mastoidectomy and in clavicular bone fracture, especially in the lateral one-third of the clavicle, for post-operative pain control (Fig. 55-4).

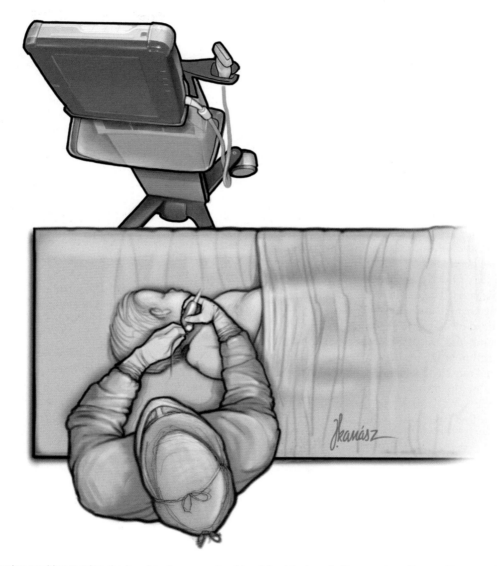

Figure 55-1. Supine position turning the head to the opposite side of the block and ultrasound position on the opposite side of the block facing the physician.

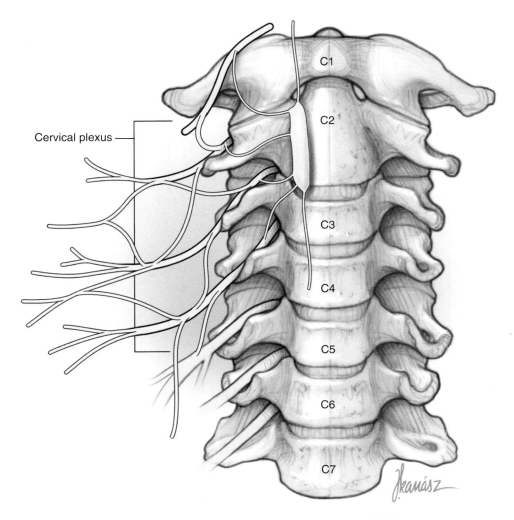

Figure 55-2. Superficial plexus block provides cutaneous innervation to C1-C4.

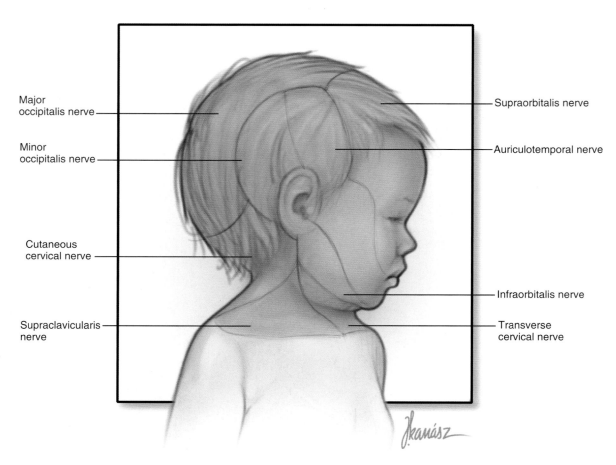

Major
occipitalis nerve

Minor
occipitalis nerve

Cutaneous
cervical nerve

Supraclavicularis
nerve

Supraorbitalis nerve

Auriculotemporal nerve

Infraorbitalis nerve

Transverse
cervical nerve

Figure 55-3. The superficial plexus block will cover the following: lesser occipital, greater auricular, transverse cervical and supraclavicular nerves.

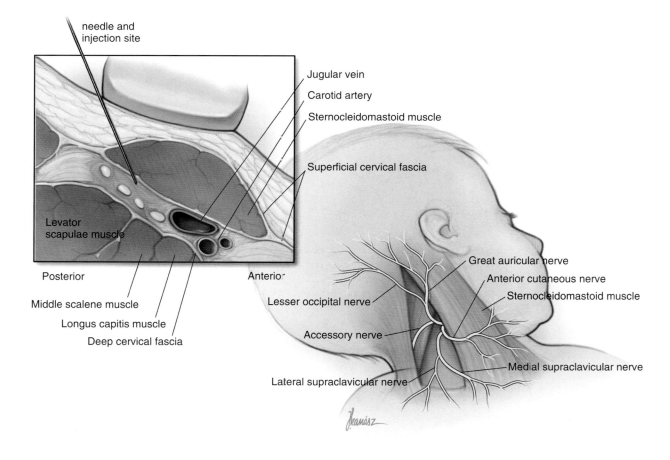

needle and
injection site

Jugular vein

Carotid artery

Sternocleidomastoid muscle

Superficial cervical fascia

Levator
scapulae muscle

Posterior

Anterior

Middle scalene muscle

Longus capitis muscle

Deep cervical fascia

Great auricular nerve

Anterior cutaneous nerve

Sternocleidomastoid muscle

Lesser occipital nerve

Accessory nerve

Medial supraclavicular nerve

Lateral supraclavicular nerve

Figure 55-4. Visualizing the needle advancement in linear approach, targeting the posterior border of the sternocleidomastoid muscle and infiltrating the area with local anesthetic.

Rectus Sheath Block in Pediatrics

56

John Seif

POSITION

The patient should be positioned in the supine position with full exposure of the abdomen.

ANATOMY

The rectus abdominis muscle forms a layer on each side of the midline by the linea alba. It also lies medially to the external oblique, internal oblique, and transversus abdominis muscles. The xiphoid process and the costal margins lie superiorly, and the ilioinguinal ligament and the symphysis pubis lie inferiorly (Fig. 56-1).

SONOANATOMY AND TECHNIQUE

Ultrasound guidance for this procedure is very helpful in identifying the rectus muscle on both sides of the linea alba. Place the ultrasound probe in the transverse view parallel to the rectus muscle and lateral to the umbilicus. Pass the injecting needle or Tuohy needle (for catheter use) in the in-plane position and penetrate the anterior rectus sheath to the posterior border of the rectus abdominis muscle. Inject the local anesthetic peeling the rectus abdominis muscle superiorly and pushing the posterior rectus sheath inferiorly (Fig. 56-2).

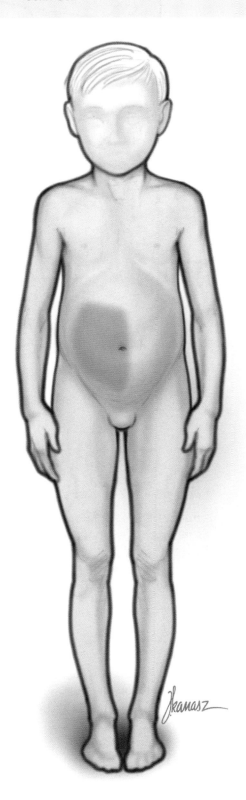

Figure 56-1. The area highlighted in the figure is the area covered by rectus sheath block.

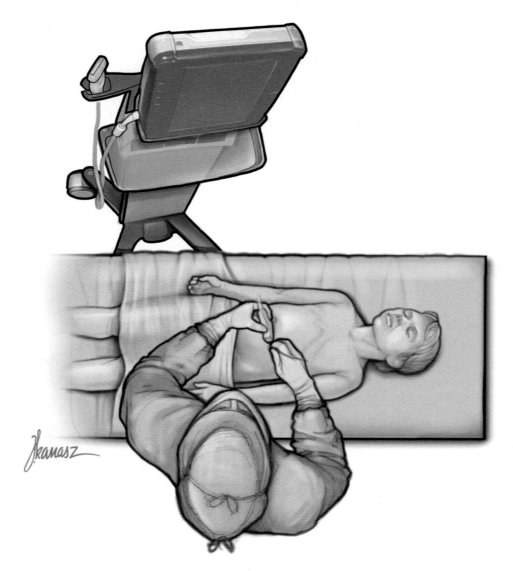

Figure 56-2. **The ultrasound screen is placed on the opposite side of the block. Advancing the needle in plane with the linear ultrasound probe.**

KEY POINTS

- Identify the rectus muscle under ultrasound, and track it with the ultrasound probe in transverse view until the muscle tapers laterally. At this point, the anterior and posterior rectus sheaths meet (Fig. 56-3).
- Slowly advance the blunt injecting needle to avoid penetrating the bowels.

PEARLS

- Real-time imaging provides direct visualization of the needle advancement beyond the rectus muscle

and can prevent penetrating the posterior rectus sheath.
- A "pop" will be felt after passing through the anterior rectus sheath.
- This block should be done bilaterally on separate levels to cover the cutaneous branches from T9 to T12, depending on the surgical incision level.

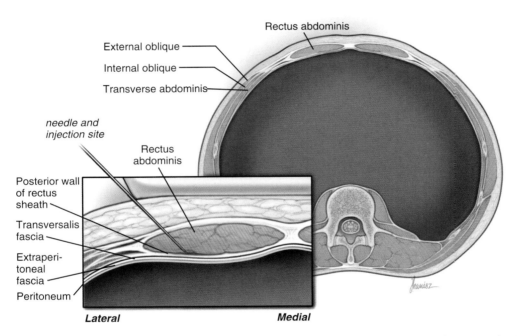

External oblique

Internal oblique

Transverse abdominis

Rectus abdominis

needle and injection site

Rectus abdominis

Posterior wall of rectus sheath

Transversalis fascia

Extraperitoneal fascia

Peritoneum

Lateral

Medial

Figure 56-3. The local anesthetic elevates the rectus abdominis muscle superiorly and pushes the posterior rectus sheath inferiorly.

Index

Page numbers followed by "*f*" indicate figures, "*b*" indicate boxes, and "*t*" indicate tables.